# ECG Workout

## Exercises in Arrhythmia Interpretation

# ECG Workout

## Exercises in Arrhythmia Interpretation

## 4th Edition

**Jane Huff, RN, CCRN**

Education Coordinator, Critical Care Unit
Arrhythmia Instructor
Advanced Cardiac Life Support (ACLS) Instructor
White County Medical Center
Searcy, Arkansas

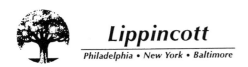
*Lippincott*
Philadelphia • New York • Baltimore

*Acquisitions Editor:* Alan Sorkowitz
*Senior Project Editor:* Erika Kors
*Senior Production Manager:* Helen Ewan
*Managing Editor/Production:* Barbara Ryalls
*Design Coordinator:* Brett MacNaughton
*Manufacturing Manager:* William Alberti
*Compositor:* Maryland Composition
*Printer:* Quebecor World, Dubuque

Edition 4th

9  8  7  6  5  4

**Library of Congress Cataloging-in-Publication Data**

Huff, Jane, RN.
   ECG workout : exercises in arrhythmia interpretation / Jane Huff—4th ed.
    p. cm.
   ISBN 0-7817-3192-5 (alk. paper)
   1. Arrhythmia—Diagnosis—Problems, exercises, etc. 2.
Electrocardiography—Interpretation—Problems, exercises, etc. I. Title.
   [DNLM: 1. Arrhythmia—diagnosis—problems. 2. Electrocardiography—problems.]
   RC685.A65 H84 2001
   616.1′2807547′076—dc21

                                2001050393

# *Reviewers*

**Marsha Coberly, RN, C, MSN**
Lecturer, Medical-Surgical Section
College of Nursing
University of New Mexico
Albuquerque, New Mexico

**Judith Ann Driscoll, RN, MSN**
Assistant Professor
Deaconess College of Nursing
St. Louis, Missouri

**Mary Ann O'Brien, RN**
Instructor, Practical Nursing
James Lorenzo Walker Vocational—Technical
  Center
Naples, Florida

**Cindy Roach, RN, DSN**
Associate Professor
Chair, Department of Adult Health Nursing
Beth-el College of Nursing and Health Science
Colorado Springs, Colorado

**Mary C. Shoemaker, PhD, RN**
Level Coordinator, Associate Professor
Saint Francis Medical Center College of Nursing
Peoria, Illinois

**Linda J. Ulak, RN, EdD, MS, CCRN**
Assistant Professor, College of Nursing
Seton Hall University
South Orange, New Jersey

# *Preface*

*ECG Workout: Exercises in Arrhythmia Interpretation* was written to assist physicians, nurses, medical and nursing students, paramedics, emergency medical technicians, telemetry technicians, and other allied health personnel to acquire the knowledge and skills essential for identification of basic arrhythmias. The text can also be used as a reference for ECG review for those already knowledgeable in ECG interpretation.

The text is written simply and illustrated with drawings, figures, tables, and ECG tracings. Each chapter is designed to build on the knowledge base from the previous chapters so the beginning student can quickly understand and grasp the basic concepts of electrocardiography. A great effort has been made not only to provide ECG tracings of good quality, but also to provide a sufficient number and variety of ECG practice strips so the learner feels confident in arrhythmia interpretation. There are 567 practice strips—more than any book currently on the market.

Chapter 1 provides a discussion of basic anatomy and physiology of the heart. The electrical basis of electrocardiology is discussed in Chapter 2. The components of the ECG tracing (waveforms, intervals, segments, and complexes) are described in Chapter 3. This chapter also includes practice tracings on waveform identification. Cardiac monitors, lead systems, lead placement, ECG artifacts, and troubleshooting monitor problems are discussed in Chapter 4. A step-by-step guide to rhythm strip analysis is provided in Chapter 5, in addition to practice tracings on rhythm strip analysis. The individual arrhythmia chapters (Chapters 6 through 9) include a description of each arrhythmia, arrhythmia examples, causes, and management protocols. Each arrhythmia chapter also includes 95 to 100 practice strips for self-evaluation. Chapter 10 presents a general discussion of cardiac pacemakers (types, indications, function, pacemaker terminology, malfunctions, and pacemaker analysis), along with practice tracings on pacemaker rhythm strips. Chapter 11 includes two post-tests that can be used as a self-evaluation tool or for testing purposes.

The text has been almost completely revised, including text expansion and the revision or addition of new tables and figures. An important addition to the fourth edition of ECG Workout are the new ACLS guidelines, which are incorporated into each arrhythmia chapter as applicable to the rhythm discussion. The ECG tracings are actual strips from patients. Above each rhythm strip are 3-second indicators for rapid rate calculation. For more precise rate calculation, an ECG conversion table is provided on the inside back cover. For convenience, a removable ECG conversion table is also included with the text. **The heart rates for regular rhythms listed in the answer keys were determined by the precise rate calculation method and will not always coincide with the rapid rate calculation method.** Rate calculation methods are discussed in Chapter 5.

The author and publisher have made every attempt to check the content, especially drug dosages and management protocols, for accuracy. Medicine is continually changing, and the reader has the responsibility to keep informed of local care protocols and changes in emergency care procedures.

# Contents

# 1

# ANATOMY AND PHYSIOLOGY OF THE HEART

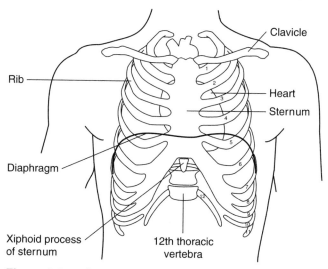

**Figure 1-1.** Thoracic projection of the boundaries of the heart on the chest wall.

## DESCRIPTION AND LOCATION OF THE HEART

The heart is a hollow, four-chambered muscular organ, which lies in the mediastinal cavity between the right and left lung, just behind the body of the sternum and in front of the spinal column (Figure 1-1). The upper heart border (the base) lies beneath the second rib. The lower heart border terminates in a blunt point known as the apex at the level of the fifth intercostal space, left midclavicular line. There, the heart's apex can be palpated during ventricular contraction. This clinical finding is called the *point of maximal impulse* or PMI and indicates the heart's position within the thorax. The heart's position is not straight up and down, but tilted to the left and rotated so the right atrium and ventricle are positioned toward the front (anteriorly) and the left atrium and ventricle are positioned to the side (laterally). About two thirds of the heart extends to the left of the body's midline, and one third extends to the right. Although heart size varies with body size, the average adult heart is 5 inches long and 3½ inches wide. This corresponds to an average man's clenched fist.

## FUNCTION OF THE HEART

The heart functions primarily as a pump to supply the body with enough blood to meet its metabolic requirements. The heart is capable of adjusting its pump performance to meet various demands. As metabolic demands increase, the heart responds by accelerating its rate to increase cardiac output. As metabolic demands decrease, the heart responds by slowing its rate, resulting in a decrease in cardiac output. As a pump, the heart has several unique properties: It expands and contracts without placing stress on the heart muscle, it can withstand continual activity without developing muscle fatigue, and it is capable of generating electrical impulses, which maintain a proper heart rhythm.

## HEART SURFACES

There are four main heart surfaces to consider when discussing the heart: anterior, posterior, inferior, and lateral (Figure 1-2). A simplified concept of the heart surfaces is listed below:

Anterior: the front
Posterior: the back
Inferior: the bottom
Lateral: the side

## STRUCTURE OF THE HEART WALL

The heart wall is arranged in three layers (Figure 1-3):

Pericardium: the outermost layer
Myocardium: the middle muscular layer
Endocardium: the inner layer

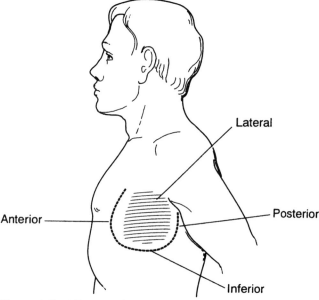

**Figure 1-2.** Heart surfaces.

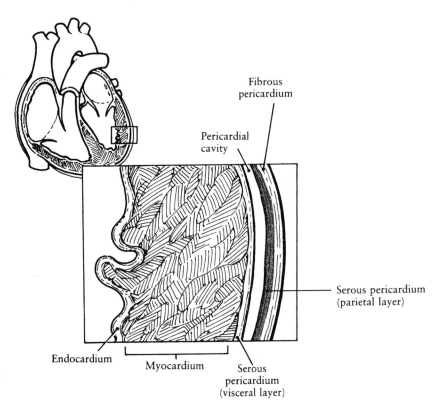

**Figure 1-3.** Heart wall. (From Bullock BL, Rosendahl PP: Pathophysiology, 3$^{rd}$ ed. Philadelphia: JB Lippincott, 1992.)

The pericardium is a saclike structure that encases the heart. The pericardium consists of an outer tough, inelastic, fibrous sac (the fibrous pericardium) and an inner thin, two-layered, fluid-secreting membrane (the serous pericardium). The outer fibrous pericardium comes in direct contact with the covering of the lung, the pleura, and is attached to the center of the diaphragm inferiorly, to the sternum anteriorly, and to the esophagus, trachea, and main bronchi posteriorly. This position anchors the heart to the chest and prevents it from shifting about. The moist serous pericardium consists of two layers: the parietal layer, which lines the inside of the fibrous pericardium, and the visceral layer, which lines the outer surface of the myocardium. Between the two layers of the serous pericardium is the pericardial space or cavity, which is usually filled with 10 to 30 cc of thin, clear, serous fluid secreted by the serous layers. This fluid provides lubrication during heart contraction and relaxation.

The myocardium is the muscular layer that makes up the bulk of the heart wall. It contains the conduction system, the blood supply, and the myocardial muscle contractile fibers responsible for contraction. Myocardial thickness varies in different regions of the heart. The two upper chambers, the atria, are thin-walled and approximately 2 mm thick. The right ventricle is approximately 4 mm thick, whereas that of the left ventricle is between 13 and 15 mm thick.

The endocardium is a thin layer of tissue that lines the heart chambers and valves. Papillary muscles originate in the ventricular endocardium and attach to chordae tendineae (Figure 1-4).

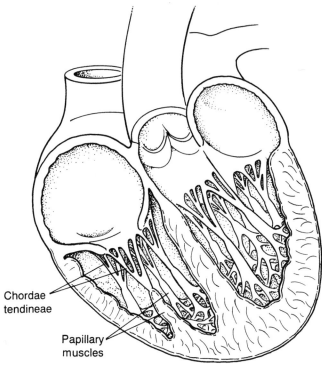

**Figure 1-4.** Papillary muscles and chordae tendineae.

## HEART CHAMBERS

The interior of the heart consists of four hollow chambers (Figure 1-5). The two upper chambers, the right atrium and the left atrium, are divided by a wall called the *interatrial septum.* The two lower chambers, the right ventricle and the left ventricle, are divided by a thicker wall called the *interventricular septum.* The two septa divide the heart into two pumping systems, a right heart and a left heart. The right heart pumps venous (deoxygenated) blood into the lungs. The left heart pumps arterial (oxygenated) blood into the systemic circulation.

The thickness of the walls in each chamber is related to the workload performed by that chamber. Both atria are low-pressure chambers serving as blood collecting reservoirs for the ventricles. Therefore, their walls are relatively thin. They add a small amount of force to the moving blood. The right ventricular wall is thicker than the walls of the atria, but much thinner than that of the left ventricle. The right chamber pumps blood a fairly short distance to the lungs against a relatively low resistance to flow. The left ventricle has the thickest wall because it must eject blood through the aorta to all parts of the body against a much greater resistance to flow.

## HEART VALVES

There are four valves in the heart: the tricuspid valve, separating the right atrium from the right ventricle; the pulmonic valve, separating the right ventricle from the pulmonary artery; the mitral valve, separating the left atrium from the left ventricle; and the aortic valve, separating the left ventricle from the aorta (Figure 1-6). The primary function of the valves is to permit blood flow in one direction only. The opening and closing of the valves depend on pressure gradients within the cardiovascular system.

The tricuspid and mitral valves separate the atria from the ventricles and are referred to as the atrioventricular valves (AV valves). The tricuspid valve orifice is larger (approximately 11 cm in circumference) and has three valve cusps or leaflets. The mitral valve is approximately 9 cm in circumference and has two valve leaflets. Fibrous cords called *chordae tendineae* attach the cusps of these valves to the papillary muscles in the ventricles. As the atria fill with blood, pressure in the atria exceeds that of the ventricles, forcing the AV valves open and allowing blood to flow passively from the atria into the ventricles. During ventricular filling, (or diastole) when the AV valves are open, the valves, the chordae tendineae, and the papillary muscles form a funnel, which helps promote blood flow into the ventricles. Toward the end of diastole, the two atria contract, pumping the rest of their contents into the ventricles. This atrial contraction, called the *atrial kick,* accounts for 10% to 30% of cardiac output. The atrial kick is lost in those arrhythmias that have asynchronous contraction between the atria and ventricles. Two examples of asynchronous rhythms include atrial fibrillation and third-degree AV block. At the end of diastole,

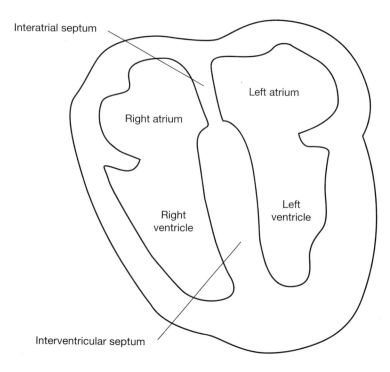

**Figure 1-5.** Chambers of the heart.

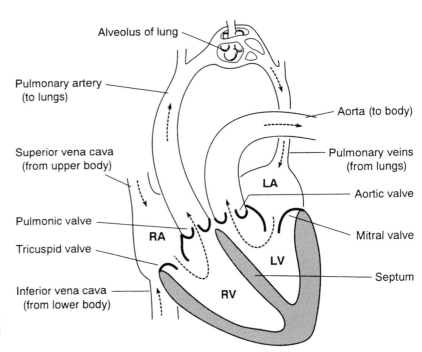

**Figure 1-6.** Chambers, valves, blood flow. *RA*, right atrium; *RV*, right ventricle; *LA*, left atrium; *LV*, left ventricle.

the increased pressure in the ventricles compared with lessening pressure in the atria helps to close the valves. During ventricular contraction (or systole), the valve cusps are prevented from being everted into the atria by contraction of the papillary muscles and tension in the chordae tendineae. Thus, blood is prevented from flowing backward into the atria despite the high ventricular pressures. A dysfunction of the chordae tendineae or papillary muscles (usually caused by myocardial infarction) can cause an incomplete closure of an AV valve, resulting in a murmur. Closure of the AV valves constitutes the first heart sound ($S_1$).

The aortic and pulmonic valves, or semilunar valves, are each composed of three cup-shaped cusps of approximately equal size. The pulmonic valve is located just inside the orifice of the pulmonary artery, and the aortic valve lies just inside the orifice of the aorta. The aortic cusps are thicker than the pulmonic; both are thicker than the AV cusps. During ventricular systole, the cusps are thrust open as blood flows from an area of greater pressure in the ventricles to an area of lesser pressure in the aorta and pulmonary artery. As the ventricular chambers empty and pressure in the chambers decreases, some blood trickles backward along the walls of the aorta and pulmonary artery filling the cup-shaped cusps with blood and forcing them shut. Backflow into the ventricles is prevented because of the cusps' strength, shape, and ability to form a tight seal. Closure of the semilunar valves constitutes the second heart sound ($S_2$).

## BLOOD FLOW THROUGH THE HEART AND LUNGS

Blood flow through the heart and lungs can be traced from the right side to the left side (see Figure 1-6). The right atrium receives unoxygenated blood from the superior vena cava, the inferior vena cava, and the coronary sinus. The superior vena cava returns venous blood from the head, upper extremities, and the chest wall. The inferior vena cava returns venous blood from the trunk, abdominal organs, and lower extremities. The coronary sinus returns venous blood from the myocardium.

As the right atrium fills with blood, the pressure in the chamber increases. When pressure in the right atrium exceeds that of the right ventricle, the tricuspid valve opens, allowing blood to flow into the right ventricle. As the right ventricle fills with blood, pressure in that chamber increases, forcing the tricuspid valve shut and the pulmonic valve open, ejecting blood into the pulmonary arteries and on to the lungs. In the lungs, the blood picks up oxygen and releases excess carbon dioxide.

The left atrium receives the oxygenated blood from the lungs by way of the pulmonary veins. As the left atrium fills with blood, the pressure in the chamber increases. When the pressure in the left atrium exceeds that of the right ventricle, the mitral valve opens, allowing blood to flow into the left ventricle. As the left ventricle fills with blood, pressure in that chamber increases, forcing the mitral valve shut and the aortic valve open, ejecting blood into the aorta.

The blood is then distributed throughout the body where the blood releases oxygen to the cells and picks up carbon dioxide.

Although blood flow can be traced, for simplicity's sake, from the right heart to the left heart, it must be remembered that right heart events and left heart events occur simultaneously. At the same time the right atrium receives unoxygenated blood from the body, the left atrium receives oxygenated blood from the lungs. Increased pressures in the filled atria force the tricuspid and mitral valves open, allowing blood to enter both ventricles. Increased pressure in the filled ventricles forces both AV valves shut and the pulmonic and aortic valves open. The ventricles contract simultaneously, ejecting blood through the pulmonary artery to the pulmonary circulation and through the aortic valve to the systemic circulation.

## CORONARY CIRCULATION

The blood supply to the heart is provided by the right and left coronary arteries, which arise from the aorta just above and behind the aortic valve (Figure 1-7). They extend over the outside surface of the heart and branch several times. These arteries plunge inward through the myocardial wall and undergo further branching. There is much individual variation in the pattern of coronary artery branching.

The right coronary artery supplies blood to the right atrium, the right ventricle, the SA node in 55% of the population, the AV node and bundle of His in

90% of the population, the inferior wall of the left ventricle, the posterior wall of the left ventricle in 90% of the population, and the posterior third of the interventricular septum in 90% of the population. The left coronary artery has a short main stem, the left main coronary artery, which branches into the left anterior descending (LAD) and the left circumflex. The LAD supplies blood to the anterior and lateral walls of the left ventricle, the anterior two thirds of the interventricular septum, and the right and left bundle branches. The left circumflex artery supplies blood to the left atrium, lateral wall of the left ventricle, posterior wall of the left ventricle in 10% of the population, the SA node in 45% of the population, the AV node and bundle of His in 10% of the population, and the posterior third of the interventricular septum in 10% of the population. Table 1-1 summarizes the major cardiac structures and their usual arterial supply.

*Vessel dominance* is a term commonly used in describing coronary vasculature and refers to the distribution of the terminal portion of the arteries. The dominant artery is the one that supplies the posterior interventricular septum and the posterior surface of the left ventricle. The left coronary artery is wider and perfuses the greatest proportion of the myocardium. However, in 90% of the population, the right coronary artery perfuses the posterior interventricular septum and posterior surface of the left ventricle and is the dominant artery.

The right and left coronary artery branches are interconnected by very small arteries, which provide the potential for cross flow from one artery to the

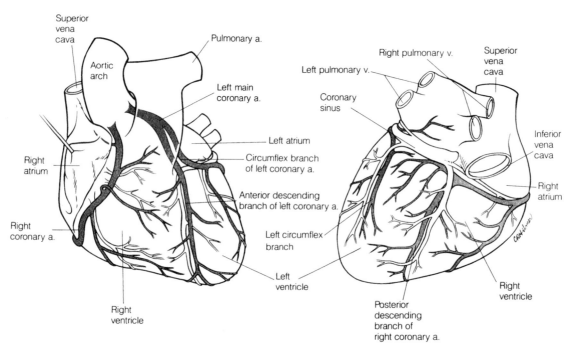

**Figure 1-7.** Coronary blood supply. (From Porth CM: Pathophysiology, 3rd ed. Philadelphia: JB Lippincott, 1990.)

**Table 1-1.  The Coronary Circulation and Heart Structures It Supplies**

| Artery | Structure Supplied |
|---|---|
| Right coronary artery | Right atrium |
| | Right ventricle |
| | SA node in 55% of population |
| | AV node and bundle of His in 90% of population |
| | Inferior wall of left ventricle |
| | Posterior wall of left ventricle in 90% of population |
| | Posterior third of interventricular septum in 90% of population |
| Left coronary artery | |
| Left anterior descending | Anterior wall of left ventricle |
| | Lateral wall of left ventricle |
| | Anterior two thirds of interventricular septum |
| | Right and left bundle branches |
| Left circumflex | Left atrium |
| | SA node in 45% of population |
| | AV node and bundle of His in 10% of population |
| | Lateral wall of left ventricle |
| | Posterior wall of left ventricle in 10% of population |
| | Posterior third of interventricular septum in 10% of population |

other. These small arteries are commonly called *collateral vessels* or *collateral circulation*. If a blockage occurs in a branch of one of the coronary arteries, the collateral vessels may provide additional blood flow to those areas of reduced blood supply.

In most body parts, arterial blood flow reaches a peak during ventricular contraction (systole). However, blood flow to the myocardium is poorest during ventricular contraction. This is because the coronary arteries are compressed when the myocardium contracts, and this action interferes with blood flow. Also, the openings of the coronary arteries are closed during ventricular contraction. Blood flow into the myocardium increases during ventricular relaxation (diastole) because the coronary arteries are no longer compressed and the orifices of the coronary arteries are open.

The blood that has passed through the capillaries of the myocardium is drained by branches of the cardiac veins whose path runs parallel to those of the coronary arteries. Some of these veins empty directly into the right atrium and right ventricle, but the majority feed into the coronary sinus, which empties into the right atrium.

## CARDIAC INNERVATION

The heart is under the control of the autonomic nervous system, which includes the sympathetic and parasympathetic nervous systems. Both systems are located in the cardiac center of the medulla oblongata, a part of the brain stem. In this area of the brain, masses of neurons function as cardioinhibitor and cardioaccelerator reflex centers. These centers receive sensory impulses from various parts of the circulatory system and, in response, relay motor impulses to the heart.

The sympathetic nervous system, a part of the cardioaccelerator center, innervates the heart through sympathetic nerve fibers arising from the upper thoracic spinal cord. Sympathetic nervous system stimulation results in the release of epinephrine and norepinephrine, which accelerates firing of the SA node, speeds conduction through the AV node, and increases the force of cardiac contraction.

The parasympathetic nervous system, a part of the cardioinhibitor center, innervates the heart through vagal nerve fibers. Parasympathetic nervous system stimulation results in the release of acetylcholine, which slows the heart rate, slows conduction through the AV node, and decreases ventricular contractile force. Normally, a balance is maintained between the inhibitory effects of the parasympathetic fibers and the excitatory effects of the sympathetic fibers.

Painful impulses originating within the heart are relayed by way of sensory nerve fibers to the nerve cell bodies located in the T1 through T5 segments of the thoracic spine. Cardiac pain tends to be referred to skin or skeletal muscles that share nerve supplies from the same or adjacent spinal segments. Therefore, cardiac pain is often referred to areas innervated by thoracic segments T1 through T5, such as the epigastric area, anterior chest wall, sternum, jaw, shoulders, scapula, arms, wrists, and hands.

# 2

# ELECTROPHYSIOLOGY

## CARDIAC CELLS

The heart is composed of cylindrical cardiac cells that branch and connect with branches of adjacent cells, forming an anastomosing network of cells. At the junctions where the branches join together is a specialized cellular membrane of low electrical resistance, which permits rapid conduction of electrical impulses from one cell to another throughout the cell network. Stimulation of one cardiac cell initiates stimulation of adjacent cells and ultimately leads to cell contraction.

There are two types of cardiac cells: electrical cells and myocardial cells. The electrical cells are specialized cells of the electrical conduction system and are responsible for impulse formation and conduction. The myocardial cells consist of contractile protein filaments called *actin* and *myosin* and are responsible for muscle contraction.

The electrical cells are distributed in an orderly fashion along the conduction system of the heart. These cells possess three specific properties:

**1.** Automaticity—the ability of the cell to spontaneously generate and discharge an electrical impulse

**2.** Excitability—the ability of the cell to respond to an electrical impulse

**3.** Conductivity—The ability of the cell to transmit an electrical impulse from one cell to another

The myocardial (or "working") cells form the thin muscular layer of the atrial wall and the much thicker muscular layer of the ventricular wall. These cells possess two specific properties:

**1.** Contractility—the ability of the cell filaments to shorten and return to their original length

**2.** Extensibility—the ability of the cell filaments to stretch

## DEPOLARIZATION AND REPOLARIZATION

The electrical cells are able to generate and conduct electrical impulses that result in depolarization (electrical activation), contraction, and repolarization (recovery) of the myocardial cells (Figure 2-1). These electrical impulses are the result of a flow of positively charged ions back and forth across the semipermeable cardiac cell membrane.

Each cardiac cell is surrounded and filled with a solution that contains positively charged ions and negatively charged ions. Intracellular and extracellular spaces have very different ionic compositions.

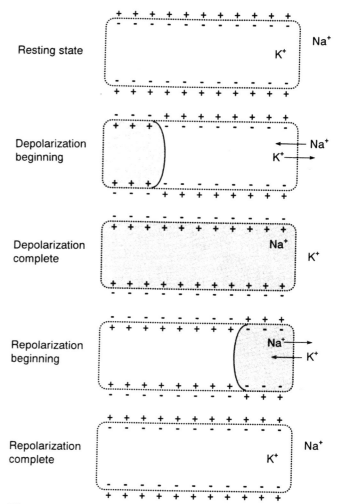

**Figure 2-1.** Depolarization and repolarization of a cardiac cell.

The intracellular space contains high concentrations of potassium ion (positively charged) and protein (negatively charged), but has low concentrations of sodium ion (positively charged). The extracellular space contains high concentrations of sodium ion and chloride ion (negatively charged), but has low concentrations of potassium ion. Electrical charges are regulated primarily by the movement of two electrolytes: potassium (the primary intracellular ion) and sodium (the primary extracellular ion).

The cycle of ion shifts continuously changes the electrical charge inside the cell, resulting in periods of activity (depolarization) and periods of rest (repolarization). The distribution of ions on either side of the membrane is determined, in part, by the presence of pores or channels in the cell membrane. Some channels are always open; others can be opened or closed; still others can be selective, allowing one kind of ion to pass through and excluding all others. Membrane channels open and close in response to a stimulus (electrical, mechanical, or chemical). Another factor affecting ion distribution across the cell membrane is the concentration gradient. Particles in solution move, or diffuse, from areas of higher concentration to areas of lower concentration. In the case of uncharged particles, movement proceeds until there is uniform distribution of particles within a solution. Charged particles also diffuse, but the diffusion of charged particles is influenced not only by the concentration gradient but also by an electrical gradient (positively charged particles tend to flow toward negatively charged particles, whereas negatively charged particles are attracted to positively charged particles). This results in an unequal distribution of charged particles across the cell membrane with an electrical difference between the intracellular and extracellular regions.

At rest, the electrical charge inside the cell is more negative and the outside of the cell is more positive. In this resting state, the cells are said to be polarized and no electrical activity is occurring. This stage is represented on the electrocardiogram (ECG) by an isoelectric line (the flat line or baseline; see Figure 2-5). Once a cell is stimulated, the membrane permeability changes, allowing sodium to enter the cell rapidly and potassium to exit. This ionic exchange causes the inside of the cell to become more positive than the outside and results in cell depolarization. Once depolarization is complete, potassium is allowed to reenter and sodium to exit, returning the inside of the cell to its resting, more negative charge. This process is called *repolarization* or *cell recovery.*

Depolarization of one cardiac cell acts as a stimulus on adjacent cells and causes them to depolarize. Propagation of the electrical impulses from cell to cell produces an electric current, which can be detected by skin electrodes and recorded as waves or deflections on a graph paper called the *electrocardiogram (ECG).*

## ELECTRICAL CONDUCTION SYSTEM OF THE HEART

The heart is supplied with an electrical conduction system that generates and conducts electrical impulses along specialized pathways to the atria and ventricles causing them to contract (Figure 2-2). The system consists of the sinoatrial (SA) node, the interatrial tract (Bachmann's bundle), the internodal tracts, the atrioventricular (AV) node, the bundle of His, the right and left bundle branches, and the Purkinje fibers.

The SA node is located in the wall of the right atrium near the inlet of the superior vena cava. Specialized electrical cells, called *pacemaker cells,* in the SA node discharge impulses at a rate of 60 to 100 times per minute in rhythmic fashion.

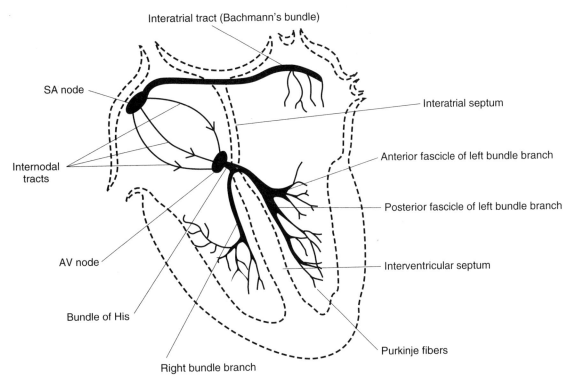

**Figure 2-2.** Electrical conduction system of the heart.

Pacemaker cells are located at other sites along the conduction system, but the SA node is normally in control and is called the "pacemaker of the heart" because it possesses the highest level of automaticity (ie, its inherent firing rate is greater than the other pacemaker sites; AV node pacemaker cells fire at 40 to 60 per minute whereas ventricular pacemaker cells fire at 30 to 40 per minute or less). If the SA node fails to generate electrical impulses at its normal rate or the conduction of these impulses is interrupted (blocked), pacemaker cells in other sites can assume control as pacemaker of the heart, but usually at a much slower rate. In general, the farther away the impulse originates from the SA node, the slower the rate.

As the electrical impulse leaves the SA node, it is conducted through the left atrium by way of Bachmann's bundle and through the right atrium by way of the internodal tracts, causing electrical activation (depolarization) and contraction of the atria. The impulse is then conducted to the AV node located in the lower right atrium near the interatrial septum. The AV node relays the electrical impulses from the atria to the ventricles in an orderly and timely way. It provides the only normal conduction pathway between the atria and the ventricles. The AV node has three main functions:

**1.** Its primary function is to slow conduction of the electrical impulse through the AV node to allow time for the atria to contract and empty their contents into the ventricles before the ventricles contract. The delay in the AV node is represented on the ECG tracing as the flat line of the PR interval.

**2.** It can function as a backup pacemaker, if the SA node fails, at a rate of 40 to 60 beats per minute.

**3.** When the atrial rate is rapid, the AV node blocks some of the impulses from being conducted to the ventricles, thus protecting the ventricles from dangerously fast rates.

After the delay in the AV node, the impulse moves rapidly through the bundle of His. The bundle of His splits into two important conducting pathways called the *right bundle branch* and the *left bundle branch.* The right bundle branch conducts the electrical impulse to the right ventricle, whereas the left bundle branch divides into an anterior fascicle and a posterior fascicle, which conduct the impulse to the left ventricle. The impulse then enters the Purkinje system where the Purkinje fibers conduct the impulse to the myocardial cells of the ventricles, causing ventricular depolarization and contraction. Repolarization then occurs.

The heart's electrical activity is represented on the monitor or ECG tracing by three basic waveforms: the P wave, the QRS complex, and the T wave (Figure 2-3). Between the waveforms are the following segments and intervals: the PR interval, the ST segment, and the QT interval. A U wave is sometimes present. Although the letters themselves have no special significance, each component represents a particular event in the depolarization–repolarization cycle. The P wave depicts atrial depolarization, or the spread of the impulse from the SA node throughout the atria. The PR interval represents the time required for the impulse to leave the SA node, travel through the atria, AV node, bundle of His, bundle branches, and Purkinje fibers. The QRS complex depicts ventricular depolarization, or the spread of the impulse throughout the ventricles. The ST segment represents the end of ventricular depolarization and the beginning of ventricular repolarization. The T wave represents the latter phase of ventricular repolarization. The U wave, which is not always present, is thought to represent further repolarization of the ventricles. The QT interval represents both ventricular depolarization and repolarization.

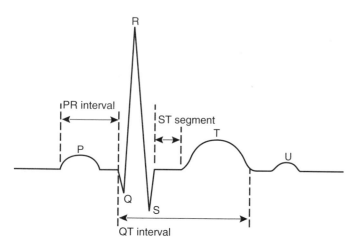

**Figure 2-3.** Relationship of the electrical conduction system to the ECG.

## THE CARDIAC CYCLE

A cardiac cycle consists of one heartbeat or one P–QRS–T sequence. It represents a sequence of atrial contraction (systole) and relaxation (diastole) followed by ventricular contraction and relaxation. The basic cycle repeats itself again and again (Figure 2-4). Regularity of the cardiac rhythm can be assessed by measuring from one heartbeat to the next (from one R wave to the next R wave—also called the R-R interval). Between cardiac cycles, the monitor or ECG recorder returns to a baseline called the isoelectric line, a flat line between the T wave and the P wave (Figure 2-5). Any waveform above the isoelectric line is considered a positive (upright) deflection and any waveform below this line is considered a negative (downward) deflection. A deflection having both a positive and negative component is called a biphasic deflection. This basic concept can be applied to the P wave, the QRS complex, and the T wave deflections.

## WAVEFORMS AND CURRENT FLOW

A monitor lead or ECG lead provides a view of the heart's electrical activity between two points or poles (a positive pole and a negative pole). The direction in which the electric current flows determines how the waveforms appear on the ECG tracing (Figure 2-6). An electric current flowing toward the positive pole will produce a positive deflection; an electric current traveling toward the negative pole will produce a negative deflection. When the current flows perpendicular to the pole, the wave-

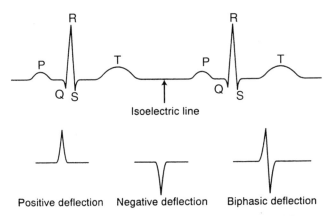

**Figure 2-5.** Relationship between waveforms and the isoelectric line.

form will be both positive and negative (biphasic). Current flowing at a 45-degree angle to the negative pole will produce a biphasic deflection that is more negative than positive; current flowing at a 45-degree angle to the positive pole will produce a biphasic deflection that is more positive than negative.

The size of the wave deflection depends on the magnitude of the electric current flowing toward the individual pole. The magnitude of the electric current is determined by how much voltage is generated by depolarization of a particular portion of the heart. The QRS complex is normally larger than the P wave because depolarization of the larger muscle mass of the ventricles generates more voltage than does depolarization of the smaller muscle mass of the atria.

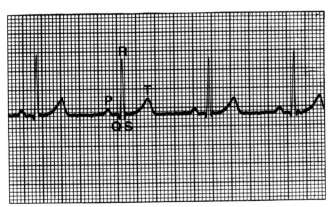

**Figure 2-4.** The cardiac cycle.

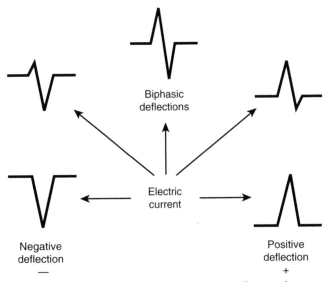

**Figure 2-6.** Relationship between current flow and waveform deflections.

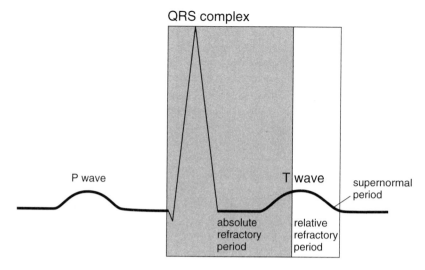

**Figure 2-7.** Refractory and supernormal periods.

## REFRACTORY AND SUPERNORMAL PERIODS OF THE CARDIAC CYCLE

There is a period of time during the cardiac cycle when the cardiac cells may or may not be depolarized by an electrical stimulus, depending on the strength of the electrical impulse. This period is called the *refractory period* and is divided into the absolute refractory period (ARP) and the relative refractory period (RRP), as shown in Figure 2-7. The absolute refractory period extends from the onset of the QRS complex to the peak of the T wave. During this time, the cardiac cells have depolarized and are in the process of repolarizing. Because the cardiac cells have not repolarized to their threshold potential (the level at which a cell must be repolarized before it can be depolarized again), they cannot be stimulated to depolarize—in other words, the electrical cells cannot conduct an impulse nor can the myocardial cells contract during the absolute refractory period. The relative refractory period begins at the peak of the T wave and ends with the end of the T wave. During this time, the cardiac cells have repolarized sufficiently to respond to a strong stimulus. This period is also called the *vulnerable period of repolarization*. A strong stimulus occurring during the vulnerable period may usurp the primary pacemaker of the heart usually the SA node) and take over pacemaker control. An exam-

ple might be a premature ventricular contraction (PVC) that falls during the vulnerable period and takes over control of the heart in the form of ventricular tachycardia. The supernormal period occurs near the end of the T wave just before the cells have completely repolarized. During this period, the cardiac cells will respond to a weak stimulus.

## ECG GRAPH PAPER

The P–QRS–T sequence is recorded on special graph paper made up of horizontal and vertical lines (Figure 2-8). The horizontal lines measure the duration of the waveforms in seconds of time. Each small square measured horizontally represents 0.04 seconds. The width of the QRS complex in Figure 2-9 extends across two squares and represents 0.08 seconds (0.04 seconds × two squares). The vertical lines measure the voltage or amplitude of the waveform in millimeters (mm). Each small square measured vertically represents 1 mm in height. The height of the QRS complex in Figure 2-9 extends upward from baseline 16 small squares and represents 16 mm voltage (1 mm × 16 squares).

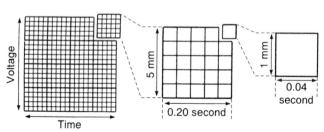

**Figure 2-8.** Electrocardiographic paper.

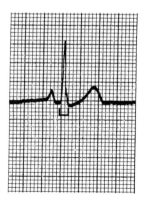

**Figure 2-9.** QRS width: 0.08 seconds; QRS height: 16 mm.

# 3

# WAVEFORMS, INTERVALS, SEGMENTS, AND COMPLEXES

Much of the information provided by the ECG tracing is obtained from the examination and/or measurement of the three principal waveforms (the P wave, the QRS complex, and the T wave) and their associated intervals and segments. Assessment of these data provides the facts necessary for an accurate cardiac rhythm interpretation.

## P WAVE

The first deflection of the cardiac cycle, the P wave, is caused by depolarization of the atria. The waveform begins as the deflection leaves baseline and ends when the deflection returns to baseline (Figure 3-1). Normal P waves are small, rounded, and positive (upright) in Lead II with an amplitude between 0.5 mm and 2.5 mm and a duration of 0.10 seconds or less. There should be one P wave preceding each QRS complex. More than one P wave before a QRS complex indicates a conduction disturbance such as occurs in second- and third-degree heart block. A P wave of normal size, shape, and direction indicates that the electrical impulse originated in the SA node and that normal depolarization of the atria has occurred.

Abnormal P waves may result from the following:

**1.** The impulse travels through damaged or abnormal atria, resulting in P waves of greater amplitude or width. A tall pointed P wave is seen in right atrial enlargement secondary to pulmonary disease or congenital heart disease. A wide notched P wave is seen in left atrial enlargement secondary to valvular heart disease or hypertensive heart disease.

**2.** The electrical impulse originated in a site outside the SA node (an occurrence known as an ectopic rhythm), resulting in P waves that are abnormal in size, shape, or direction. In some ectopic rhythms, the P wave may be absent.

**3.** The administration of quinidine causes notching and widening of the P wave.

P wave examples are shown in Figure 3-2.

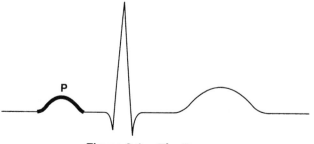

**Figure 3-1.** The P wave.

## PR INTERVAL

The PR interval represents the time required for the electrical impulse to leave the SA node and to travel through the atria, the AV node, the bundle branches, and the Purkinje network. The PR interval includes a P wave and the short, flat (isoelectric) line that follows it (Figure 3-3). The PR interval is measured from the beginning of the P wave as it leaves baseline to the beginning of the QRS complex. The duration of the normal PR interval is 0.12 to 0.20 seconds. A normal PR interval indicates that the electrical impulse was conducted from the SA node to the Purkinje fibers within a normal amount of time.

The PR interval may be shorter than normal if the electrical impulse was conducted through an accessory (faster than normal) conduction pathway that bypasses the AV node and bundle of His or if the impulse originated in an ectopic site close to or in the AV junction (junctional rhythms). The PR interval may be longer than normal if the electrical impulse is abnormally delayed traveling through the AV node (eg, first-degree AV block). A long PR is also associated with aging and may be the first sign of underlying conduction system disease. Other causes of a prolonged PR interval are hyperkalemia and the administration of certain drugs (digitalis, quinidine, and procainamide). Examples of PR intervals are shown in Figure 3-4.

## QRS COMPLEX

The QRS complex represents the time required for the electrical impulse to depolarize the ventricles. The QRS complex is measured from the beginning of the QRS (as the first wave of the complex leaves baseline) to the point where the last wave of the complex begins to flatten out into the ST segment (Figure 3-5). This point, the junction between the QRS and the ST segment, is called the *junction* or *J point*. Elevation or depression of the ST segment makes ending the QRS more difficult. The QRS ends as soon as the straight line of the ST segment begins, even though the straight line may be above or below baseline. The normal QRS complex is predominantly positive in Lead II with a duration of 10 seconds or less. The abnormal QRS is wide with duration of 0.12 seconds or more. There are wide limits to the amplitude of the R wave in the QRS complex, but it generally ranges from 2 mm to 15 mm depending on the lead.

The QRS complex is composed of three wave deflections: the Q wave, the R wave, and the S wave. The R wave is a positive deflection; the Q wave is a nega-

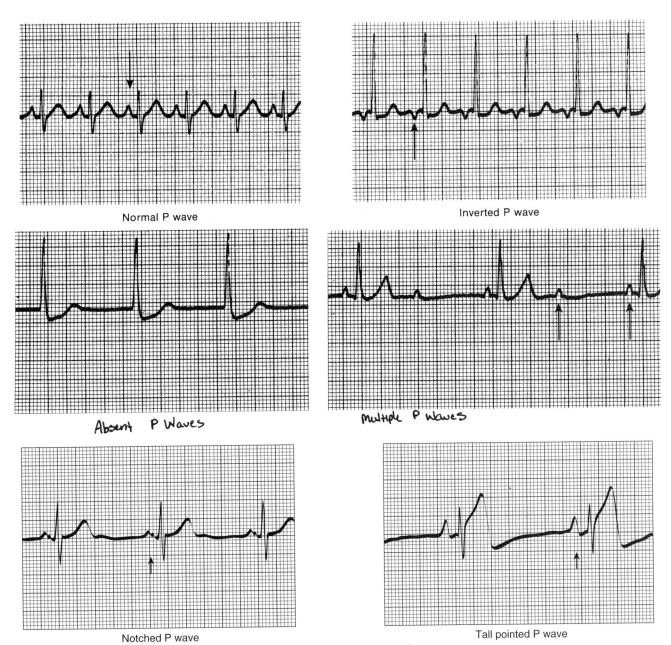

Figure 3-2. P wave examples.

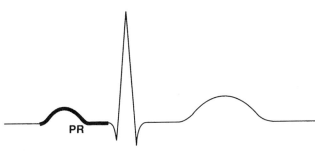

**Figure 3-3.** The PR interval.

tive deflection that precedes an R wave; the S wave is a negative deflection following an R wave. Many variations exist, however, in the configuration of the QRS, and you may not always see all three QRS waveforms (see Figure 3-6). Whatever the variation, the complex is still called the QRS complex. For example, you might see a QRS with a Q and an R wave but no S wave (Figure 3-6D), an R and S wave without a Q wave (Figure 3-6F), or an R wave without either a Q or an S wave (Figure 3-6A). If the entire complex is negative (Figure

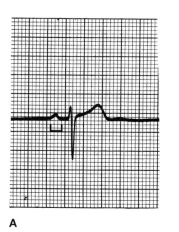

**A**

Normal PR interval of 0.20 seconds (0.04 seconds × 5 squares).

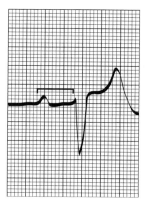

**B**

Short PR interval of 0.08 seconds (0.04 seconds × 2 squares)

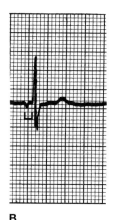

**C**

Long PR interval of 0.38 seconds (0.04 seconds × 9½ squares

**Figure 3-4.** PR interval examples.

3-6*I*), it is termed a QS complex (not a negative R wave because R waves are always positive). It is also possible to have more than one R wave (Figure 3-6*J*) and more than one S wave (Figure 3-6*M*). The second R wave is labeled R prime (R′) and the second S wave is labeled S prime (S′). To be labeled separately, a wave must cross the baseline. A wave that changes direction but does not cross the baseline is called a *notch.*

Capital letters are used to designate waves of large amplitude (5 mm or more), and lowercase letters are used to label small-amplitude waves (less than 5 mm). This can be useful in forming a mental picture of a nonillustrated complex mentioned in a textbook. For example, if a complex is described in a text as having an rS waveform, the reader can easily picture a complex with a small r wave and a big S wave.

A normal QRS complex indicates that depolarization of the ventricles occurred within a normal amount of time. An abnormally wide QRS may result from the following:

**1.** A block in the conduction of impulses through one of the bundle branches (right or left bundle branch block).

**2.** An electrical impulse that arrives early at the bundle branches (before the bundle branches have sufficiently repolarized) causing the impulse to be conducted abnormally and resulting in a wide QRS complex (aberrant ventricular conduction).

**3.** The electrical impulse is conducted from the atria to the ventricles through an abnormal conduc-

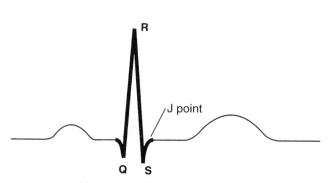

**Figure 3-5.** The QRS complex.

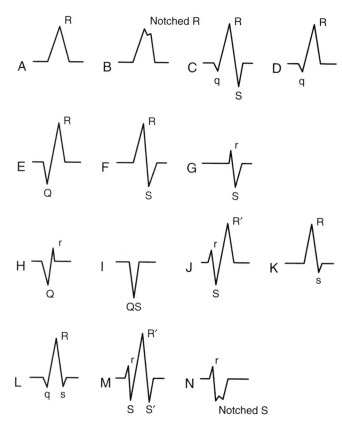

**Figure 3-6.** QRS variations.

tion pathway that bypasses the AV node and bundle of His (preexcitation syndrome).

**4.** The electrical impulse originated in an ectopic site in the ventricles.

**5.** Hyperkalemia or the administration of certain drugs (quinidine, procainamide, and disopyramide).

Tall R waves are associated with ventricular enlargement. Very low QRS complexes are seen with obesity, emphysema, hypothyroidism, pericardial effusion, amyloidosis, extensive myocardial infarction, and myocardial fibrosis. Examples of QRS complexes are shown in Figure 3-7.

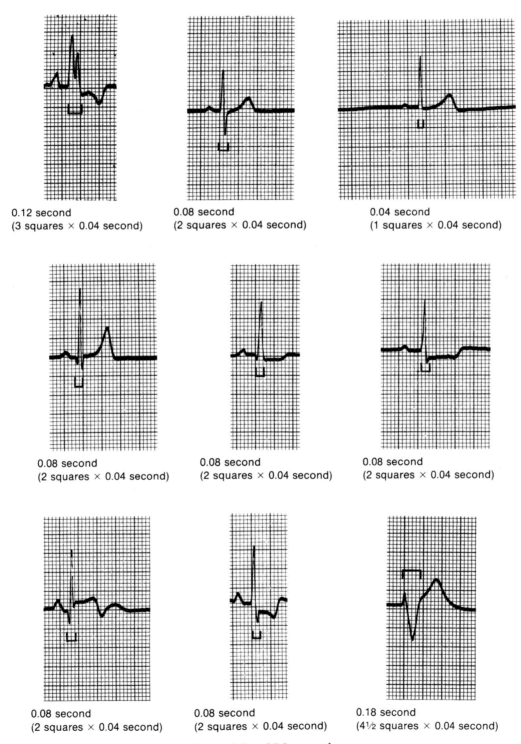

0.12 second
(3 squares × 0.04 second)

0.08 second
(2 squares × 0.04 second)

0.04 second
(1 squares × 0.04 second)

0.08 second
(2 squares × 0.04 second)

0.08 second
(2 squares × 0.04 second)

0.08 second
(2 squares × 0.04 second)

0.08 second
(2 squares × 0.04 second)

0.08 second
(2 squares × 0.04 second)

0.18 second
(4½ squares × 0.04 second)

**Figure 3-7.** QRS examples.

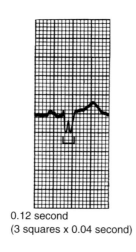
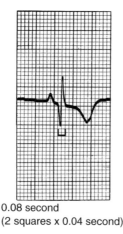
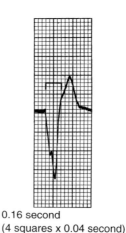

| 0.12 second | 0.08 second | 0.16 second |
| (3 squares x 0.04 second) | (2 squares x 0.04 second) | (4 squares x 0.04 second) |

**Figure 3-7.** *(Continued)*

## ST SEGMENT

The ST segment represents the end of ventricular depolarization and the beginning of ventricular repolarization. The ST segment begins with the end of the QRS complex and ends with the onset of the T wave (Figure 3-8). The point marking the end of the QRS is known as the *J point*. The normal ST segment is flat (isoelectric). Elevation or depression of the ST segment by 1 mm or more above or below baseline (measured 0.08 seconds or two squares past the J point) is considered abnormal. One way to estimate deviation from the baseline is to draw a line through the PR interval extending it through the T wave. If elevated, the ST segment may be horizontal (straight across), convex (arched upward), or concave (arched inward). If depressed, the ST segment may be horizontal, downsloping, or sagging.

An elevated ST segment is an ECG sign of myocardial injury, as seen in acute myocardial infarction. Other causes of ST segment elevation include coronary vasospasm (Prinzmetal's angina), pericarditis, and ventricular aneurysm. Sometimes, the ST segment may be slightly elevated above the baseline across the entire 12-lead ECG tracing in perfectly healthy people. This finding is the result of early repolarization changes and reflects a phase of ventricular repolarization that occurs earlier in the cardiac cycle than in most people. This is particularly common in young males. A depressed ST segment is an ECG sign of myocardial ischemia. Although ST segment depression is most often associated with myocardial ischemia, other common causes include left and right ventricular hypertrophy, left and right bundle branch block, hypokalemia, and the administration of certain drugs (quinidine, procainamide, and digitalis). Digitalis causes a sagging ST segment depression with a characteristic "scooped-out" appearance. Examples of ST segments are shown in Figure 3-9.

## T WAVE

The T wave represents the latter phase of ventricular repolarization. The normal T wave begins as the deflection slopes upward from the ST segment and ends when the waveform returns to baseline (Figure 3-10). Normal T waves are rounded, asymmetric (the peak is closer to the end of the wave than to the beginning), positive in Lead II, with an amplitude less than 5 mm. Abnormal T waves tend to be symmetric and may be abnormally tall or low, flattened, biphasic, or inverted. Abnormal T waves are seen in myocardial ischemia, myocardial infarction, hypokalemia, hyperkalemia, pericarditis, ventricular hypertrophy, bundle branch block, and in the administration of certain drugs (digitalis, procainamide, quinidine, and phenothiazines). Examples of T waves are shown in Figure 3-11.

## QT INTERVAL

The QT interval represents the time between the onset of ventricular depolarization and the end of ventricular repolarization. The QT interval is mea-

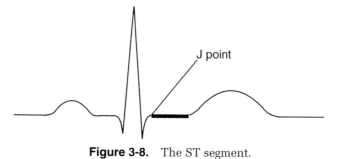

**Figure 3-8.** The ST segment.

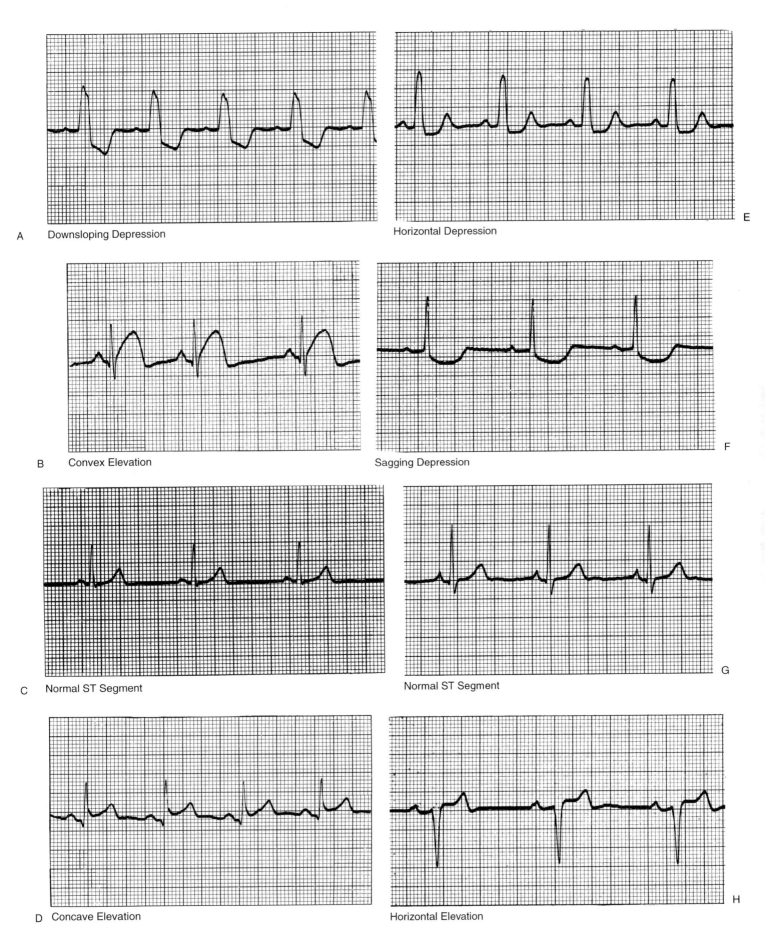

A   Downsloping Depression

B   Convex Elevation

C   Normal ST Segment

D   Concave Elevation

E   Horizontal Depression

F   Sagging Depression

G   Normal ST Segment

H   Horizontal Elevation

**Figure 3-9.**   ST segment examples.

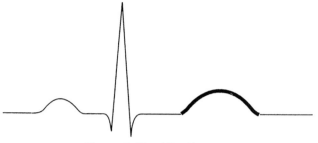

**Figure 3-10.** The T wave.

sured from the beginning of the QRS complex to the end of the T wave (Figure 3-12). The length of the QT interval normally varies according to age, gender, and especially heart rate. As the heart rate increases, the QT interval decreases; conversely, as the heart rate decreases, the QT interval increases. Therefore, the QT interval can be measured more accurately if it is corrected for heart rate. The normal QT interval corrected for heart rate ($QT_c$) is found in Table 3-1. Generally speaking, the normal QT should be less than half the distance between two consecutive R

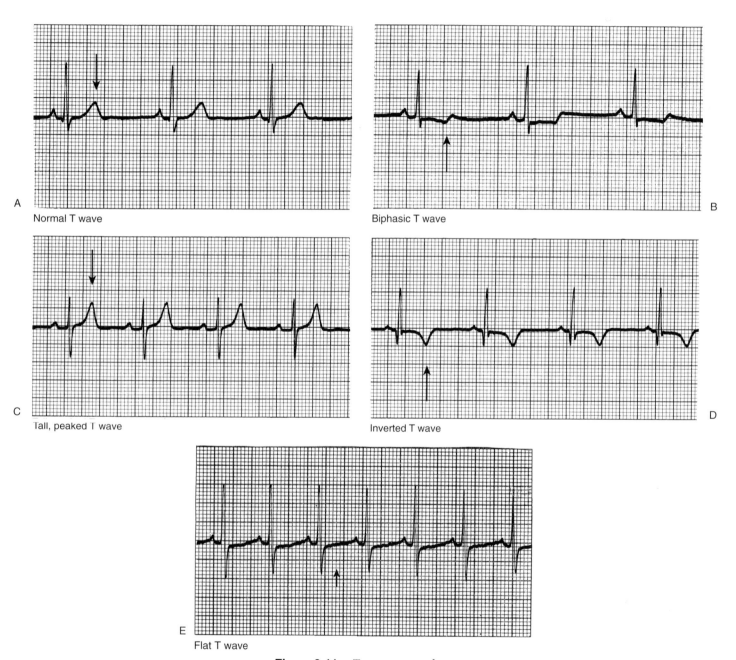

A    Normal T wave

B    Biphasic T wave

C    Tall, peaked T wave

D    Inverted T wave

E    Flat T wave

**Figure 3-11.** T wave examples.

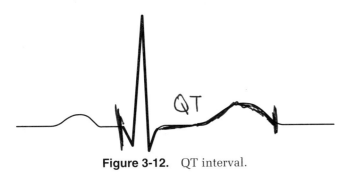

**Figure 3-12.** QT interval.

**Table 3-1.** QT$_c$ Interval normals

| Heart Rate (per minute) | QT$_c$ Normal Range (seconds) |
|---|---|
| 40 | 0.41–0.51 |
| 50 | 0.38–0.46 |
| 60 | 0.35–0.43 |
| 70 | 0.33–0.41 |
| 80 | 0.32–0.39 |
| 90 | 0.30–0.36 |
| 100 | 0.28–0.34 |
| 120 | 0.26–0.32 |
| 150 | 0.23–0.28 |
| 180 | 0.21–0.25 |
| 200 | 0.20–0.24 |

waves (called the R-R interval) when the rhythm is regular. The determination of the QT interval should be made in a lead where the T wave is most prominent and should not include the U wave. Also, accurate measurement of the QT can be done only when the rhythm is regular for at least two cardiac cycles before the measurement.

A normal QT interval indicates that ventricular depolarization and repolarization have occurred within a normal amount of time. A short QT interval represents an increase in the rate of repolarization of the ventricles and is not significant. This occurs with digitalis therapy and hypercalcemia. The importance of measuring the QT interval is to determine if it is prolonged. A prolonged QT interval indicates that ventricular repolarization time is delayed. This lengthens the relative refractory period (or vulnerable period) of the cardiac cycle, a situation that predisposes people to life-threatening arrhythmias (see discussion of torsade de pointes in Chapter 9). The most common causes of a prolonged QT interval include electrolyte imbalances (hypokalemia, hypocalcemia, hypomagnesemia), liquid protein diets, bradyarrhythmias, myocardial ischemia, acute myocardial infarction, left ventricular hypertrophy, subarachnoid hemorrhage, hypothermia, hereditary long-QT syndromes, and the administration of certain drugs (quinidine, procainamide, disopyramide, tricyclic antidepressants, amiodarone, phenothiazines, flecainide, ibutilide, and sotalol). It can also occur without a known cause (idiopathic). Examples of QT intervals are shown in Figure 3-13.

## U WAVE

The U wave is a small wave deflection that may occasionally follow the T wave. Neither its presence nor its absence is considered abnormal. The U wave is thought to be part of the ventricular repolarization process. The waveform begins as the deflection leaves baseline and ends when the deflection returns to baseline (Figure 3-14). Normal U waves are small, rounded, less than 2 mm in height, and in the same direction as the T wave. The U wave is larger at slow heart rates and smaller with fast heart rates.

Prominent U waves (taller than 2 mm) may be caused by left ventricular hypertrophy, exercise,

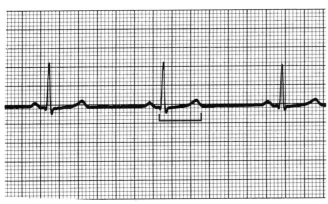

Normal QT interval of 0.44 sec (11 squares × .04 sec = 0.44 sec). Heart rate of 48 (31 small squares between consecutive R waves = 48)

**A**

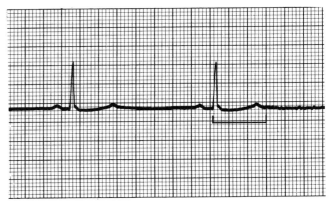

Prolonged QT interval of 0.56 sec (14 squares × .04 sec = 0.56 sec). Heart rate of 40 (38 small squares between consecutive R waves = 40)

**B**

**Figure 3-13.** QT interval examples.

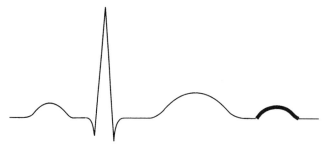

**Figure 3-14.** The U wave.

cerebrovascular accident, hypomagnesemia, hypokalemia, or in patients taking digitalis, quinidine, procainamide, disopyramide, amiodarone, sotalol, or phenothiazines. A prominent U wave is indicative of delayed ventricular repolarization and (like a prolonged QT interval) predisposes the person to development of a specific type of polymorphic ventricular tachycardia called *torsade de pointes* (see discussion of torsade de pointes in Chapter 9). Examples of U waves are shown in Figure 3-15.

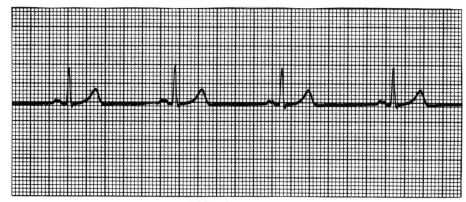

ECG without U wave

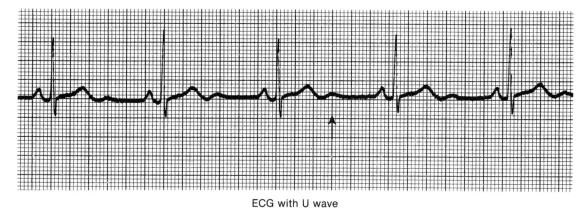

ECG with U wave

**Figure 3-15.** U wave examples.

# Waveform Practice: Labeling Waves

**Directions:** For each of the following rhythm strips (strips 3-1 through 3-14) label the P, Q, R, S, T, and U waves. Some of the strips may not have all of these waveforms. Check your answers with the answer keys in the Appendix.

Q – 1st neg. defl.
R – 1st pos.
S – 1st neg after pos.

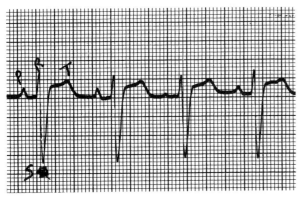

**Strip 3-1.**

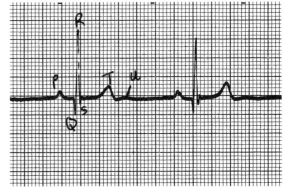

**Strip 3-2.**

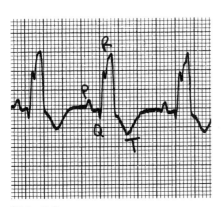

**Strip 3-3.**

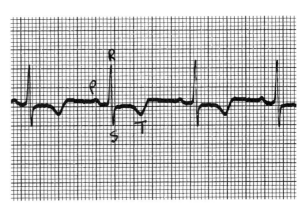

**Strip 3-4.**

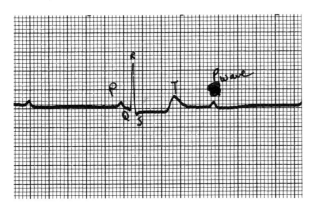

**Strip 3-5.**

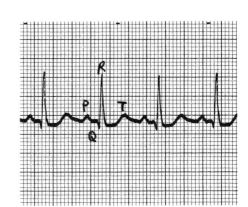

**Strip 3-6.**

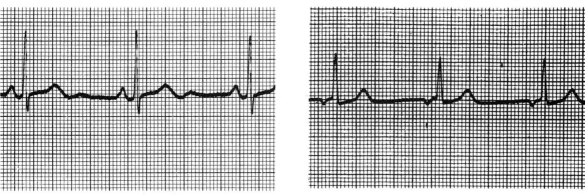

**Strip 3-7.**

**Strip 3-8.**

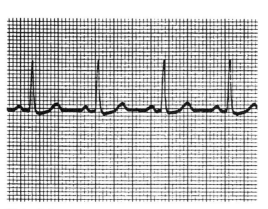

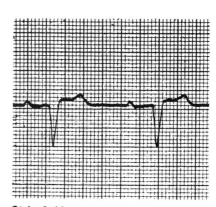

**Strip 3-9.**

**Strip 3-10.**

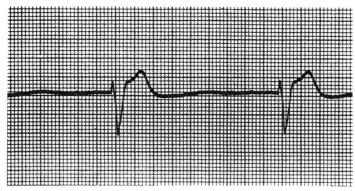

**Strip 3-11.**

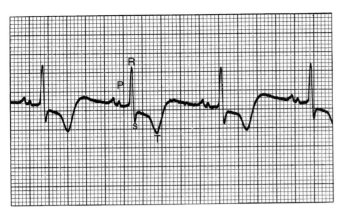

**Strip 3-12.**

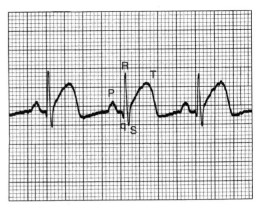

**Strip 3-13.**

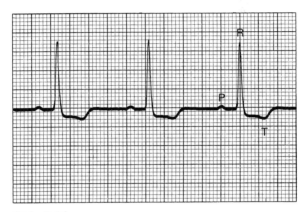

**Strip 3-14.**

# 4

# CARDIAC MONITORS

## PURPOSE OF ECG MONITORING

The electrocardiogram (ECG) is a recording of the electrical activity of the heart. The ECG records two basic electrical processes:

**1.** Depolarization (the spread of the electrical stimulus through the heart muscle), producing the P wave from the atria and the QRS from the ventricles

**2.** Repolarization (the return of the stimulated muscle to the resting state), producing the ST segment, the T wave, and the U wave

The depolarization–repolarization process produces electric currents, which are transmitted to the surface of the body. This electrical activity is detected by electrodes attached to the skin. After the electric current is detected, it is amplified, displayed on a monitor screen (oscilloscope), and recorded on ECG graph paper as waves and complexes. The waveforms can then be analyzed in a systematic manner, and the "cardiac rhythm" can be identified.

Bedside monitoring allows continuous observation of the heart's electrical activity and is used to identify arrhythmias (disturbances in rate, rhythm, or conduction) and to evaluate the effects of therapy. Continuous monitoring is used to monitor patients in critical care units, cardiac stepdown units, surgery suites, outpatient surgery departments, emergency rooms, postanesthesia recovery units, and so forth.

## TYPES OF BEDSIDE MONITORING

There are two types of bedside monitoring: hardwire and telemetry. With hardwire monitoring, conductive gel discs (electrodes) are placed on the patient's chest and attached to a lead-cable system, which is then connected to a bedside monitor. With telemetry (wireless monitoring), electrodes are attached to the patient's chest and the leads are connected to a portable monitor transmitter.

### Hardwire Monitoring

Hardwire monitoring will use either a five-leadwire system or a three-leadwire system:

**1. Five-leadwire system** (Figure 4-1). With the five-leadwire system, five electrodes and five leadwires are used. One electrode is placed below the right clavicle (2$^{nd}$ interspace, right midclavicular line), one below the left clavicle (2$^{nd}$ interspace, left midclavicular line), one on the right lower rib cage (8$^{th}$ interspace, right midclavicular line), one on the

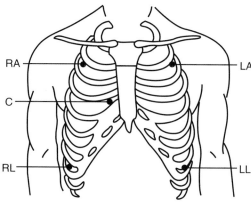

**Figure 4-1.** Hardwire monitoring—Five leadwire system. This illustration shows you where to place the electrodes and attach leadwires using a five-leadwire system. The leadwires are color-coded as follows:
  white—right arm (RA)
  black—left arm (LA)
  green—right leg (RL)
  red—left leg (LL)
  brown—chest (C)
Leads placed in the arm and leg positions as shown allow you to view leads I, II, III, aVR, aVL, and aVF. To view chest leads V$_1$–V$_6$, the chest lead must be placed in the specific chest lead position desired (see Figure 4-2). In this example, the brown chest lead is in V$_1$ position.

left lower rib cage (8$^{th}$ interspace, left midclavicular line), and one in a chest lead position (V$_1$–V$_6$). The six chest lead positions (Figure 4-2) include:

V$_1$  4$^{th}$ intercostal space, right sternal border
V$_2$  4$^{th}$ intercostal space, left sternal border
V$_3$  Midway between V$_2$ and V$_4$
V$_4$  5$^{th}$ intercostal space, left midclavicular line
V$_5$  5$^{th}$ intercostal space, left anterior axillary line
V$_6$  5$^{th}$ intercostal space, left midaxillary line

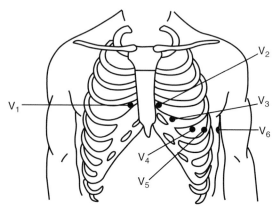

**Figure 4-2.** Chest lead positions.

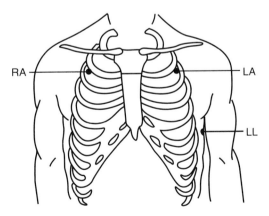

**Figure 4-3.** Hardwire monitoring—Three-leadwire system.

This illustration shows you where to place the electrodes and attach leadwires using a three-leadwire system. The lead wires are color-coded as follows:

white—right arm (RA)
black—left arm (LA)
red—left leg (LL)

Leads placed in this position will allow you to monitor leads I, II, or III using the lead selector on the monitor.

The right arm (RA) lead is attached to the electrode below the right clavicle, the left arm (LA) lead is attached to the electrode below the left clavicle, the right leg (RL) lead is attached to the electrode on the right lower rib cage, the left leg (LL) lead is attached to the electrode on the left lower rib cage, and the chest lead is attached to the chest electrode.

With the five-leadwire system for hardwire monitoring, you can continuously monitor two leads using a lead selector on the monitor. Leads placed in the arm and leg positions as shown in Figure 4-1 allow you to view leads I, II, III, aVR, aVL, and aVF. To view chest leads $V_1$ through $V_6$, you must place the chest lead in the specific chest lead position desired.

Generally, one of the limb leads (usually I, II, or III) and one of the chest leads (usually $V_1$ or $V_6$) are chosen to be monitored.

**1. Three-leadwire system** (Figure 4-3). With the three-leadwire system, three electrodes and three leadwires are used. One electrode is placed below the right clavicle ($2^{nd}$ interspace, right midclavicular line), one below the left clavicle ($2^{nd}$ interspace, left midclavicular line), and one on the left lower rib cage ($8^{th}$ interspace, left midclavicular line). The right arm (RA) lead is attached to the electrode below the right clavicle, the left arm (LA) lead is attached to the electrode below the left clavicle, and the left leg (LL) lead is attached to the electrode on the left lower rib cage. You can monitor limb leads I, II, or III by turning the lead selector on the monitor. Although you can't monitor chest leads ($V_1$–$V_6$) with a three-leadwire system, you can monitor modified chest leads, which provide similar information. To monitor any of these leads, reposition the left leg (LL) lead to the appropriate position for the chest lead you want to monitor, and turn the lead selector on the monitor to Lead III. Examples of modified chest lead $V_1$ ($MCL_1$) and modified chest lead $V_6$ ($MCL_6$) are shown in Figure 4-4.

### Telemetry Monitoring

Wireless monitoring, or telemetry, gives the patient more freedom than the hardwire monitoring system. Instead of being connected to a bedside monitor, the patient is connected to a portable monitor transmitter, which can be placed in a pajama pocket or in a telemetry pouch. Telemetry monitoring systems are available in a five-leadwire system and a three-leadwire system.

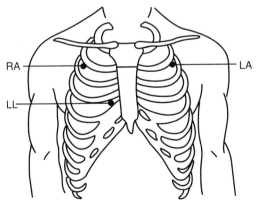

Modified Chest Lead $V_1$ ($MCL_1$)

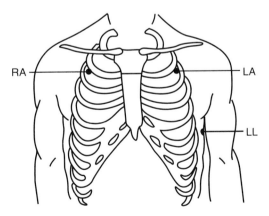

Modified Chest Lead $V_6$ ($MCL_6$)

**Figure 4-4.** Hardwire monitoring—Three-leadwire system: Leads $MCL_1$ and $MCL_6$. Modified chest leads can be monitored with the three-leadwire system by repositioning the left leg (LL) lead to chest position desired and turning the lead selector on the monitor to Lead III.

**1. Five-leadwire system** (Figure 4-5). The five-leadwire system for telemetry is connected in the same manner as the five-leadwire system for hardwire monitoring with the four limb positions (RA, LA, RL, LL) in the conventional locations and the chest leads placed in the desired $V_1$–$V_6$ location. With this system, you can monitor any one of the 12 leads using a lead selector on the monitor. Leads placed in the limb positions as shown in Figure 4-5 allow you to view leads I, II, III, $aV_R$, $aV_L$, and $aV_F$. To view chest leads $V_1$–$V_6$, you must place the chest lead in the specific chest lead position desired.

**2. Three-leadwire system** (Figure 4-6). The three-leadwire system for telemetry uses three electrode pads and three leadwires. The leadwires are connected to positive, negative, and ground connections on the telemetry transmitter and placed in limb and chest positions similar to those used with the 12-lead ECG. These leads record electrical forces viewed between two electrodes, one designated negative and one designated positive. One limb lead (I, II, III) at a time may be monitored or one of the modified chest leads ($MCL_1$ or $MCL_6$).

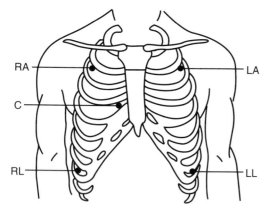

**Figure 4-5.** Telemetry monitoring—Five-leadwire system.
This illustration shows you where to place the electrodes and attach leadwires using a five-leadwire system. The leadwires are color-coded as follows:

  white—right arm (RA)
  black—left arm (LA)
  green—right leg (RL)
  red—left leg (LL)
  brown—chest (C)

With the 5 leadwire system for telemetry monitoring you can monitor any one of the 12 leads using a lead selector on the monitor. Leads placed in the conventional limb positions allow you to view leads I, II, III, $aV_R$, $aV_L$, and $aV_F$. To view chest lead $V_1$–$V_6$ the chest lead must be placed in the specific chest lead desired.

# APPLYING THE ELECTRODE PADS

Proper attachment of the electrodes to the skin is the most important step in obtaining a good quality ECG tracing. Unless there is good contact between the skin and the electrode pad, distortions of the ECG tracing (artifacts) may appear. An *artifact* is any abnormal wave, spike, or movement on the ECG tracing that is not generated by the electrical activity of the heart. The procedure for attaching the electrodes is as follows:

**1. Choose monitor lead position.** It is helpful to assess the 12-lead ECG to ascertain which lead provides the best QRS voltage and P wave identification.

**2. Prepare the skin.**
  **a.** Shave the sites, if necessary, with a razor. Hair interferes with good contact between the electrode pad and the skin.
  **b.** Wipe sites with alcohol or acetone pad to remove skin oil. Allow to dry.
  **c.** Gently abrade skin. A dry washcloth may be used. Some companies produce electrode pads with a small amount of abrasive material attached to the pad's peel-off section—these work extremely well.
  **d.** If the patient is perspiring, apply a thin coat of tincture of benzoin and allow it to dry.

**3. Attach electrode pads.**
  **a.** Avoid placing pads over bony areas, such as the clavicles or prominent rib markings.
  **b.** Remove pads from packaging. Check electrode disc for presence of moist conductive gel. Dried gel can cause loss of the ECG signal.
  **c.** Place electrode pad on prepared sites, pressing firmly around periphery of the pad.

**4. Connect leadwires.** Attach appropriate leadwires to the electrode pads according to established electrode-lead positions.

# TROUBLESHOOTING MONITOR PROBLEMS

Many problems may be encountered during cardiac monitoring. The most common problems are related to patient movement, interference from equipment in or near the patient room, weak ECG signals, poor choice of monitor lead or electrode placement,

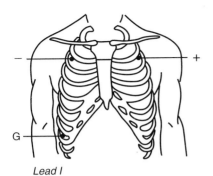

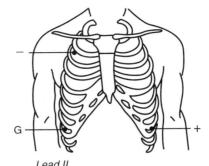

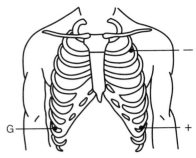

*Lead I*

Negative lead — 2nd interspace
right midclavicular line

Positive lead — 2nd interspace
left midclavicular line

Ground lead — 8th interspace
right midclavicular line

*Lead II*

Negative lead — 2nd interspace
right midclavicular line

Positive lead — 8th interspace
left midclavicular line

Ground lead — 8th interspace
right midclavicular line

*Lead III*

Negative lead — 2nd interspace
left midclavicular line

Positive lead — 8th interspace
left midclavicular line

Ground lead — 8th interspace
right midclavicular line

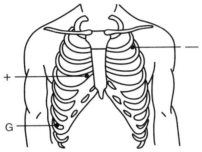

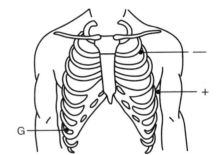

*Modified Chest Lead V$_1$ (MCL$_1$)*

Negative lead — 2nd interspace
left midclavicular line

Positive lead — 4th interspace
right sternal border

Ground lead — 8th interspace
right midclavicular line

*Modified Chest Lead V$_6$ (MCL$_6$)*

Negative lead — 2nd interspace
left midclavicular line

Positive lead — 5th interspace
left midaxillary line

Ground lead — 8th interspace
right midclavicular line

**Figure 4-6.** Telemetry monitoring—Three-leadwire system.
The three-leadwire system for telemetry uses one electrode designated as positive, one electrode designated as negative, and the third electrode as a ground. These leads record electrical forces viewed between the positive and negative electrodes. One limb lead (I, II, III) at a time may be monitored or one of the modified chest leads (MCL$_1$ or MCL$_6$).

and poor contact between the skin and electrode-lead attachments. Monitor problems can cause artifacts on the ECG tracing, making identification of the cardiac rhythm difficult or triggering false monitor alarms (high rate alarms and low rate alarms). Some problems are potentially serious and require intervention, whereas others are transient, non–life-threatening occurrences that will correct themselves. The nurse and monitor technician need to develop proficiency in recognizing monitoring problems, identifying probable causes, and seeking solutions to correct the problems. The most common monitoring problems are discussed below:

### False High Rate Alarms

High-voltage artifact potentials are often interpreted by the monitor as QRS complexes and activate the high rate alarm (Figure 4-7). Most high-voltage artifacts are related to muscle movements from turning in bed or moving the extremities. Seizure activity can also produce high-voltage artifact potentials.

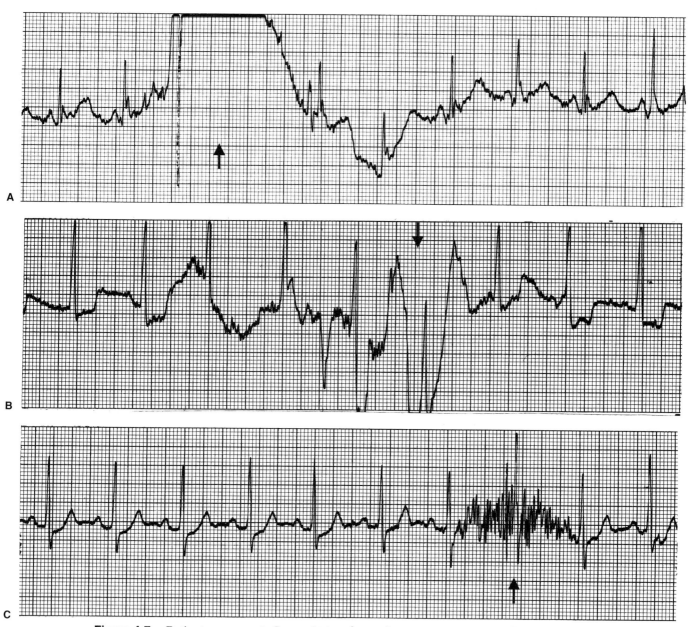

**Figure 4-7.** Patient movement. *Cause*: Strips above show patient turning in bed or extremity movement. *Solution*: Problem is usually intermittent and no correction is necessary. Movement artifact can be reduced by avoiding placement of electrode pads in areas where extremity movement is greatest (bony areas such as the clavicles).

### False Low Rate Alarms

Any disturbance in the transmission of the electrical signal from the skin electrode to the monitoring system can activate a false low rate alarm (Figures 4-8 through 4-10). This problem is usually caused by ineffective contact between the skin and the electrode or leadwire due to dried conductive gel, a loose electrode, or a disconnected leadwire. Low-voltage QRS complexes can also activate the low rate alarm.

If the ventricular waveforms are not tall enough, the monitor detects no electrical activity and will sound the low rate alarm.

### Muscle Tremors

Muscle tremors (Figures 4-11 and 4-12) can occur in tense, nervous patients or those shivering from cold or having a chill. The ECG baseline has an uneven, coarsely jagged appearance, obscuring

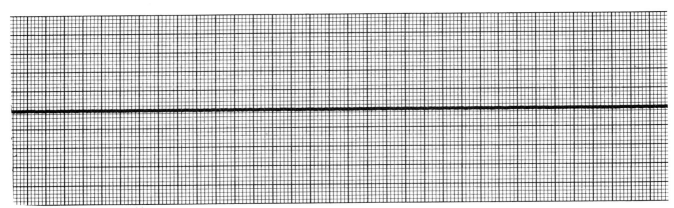

**Figure 4-8.** Continuous straight line. *Cause*: dried conductive gel, disconnected lead wire, or disconnected electrode pad. *Solution*: Check electrode/lead system: re-prep and re-attach electrodes and leads as necessary. Note: A straight line may also indicate the absence of electrical activity in the heart—the patient must be evaluated immediately for the presence of a pulse.

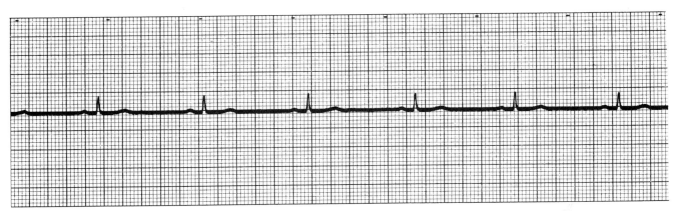

**Figure 4-9.** Continuous low waveform voltage. *Cause*: Low voltage QRS complexes. *Solution*: Turn up amplitude (gain) knob on monitor or change lead positions.

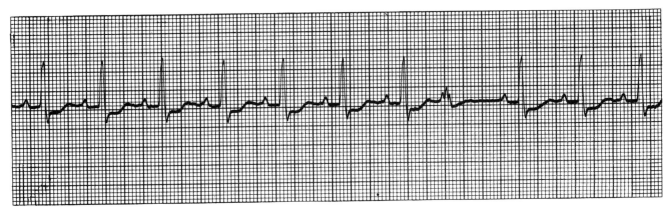

**Figure 4-10.** Intermittent low waveform voltage. *Cause*: Intermittent low voltage QRS complexes are seen in both strips above. *Solution*: If problem is frequent and activates the low rate alarm, change lead positions.

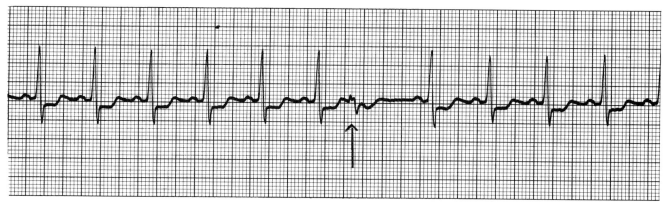

**Figure 4-10.** *(Continued)*

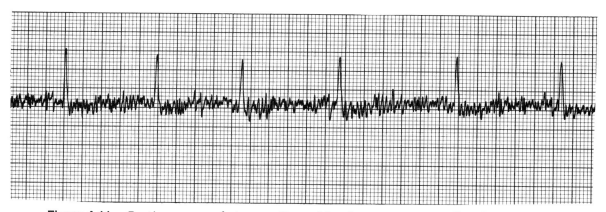

**Figure 4-11.** Continuous muscle tremor. *Cause*: Muscle tremors are usually related to tense or nervous patients or those shivering from cold or a chill. *Solution*: Treat cause.

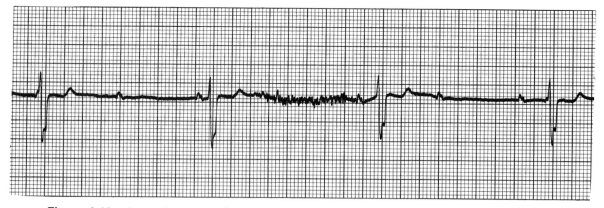

**Figure 4-12.** Intermittent muscle tremor. *Cause*: Muscle tremors that occur intermittently. *Solution*: Correction is usually not necessary.

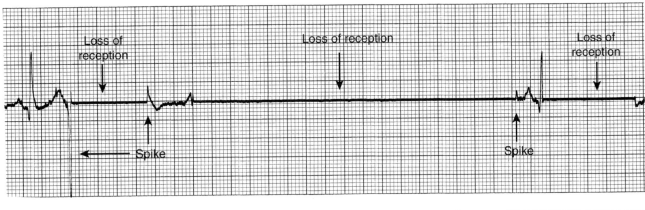

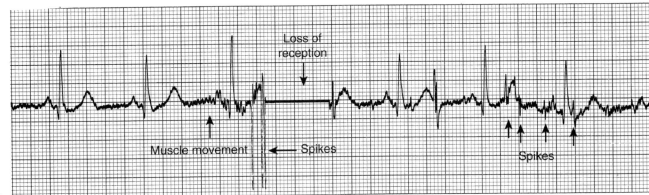

**Figure 4-13.** Telemetry-related interference. *Cause*: ECG signals are poorly received over the telemetry system causing sharp spikes and sometimes loss of signal reception. This problem is usually related to weak batteries or the transmitter being used in the outer fringes of the reception area for the base station receiver. *Solution*: Change batteries; keep patient in reception area of base station receivers.

the components of the ECG tracing. The problem may be continuous or intermittent.

### Telemetry-Related Interference

Telemetry-related artifacts occur when the ECG signals are poorly received over a telemetry monitoring system (Figure 4-13). Weak ECG signals are caused by weak batteries or by the transmitter being used in the outer fringes of the reception area of the base station receiver, resulting in sharp spikes or straight lines on the ECG tracing.

### Electrical Interference (AC Interference)

Electrical interference (Figure 4-14) can occur when multiple pieces of electric equipment are in

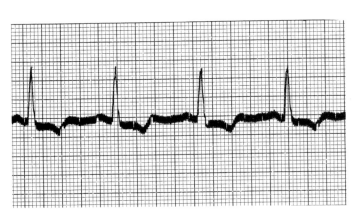

**Figure 4-14.** Electrical interference (AC interference). *Cause*: Patient using electrical equipment (electric razor, hair dryer); multiple electrical equipment in use in room; improperly grounded equipment; loose electrical connections or exposed wiring. *Solution*: If patient is using electrical equipment, problem is transient and will correct itself. If patient is not using electrical equipment: a) unplug all equipment not in continuous use b) remove from service and report any equipment with breaks or wires showing c) ask the electrical engineer to check the wiring.

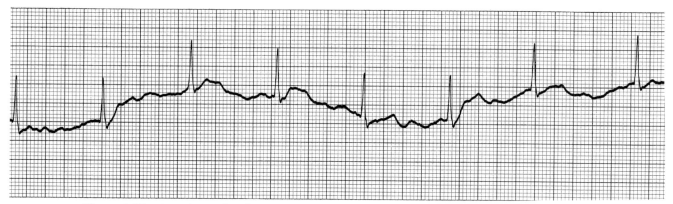

**Figure 4-15.** Wandering baseline. *Cause*: Exaggerated respiratory movements usually seen in patients in respiratory distress (COPD patients). *Solution*: Avoid placing electrode pads in areas where movements of the accessory muscles are most exaggerated (which can be anywhere on the anterior chest wall). Place the pads on the upper back or top of the shoulders if necessary.

use in the patient room, when the patient is using an electric appliance such as an electric razor or hair dryer, when improperly grounded equipment is in use, or when loose or exposed wiring is present. This type of interference results in an artifact with a wide baseline consisting of a continuous series of fine, even, rapid spikes, which can obscure the components of the ECG tracing.

## Wandering Baseline

A wandering baseline (Figure 4-15) is a monitor pattern that wanders up and down on the monitor screen or ECG tracing and is caused by exaggerated respiratory movements commonly seen in patients with respiratory distress. This type of artifact makes it difficult to identify the cardiac rhythm as well as changes in the ST segment and T wave.

# 5

# ANALYZING A RHYTHM STRIP

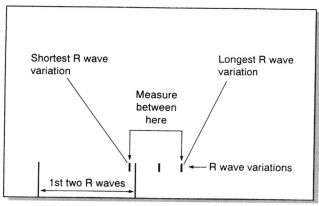

**Figure 5-1.** Index card.

Five basic steps are followed in analyzing a rhythm strip. Each step should be performed in sequence. Eventually, this will become a habit and you will be able to identify a strip quickly and accurately.

## STEP 1: DETERMINE THE REGULARITY (RHYTHM) OF THE R WAVES

Starting at the left side of the rhythm strip, place an index card above the first two R waves (Figure 5-1). Using a sharp pencil, mark on the index card above the two R waves. Measure from R wave to R wave across the rhythm strip, marking on the index card any variation in R wave regularity. If the rhythm varies by 0.12 seconds (three squares) or more between the shortest and longest R wave variation marked on the index card, the rhythm is irregular. If the rhythm does not vary, or varies by less than 0.12 seconds, the rhythm is considered regular.

Calipers may also be used, instead of an index card, to determine regularity of the rhythm strip. The R wave regularity is assessed in the same manner as with the index card, by placing the two caliper points on top of two consecutive R waves and pro-ceeding left to right across the rhythm strip, noting any variation in the R–R regularity.

The author prefers the index card method, because each R wave variation (however slight) can be marked and a specific measurement can be done to determine if a 0.12-second or greater variance exists between the shorter and longer R wave variations. With calipers, a variation in the R wave regularity may be noted, but, without marking and measuring between the shortest and longest R wave variations, there is no way to determine how irregular the rhythm is. Examples of rhythm measurements are shown in Figures 5-2 through 5-4.

## STEP 2 : CALCULATE THE HEART RATE

This measurement will always refer to the ventricular rate unless the atrial and ventricular rates differ, in which case both will be given. The ventricular rate is usually determined by looking at a 6-second rhythm strip. The top of the electrocardiogram paper is marked at 3-second intervals; two intervals equals 6 seconds (Figure 5-5). Several methods can be used to calculate heart rate. These methods differ according to the regularity or irregularity of the rhythm.

### Regular Rhythms

Two methods can be used to calculate heart rate in regular rhythms:

**1.** Rapid Rate Calculation—Count the number of R waves in a 6-second strip, and multiply by 10 (6 seconds × 10 = 60 seconds, or the heart rate per minute). This method provides an approximate heart rate in beats per minute, is fast and simple, and can be used with both regular and irregular rhythms.

**2.** Precise Rate Calculation—Count the number of small squares between two consecutive R waves

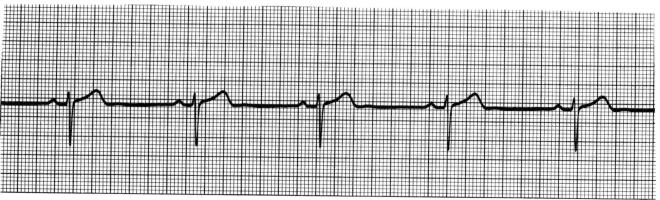

**Figure 5-2.** Regular rhythm; R-R intervals do not vary.

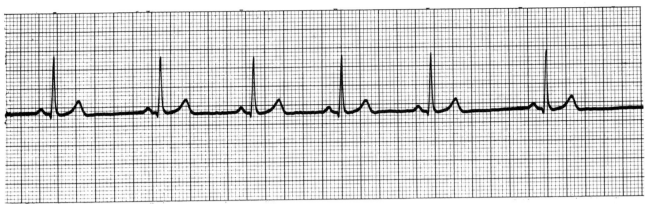

**Figure 5-3.** Irregular rhythm; R-R intervals vary by 0.32 seconds.

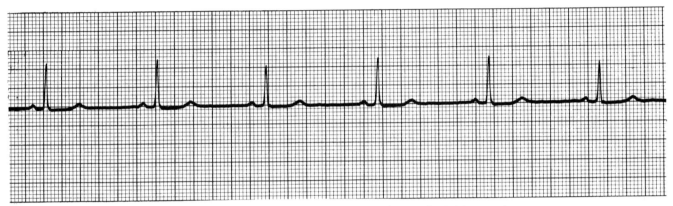

**Figure 5-4.** Regular rhythm; R-R intervals vary by 0.04 seconds.

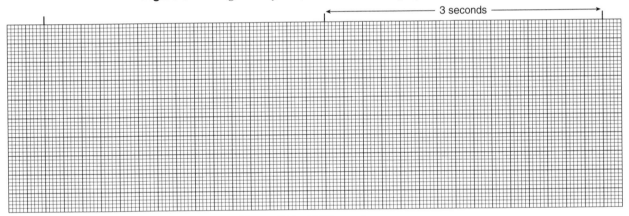

**Figure 5-5.** ECG graph paper.

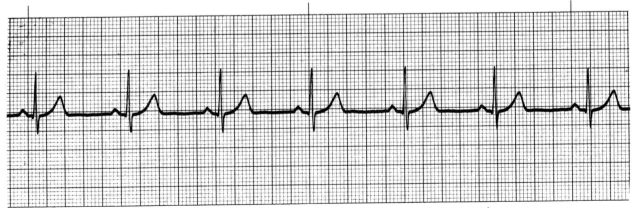

**Figure 5-6.** Regular rhythm; 25 small squares between R waves = 60 heart rate.

(Figure 5-6), and refer to the conversion table printed on the back inside cover of this book. This method is very accurate but can only be used for regular rhythms. If a conversion table is not available, divide the number of small squares between the two consecutive R waves into 1500 (the number of small squares in a 1-minute rhythm strip). The heart rates for regular rhythms in the answer keys were determined by the precise rate calculation method.

### Irregular Rhythms

Only one method is used to calculate heart rate in irregular rhythms:

Rapid Rate Calculation—Count the number of R waves in a 6-second strip and multiply by 10 (Figure 5-7), or count the number of R waves in a 3-second strip and multiply by 20 (3 seconds × 20 = 60 seconds or the heart rate per minute.)

### Other Hints

When interpreting the rhythm strip, describe the basic underlying rhythm first, then add additional information, such as normal sinus rhythm (the underlying rhythm) with frequent premature ventricular contractions (PVCs).

When rhythm strips have premature beats (Figure 5-8), the premature beats are not included in the calculation of the rate. Count the rate in the uninterrupted section—this is the underlying rhythm. In this example, the uninterrupted section is regular and the heart rate is 68 (22 squares between R waves = 68).

When rhythm strips have more than one rhythm on a 6-second strip (Figure 5-9), rates must be calculated for each rhythm. This will aid in the identification of each rhythm. In the example, the first rhythm is irregular and the heart rate is 180 (nine R waves in 3 seconds × 20 = 180). The second rhythm is regu-

lar, and the heart rate is 214 (seven squares between R waves = 214).

When a rhythm covers less than 3 seconds on a rhythm strip (Figure 5-10), rate calculation is difficult but not impossible. In the example shown in Figure 5-10, the first rhythm takes up half of a 3-second interval. There are only two R waves. Therefore, you can't determine if the rhythm is regular or irregular. In this situation, multiply the two R waves by 40 (1.5 seconds × 40 = 60 seconds, or the heart rate per minute) to obtain an approximate heart rate of 80. The second rhythm is regular, with a heart rate of 167 (9 small squares between R waves = 167).

## STEP 3: IDENTIFY AND EXAMINE P WAVES

Analyze the P waves. One P wave should precede each QRS complex. All P waves should be identical (or near identical) in size, shape, and position. In Figure 5-11, there is one P wave to each QRS complex, and all P waves are identical in size, shape, and position. In Figure 5-12, there is one P wave to each QRS, but the P waves vary in size, shape, and position.

## STEP 4: MEASURE THE PR INTERVAL

Measure from the beginning of the P wave as it leaves baseline to the beginning of the QRS complex. Count the number of squares contained in this interval, and multiply by 0.04 seconds. In Figure 5-13, the PR interval is 0.16 seconds (four squares × 0.04 seconds = 0.16 seconds).

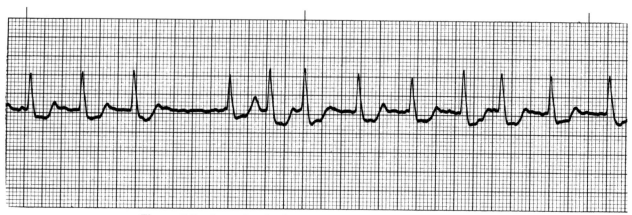

**Figure 5-7.** Irregular rhythm-11 R waves × 10 = 110 heart rate.

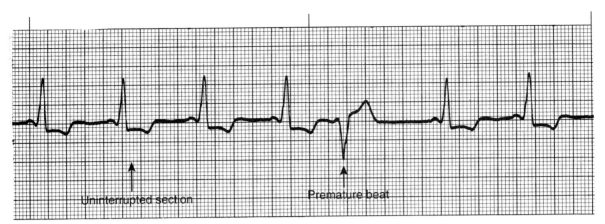

**Figure 5-8.** Rhythm with premature beat.

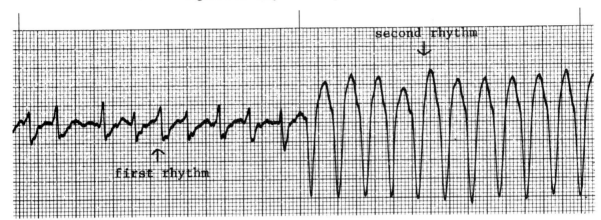

**Figure 5-9.** Rhythm strip with two different rhythms.

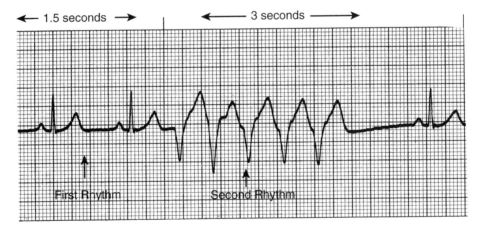

**Figure 5-10.** Calculating rate when a rhythm covers less than 3 seconds.

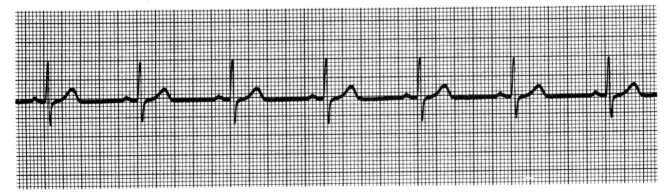

**Figure 5-11.** Normal P waves.

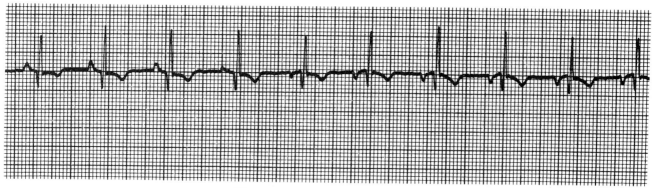

**Figure 5-12.** Abnormal P waves.

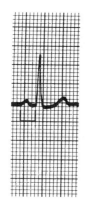

**Figure 5-13.** PR 0.16 seconds.

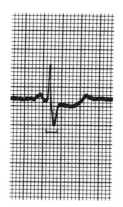

**Figure 5-14.** QRS 0.12 seconds.

## STEP 5: MEASURE THE QRS COMPLEX

Measure from the beginning of the QRS as it leaves baseline until the end of the QRS when the ST segment begins. Count the number of squares in this measurement, and multiply by 0.04 seconds. In Figure 5-14, the QRS takes up three squares and represents 0.12 seconds (three squares × 0.04 seconds = 0.12 seconds). In Figure 5-15, the QRS takes up 2½ squares and represents 0.10 seconds (2½ squares × 0.04 seconds = 0.10 seconds).

If rhythm strips are analyzed using a systematic step-by-step approach (Box 5-1), accurate interpretation will be achieved most of the time.

**Box 5-1.   Rhythm Strip Analysis**
1. Determine regularity (rhythm).
2. Calculate rate.
3. Examine P waves.
4. Measure PR interval.
5. Measure QRS complex.

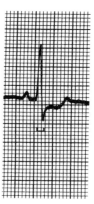

**Figure 5-15.** QRS 0.10 seconds.

# Waveform Practice—
# Analyzing Rhythm Strips

**Directions:** Analyze the following rhythm strips using the 5-step process discussed in this chapter. Check your answers with the answer keys in the appendix.

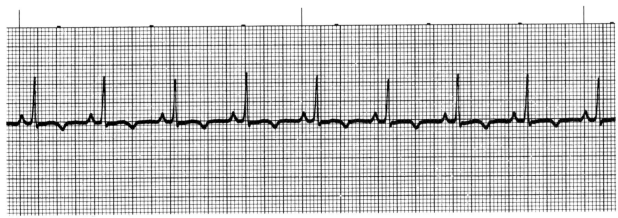

**Strip 5-1.** Rhythm: _Regular_     Rate: _79_     P wave: _Regular_
PR interval: _.16_     QRS: _.04_

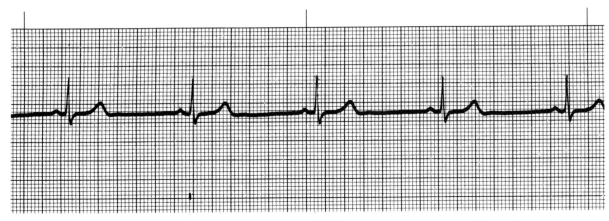

**Strip 5-2.** Rhythm: _Regular_     Rate: _45_     P wave: _Regular_
PR interval: _.~~B~~ 16_     QRS: _.06_

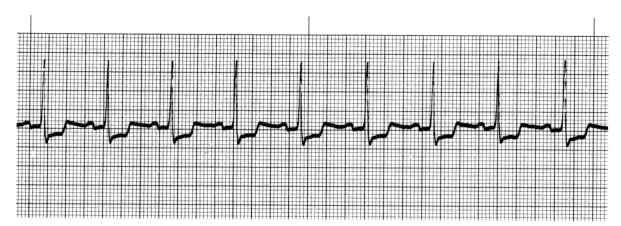

**Strip 5-3.** Rhythm: Regular    Rate: 84    P wave: Regular
PR interval: .20    QRS: .08

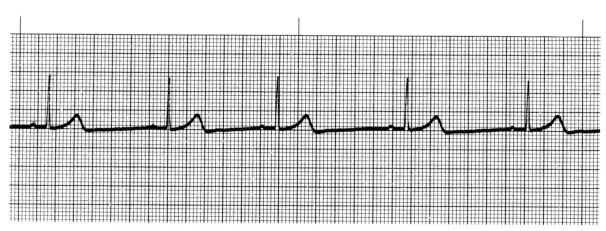

**Strip 5-4.** Rhythm: Irregular    Rate: 50    P wave: Irregular
PR interval: .16    QRS: .04

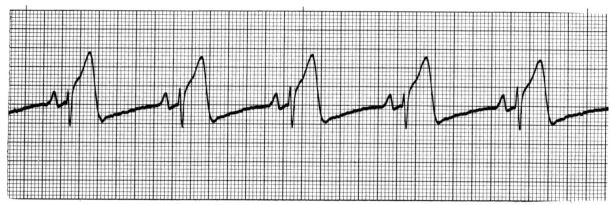

**Strip 5-5.** Rhythm: Regular    Rate: 50    P wave: Regular
PR interval: .20    QRS: .08

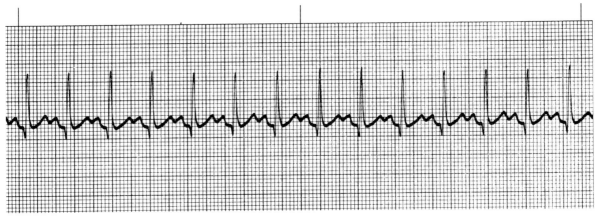

**Strip 5-6.** Rhythm:_____ Rate:_____ P wave:_____

PR interval:_____ QRS:_____

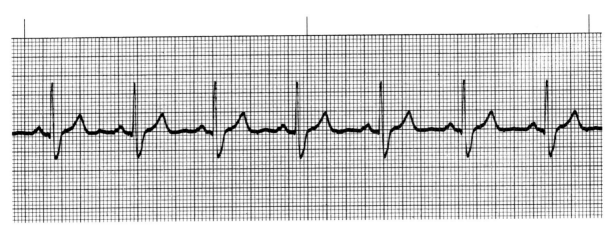

**Strip 5-7.** Rhythm:_____ Rate:_____ P wave:_____

PR interval:_____ QRS:_____

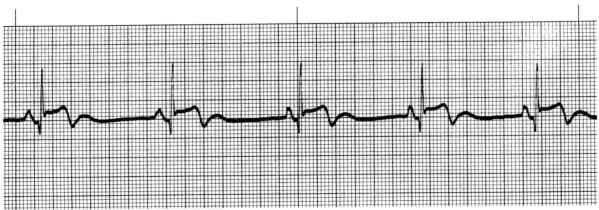

**Strip 5-8.** Rhythm:_____ Rate:_____ P wave:_____

PR interval:_____ QRS:_____

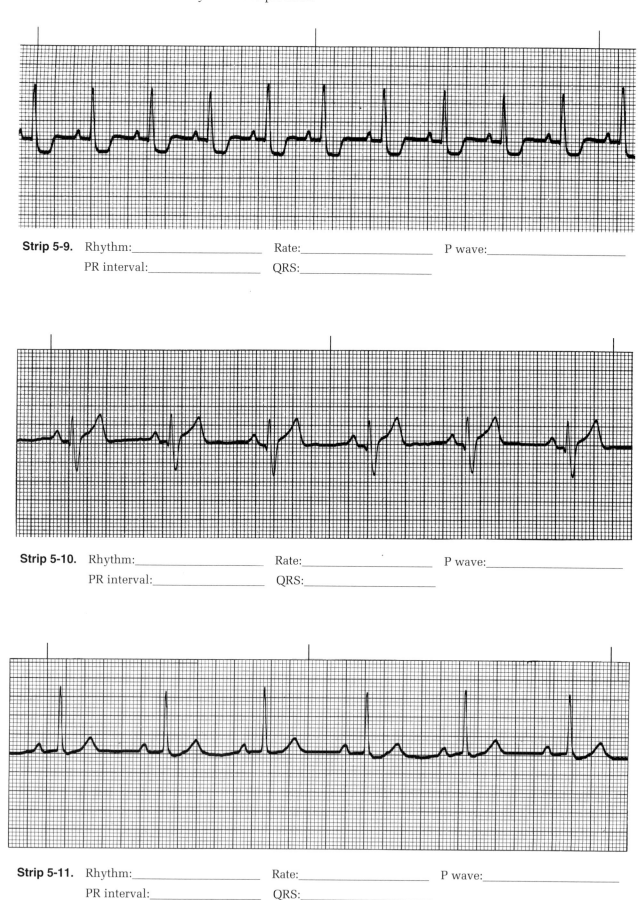

**Strip 5-9.** Rhythm:_____ Rate:_____ P wave:_____

PR interval:_____ QRS:_____

**Strip 5-10.** Rhythm:_____ Rate:_____ P wave:_____

PR interval:_____ QRS:_____

**Strip 5-11.** Rhythm:_____ Rate:_____ P wave:_____

PR interval:_____ QRS:_____

# 6

## SINUS ARRHYTHMIAS

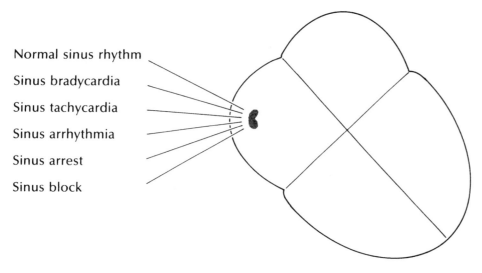

Normal sinus rhythm
Sinus bradycardia
Sinus tachycardia
Sinus arrhythmia
Sinus arrest
Sinus block

**Figure 6-1.** Sinus arrhythmias.

The term *arrhythmia* is very general, referring to all rhythms other than the normal rhythm of the heart (normal sinus rhythm). Sinus arrhythmias (Figure 6-1) result from disturbances in impulse discharge or impulse conduction from the sinus node. The sinus node retains its role as pacemaker of the heart but discharges impulses too fast (sinus tachycardia) or too slow (sinus bradycardia); discharges impulses irregularly (sinus arrhythmia); fails to discharge an impulse (sinus arrest); or the impulses discharged are blocked as they exit the SA node (sinus exit block), thus preventing conduction to the atria. Sinus bradycardia, sinus tachycardia, sinus arrhythmia, sinus arrest, and sinus block are all considered arrhythmias. However, sinus bradycardia at rest, sinus tachycardia with exercise, and

respiratory sinus arrhythmia are all normal findings.

The regulation of the heart rate is controlled by the autonomic nervous system. The autonomic nerve supply to the heart consists of two opposing groups of fibers: the sympathetic nerves and the parasympathetic nerves. Sympathetic stimulation produces an increase in heart rate, an increase in conduction through the AV node, and an increase in the strength of myocardial contraction. Parasympathetic stimulation (from the vagus nerve) produces a slowing of the heart rate, a decrease in conduction through the AV node, and a decrease in the strength of myocardial contraction. Thus, the sympathetic nervous system acts as a cardiac accelerator whereas the parasympathetic system acts as a cardiac inhibitor. Normally,

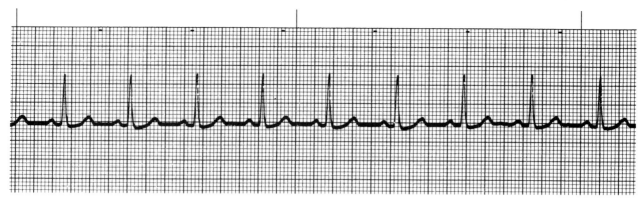

**Figure 6-2.** **Normal Sinus Rhythm**

*Rhythm:*   Regular

*Rate:*   84

*P waves:*   Normal and precede each QRS

*PR:*   0.14 to 0.16 seconds

*QRS:*   0.06 to 0.08 seconds

these systems are balanced, maintaining a heart rate between 60 and 100 times a minute.

## NORMAL SINUS RHYTHM

In a normal sinus rhythm (Figure 6-2; Box 6-1), the electrical impulses are formed in the sinoatrial (SA) node and discharged regularly at a rate of 60 to 100 times per minute. The P waves are normal in configuration and direction and precede each QRS complex. The PR interval and QRS duration are within normal limits. Normal sinus rhythm (NSR) is the normal rhythm of the heart and is of no clinical significance. No treatment is indicated.

| Box 6-1. | Normal Sinus Rhythm: Identifying ECG Features |
| --- | --- |
| Rhythm: | Regular |
| Rate: | 60–100 |
| P waves: | Normal in configuration and direction; one P wave precedes each QRS complex |
| PR: | Normal (0.12–0.20 seconds) |
| QRS: | Normal (0.10 seconds or less) |

## SINUS TACHYCARDIA

Sinus tachycardia (Figure 6-3; Box 6-2) originates in the SA node and discharges impulses regularly at a rate between 100 and 160 times per minute. The P waves are normal in configuration and direc-tion and precede each QRS complex. The PR interval and QRS duration are within normal limits. The distinguishing feature of this rhythm is the sinus origin and the rate between 100 and 160.

| Box 6-2. | Sinus Tachycardia: Identifying ECG Features |
| --- | --- |
| Rhythm: | Regular |
| Rate: | 100–160 |
| P waves: | Normal in configuration and direction; one P wave precedes each QRS complex |
| PR: | Normal (0.12–0.20 seconds) |
| QRS: | Normal (0.10 seconds or less) |

Sinus tachycardia is the normal response of the heart to the body's demand for an increase in blood flow. The sinus node gradually increases its rate in response to the needs of the body. When these needs no longer exist, the heart rate gradually slows down. Sinus tachycardia begins and ends gradually in contrast to other tachycardias, which begin and end suddenly.

Sinus tachycardia can be caused by anything that stimulates the sympathetic nervous system or anything that inhibits the parasympathetic nervous system. Conditions commonly associated with sinus tachycardia are:

1. Excitement, exertion, exercise
2. Fever, infections, septic shock
3. Hypoxia, hypovolemia, hypotension, heart failure, hyperthyroidism

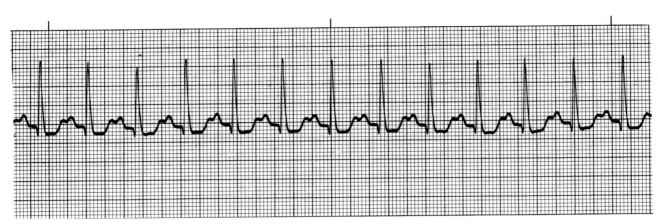

**Figure 6-3.** **Sinus Tachycardia**

| | |
| --- | --- |
| *Rhythm:* | Regular |
| *Rate:* | 115 |
| *P waves:* | Sinus |
| *PR:* | 0.16 to 0.18 seconds |
| *QRS:* | 0.08 to 0.10 seconds |

**4.** Pain, pulmonary embolism (sinus tachycardia is the most common arrhythmia seen with pulmonary embolism)

**5.** Anxiety, anemia

**6.** Myocardial ischemia, myocardial infarction (sinus tachycardia persisting after an acute infarct implies extensive heart damage and is generally a bad prognostic sign)

**7.** Drugs that increase sympathetic tone (epinephrine, norepinephrine, dopamine, dobutamine, tricyclic antidepressants, isuprel, cocaine, nitroprusside)

**8.** Drugs that decrease parasympathetic tone (atropine)

**9.** Ingestion of stimulants (coffee, tea, alcohol) or smoking

Sinus tachycardia in healthy people is a benign arrhythmia and does not require aggressive treatment. When its cause is removed or treated (fever, anxiety, and so forth), sinus tachycardia resolves gradually on its own. However, because this arrhythmia is a physiologic response of the heart to the demand for increased blood flow, it should serve as a warning sign and should never be ignored, especially in the cardiac patient. A rapid heart rate increases the workload of the heart, and the oxygen requirements of the heart are increased. Persistent tachycardia can cause decreased stroke volume, decreased cardiac output, and decreased coronary perfusion secondary to the decreased diastolic filling

time that occurs with rapid heart rates. Treatment of sinus tachycardia should be directed not at the rapid heart rate but to correcting the underlying cause of the arrhythmia.

## SINUS BRADYCARDIA

Sinus bradycardia (Figure 6-4; Box 6-3) originates in the SA node and discharges impulses regularly at a rate between 40 and 60 times per minute. The P waves are normal in configuration and direction and precede each QRS complex. The PR interval and QRS duration are within normal limits. The distinguishing feature of this rhythm is the sinus origin

| Box 6-3. | Sinus Bradycardia: Identifying ECG Features |
|---|---|
| Rhythm: | Regular |
| Rate: | 40–60 |
| P waves: | Normal in configuration and direction; one P wave precedes each QRS complex |
| PR: | Normal (0.12–0.20 seconds) |
| QRS: | Normal (0.10 seconds or less) |

and a rate between 40 and 60 times per minute.

Sinus bradycardia is the normal response of the heart to relaxation or sleeping when the parasympathetic effect on cardiac automaticity dominates over the sympathetic effect. It's common among trained

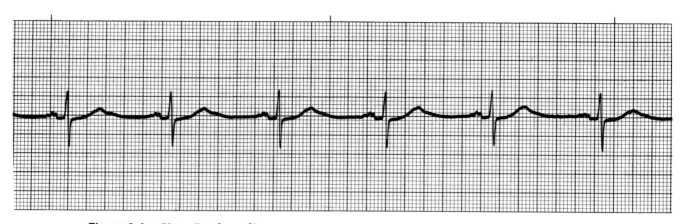

**Figure 6-4.** **Sinus Bradycardia**

*Rhythm:* Regular

*Rate:* 54

*P waves:* Sinus

*PR:* 0.20 seconds

*QRS:* 0.06 to 0.08 seconds

*Note:* A notched P wave is usually indicative of left atrial hypertrophy athletes who may have a resting or sleeping pulse rate as low as 35 beats per minute.

Sinus bradycardia can be caused by anything that increases parasympathetic tone or decreases sympathetic tone. It commonly occurs in the following conditions:

**1.** As a normal variant. Many people have resting heart rates less than 60.

**2.** In acute inferior wall myocardial infarction involving the right coronary artery, which usually supplies blood to the SA node.

**3.** As a "reperfusion rhythm" during and/or after treatment with thrombolytics.

**4.** Vagal stimulation from vomiting, straining (Valsalva maneuver), or carotid sinus massage.

**5.** Vasovagal reactions (a sudden increase in vagal tone accompanied by vascular dilation) are seen with pain, nausea, vomiting, fright, or sudden stressful situations. These reactions may result in marked bradycardia (heart rates less than 30) and hypotension. The combination of these two components results in a decrease in cardiac output so severe that it may cause fainting (vasovagal syncope). The situation is usually reversed when the person is placed in a recumbent position, thereby increasing venous return to the heart. If fainting occurs with the person in the recumbent position, it can usually be reversed by leg elevation.

**6.** Carotid sinus hypersensitivity syndrome, sleep apnea syndrome.

**7.** Hypothyroidism, hypothermia, hyperkalemia.

**8.** Sudden movement from recumbent to an upright position.

**9.** Increased intracranial pressure. Sudden appearance of sinus bradycardia in a patient with cerebral edema or subdural hematoma is an important clinical observation.

**10.** Drugs such as digitalis, calcium channel blockers, beta blockers.

**11.** Degenerative disease of the sinus node (sick sinus syndrome). Persistent sinus bradycardia is the most common and often the earliest manifestation of sick sinus syndrome. Sick sinus syndrome is a dysfunctioning sinus node, which is manifested on the ECG by marked bradyarrhythmias alternating with episodes of tachyarrhythmias and is often accompanied by symptoms of hemodynamic compromise (dizziness, syncope, chest pain, heart failure, and so forth). This syndrome has also been called the *tachy-brady syndrome*. Permanent pacemaker implantation is recommended once patients become symptomatic.

Sinus bradycardia does not require treatment unless the patient becomes symptomatic. If the arrhythmia is accompanied by significant hypotension (systolic blood pressure less than 90 mmHg), restlessness, diaphoresis, chest pain, dyspnea, decreased level of consciousness, or other signs of hemodynamic compromise, treatment is necessary. A simple maneuver such as asking the patient to cough, which decreases vagal tone, might be tried initially in an attempt to increase the heart rate. If sinus bradycardia persists, the treatment of choice is atropine, a parasympatholytic drug that prevents the vagus nerve from slowing the heart rate. The usual dose is 0.5 mg IV push every 5 min until the bradycardia is resolved or a maximum dose of 0.04 mg/kg (usually 2 to 3 mg) is given. Atropine must be administered correctly. Atropine administered too slowly or in doses less than 0.5 mg exerts a sympatholytic effect and can further decrease the heart rate. If the arrhythmia still does not resolve after the administration of atropine, a transcutaneous (external) or transvenous pacemaker may be needed. All medications that cause a decrease in heart rate should be reviewed and discontinued if indicated. For chronic bradycardia, permanent pacing may be indicated.

## SINUS ARRHYTHMIA

Sinus arrhythmia (Figure 6-5; Box 6-4) originates in the sinus node and discharges impulses irregularly. The heart rate may be normal (60 to 100) but is often associated with sinus bradycardia. The P waves are normal in configuration and direction and precede each QRS. The PR interval and QRS duration are within normal limits. The distinguishing feature of this rhythm is the sinus origin and the rhythm irregularity.

| Box 6-4. | Sinus Arrhythmia: Identifying ECG Features |
|---|---|
| Rhythm: | Irregular |
| Rate: | Normal (60–100) or slow (less than 60) |
| P waves: | Normal in configuration and direction; one P wave precedes each QRS complex |
| PR: | Normal (0.12–0.20 seconds) |
| QRS: | Normal (0.10 seconds or less) |

Sinus arrhythmia is a normal phenomenon thought to be the result of variations in autonomic tone and is commonly associated with the phases of respiration. Heart rate tends to increase gradually with in-

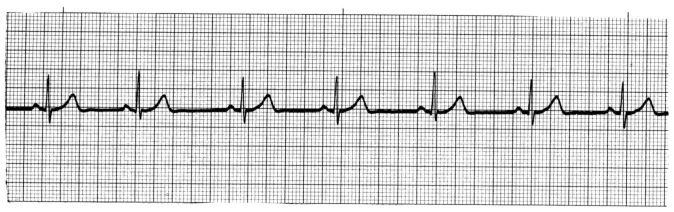

**Figure 6-5.** **Sinus Arrhythmia**

| | |
|---|---|
| *Rhythm:* | Irregular |
| *Rate:* | 60 |
| *P waves:* | Normal in configuration; precede each QRS |
| *PR:* | 0.12 to 0.14 seconds |
| *QRS:* | 0.06 to 0.08 seconds |

spiration and decrease gradually with expiration. Sinus arrhythmia is an extremely common finding among children and young adults. Although sinus arrhythmia may also occur in the elderly, it is usually not related to the phases of respiration in this age group and sometimes is the precursor of sick sinus syndrome.

## SINUS ARREST AND SINUS EXIT BLOCK

Sinus arrest and sinus exit block (two separate arrhythmias with different pathophysiologies) (Fig-

ures 6-6 and 6-7; Box 6-5) are discussed together here because distinguishing between them is at times difficult, and because their treatment and clinical significance are the same. Both sinus arrest and sinus exit block originate in the sinus node and are characterized by a pause in the sinus rhythm in which one or more beats (cardiac cycles) is missing. The P waves in the underlying rhythm will be normal in configuration and direction with one P wave preceding each QRS complex. The PR interval and QRS duration in the underlying rhythm are within normal limits. The distinguishing feature of both rhythms is the abrupt pause in the underlying sinus rhythm in

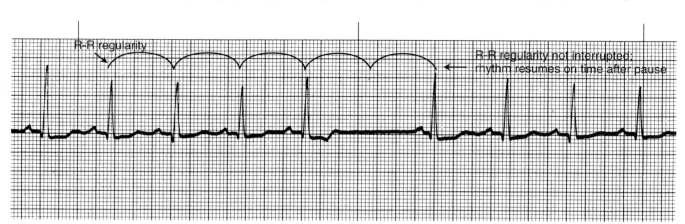

**Figure 6-6.** **Normal Sinus Rhythm with Sinus Block**

| | |
|---|---|
| *Rhythm:* | Basic rhythm regular, irregular during pause |
| *Rate:* | Basic rhythm 84 |
| *P waves:* | Normal in basic rhythm, absent during pause |
| *PR:* | 0.16 to 0.18 seconds in basic rhythm, absent during pause |
| *QRS:* | 0.08 to 0.10 seconds in basic rhythm, absent during pause |
| *Comment:* | ST segment depression is present. |

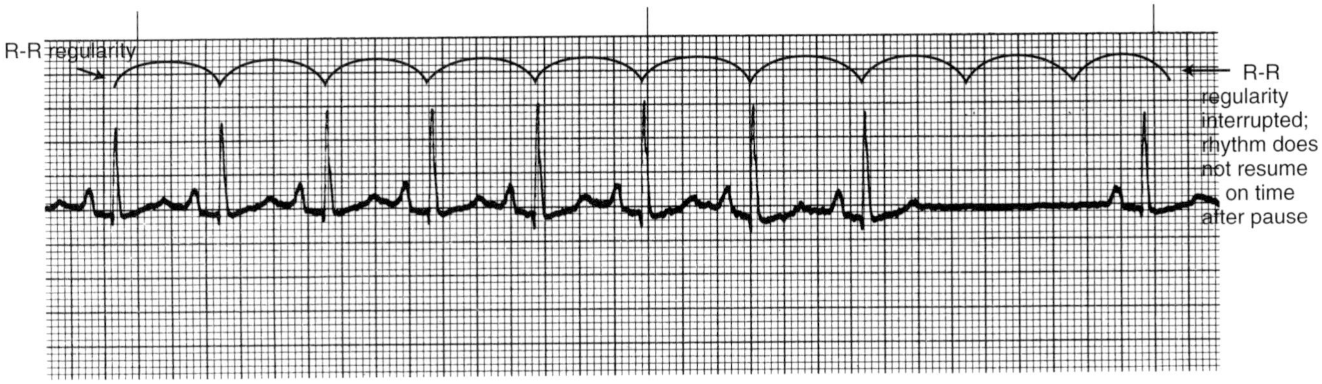

**Figure 6-7. Normal Sinus Rhythm with Sinus Arrest**

*Rhythm:* Basic rhythm regular, irregular during pause

*Rate:* Basic rhythm 94

*P waves:* Normal in basic rhythm, absent during pause

*PR:* 0.16 to 0.18 seconds in basic rhythm, absent during pause

*QRS:* 0.06 to 0.08 seconds in basic rhythm, absent during pause

which one or more P–QRS–T sequences is missing, followed by a resumption of the basic rhythm after the pause.

| Box 6-5. | **Sinus Arrest and Sinus Exit Block: Identifying ECG Features** |
|---|---|
| Rhythm: | Underlying rhythm usually regular; irregular during pause |
| Rate: | Underlying rhythm may be normal (60–100) or slow (less than 60) |
| P waves: | Sinus P waves present with underlying rhythm; P waves absent during pause |
| PR: | Normal duration (0.12–0.20 seconds) with underlying rhythm; PR absent during pause |
| QRS: | Normal (0.10 seconds or less) with underlying rhythm; QRS absent during pause |

*Differentiating Features*

Sinus block: Underlying rhythm resumes on time after the pause, with the length of the pause being a multiple of the underlying P-P (or R-R) interval

Sinus arrest: Underlying rhythm does not resume on time after the pause; the length of the pause is not a multiple of the underlying P-P (or R-R) interval

Sinus arrest is caused by a failure of the SA node to discharge an impulse. This failure in the automaticity of the SA node upsets the timing of the sinus node discharge, and the underlying rhythm will not resume on time after the pause. Therefore, the length of the pause will not be a multiple of the un-

derlying P-P or R-R interval. With sinus exit block, an electrical impulse is generated by the SA node but is blocked as it exits the sinus node, preventing conduction of the impulse to the atria. Because the regularity of the sinus node discharge is not interrupted (just blocked), the underlying rhythm will resume on time after the pause, and the length of the pause will be a multiple of the underlying P-P or R-R interval. Once the rhythm resumes after the pause (in both sinus arrest and sinus exit block), it is common for the rate to be slower for several cycles (temporary rate suppression). This will cause a brief irregularity in rhythm, but, after several cycles, the basic rate and rhythm will return.

Differentiating between the two rhythms involves comparing the length of the pause with the underlying P-P or R-R interval to determine if the underlying rhythm resumes on time after the pause. This is only useful if the underlying rhythm is regular. If the underlying rhythm is irregular, as in sinus arrhythmia (Figure 6-8), it is impossible to distinguish sinus arrest from sinus exit block on the surface electrocardiogram. In this case, the rhythm would best be interpreted as sinus arrest/block, indicating that either rhythm could be present. From a clinical viewpoint, distinguishing between sinus arrest and sinus block is usually not essential.

Sinus arrest or sinus exit block can be caused by numerous factors including:

**1.** Increase in vagal tone (nausea, vomiting, Valsalva maneuver, carotid sinus massage, carotid sinus hypersensitivity syndrome, and so forth)

**2.** Damage to the sinus node from acute inferior wall myocardial infarction, myocarditis, or degenerative forms of fibrosis

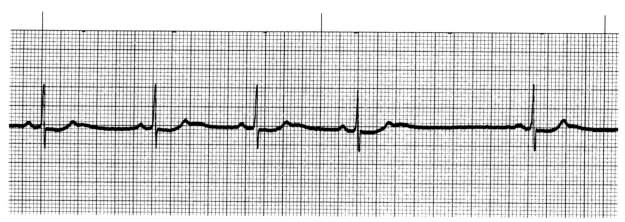

**Figure 6-8.** **Sinus Arrhythmia with Sinus Arrest/Block**

*Rhythm:*      Basic rhythm irregular

*Rate:*       Basic rhythm 60

*P waves:*     Normal in basic rhythm, absent during pause

*PR:*        0.16 to 0.18 seconds in basic rhythm, absent during pause

*QRS:*       0.06 seconds in basic rhythm, absent during pause

*Comment:*     Due to the irregularity of the basic rhythm, sinus arrest cannot be differentiated from sinus block, and the rhythm is interpreted as sinus arrest/block.

*Comment:*     ST segment depression and a U wave are present.

**3.** In association with sick sinus syndrome

**4.** Hyperkalemia, hypoxia

**5.** Use of certain drugs (digitalis, beta blockers, calcium channel blockers)

The pauses associated with sinus arrest or sinus block may be short and produce no symptoms, or long and produce symptoms of hypotension, dizziness, or syncope. Another danger to long pauses is that the SA node may lose pacemaker control. When the sinus node slows down below its minimum firing rate of 60, because of bradycardia or a pause in the underlying rhythm, an opportunity is provided for pacemaker cells in other areas of the conduction system to usurp control from the sinus node and become the dominant pacemaker of the heart. The term *ectopic* is often applied to rhythms that originate from any site other than the SA node. Ectopic sites in the atria, AV node, or ventricles (secondary pacemaker sites) may assume pacemaker control for one beat, several beats, or continuously. As in sinus bradycardia, asking the patient to cough might cause a decrease in vagal tone and result in sinus node recovery. If sinus arrest or sinus exit block produce symptoms, the arrhythmias are treated the same as in symptomatic sinus bradycardia. In addition, all medications that depress sinus node discharge or conduction should be stopped.

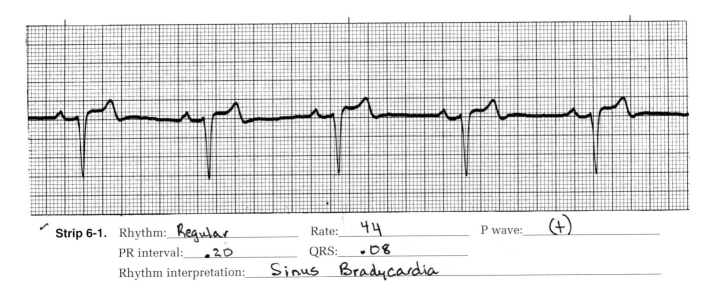

✓ **Strip 6-1.** Rhythm: _Regular_          Rate: _44_          P wave: _(+)_

PR interval: _.20_          QRS: _.08_

Rhythm interpretation: _Sinus Bradycardia_

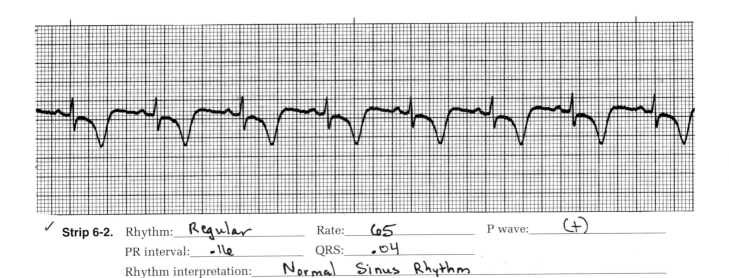

✓ **Strip 6-2.** Rhythm: _Regular_          Rate: _65_          P wave: _(+)_

PR interval: _.16_          QRS: _.04_

Rhythm interpretation: _Normal Sinus Rhythm_

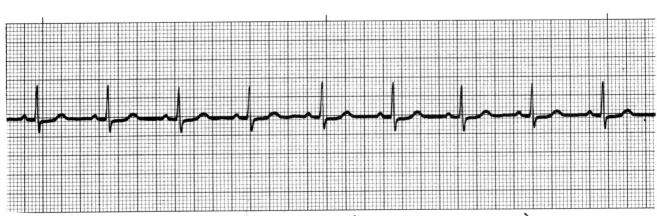

✓ **Strip 6-3.** Rhythm: _Regular_          Rate: _79_          P wave: _(+)_

PR interval: _.16_          QRS: _.04_

Rhythm interpretation: _Normal Sinus Rhythm_

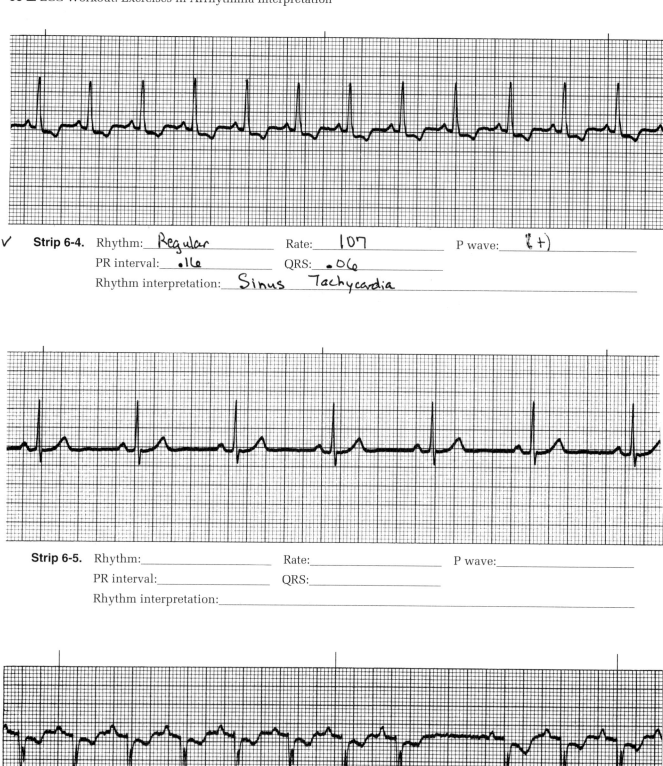

✓ **Strip 6-4.** Rhythm: _Regular_          Rate: _107_          P wave: _(+)_
PR interval: _.16_          QRS: _.06_
Rhythm interpretation: _Sinus Tachycardia_

**Strip 6-5.** Rhythm:_____          Rate:_____          P wave:_____
PR interval:_____          QRS:_____
Rhythm interpretation:_____

✓ **Strip 6-6.** Rhythm: _Regular_          Rate: _100_          P wave: _(+)_
PR interval: _.20_          QRS: _.08_
Rhythm interpretation: _Sinus Rhythm c̄ a Sinus Exit Block_

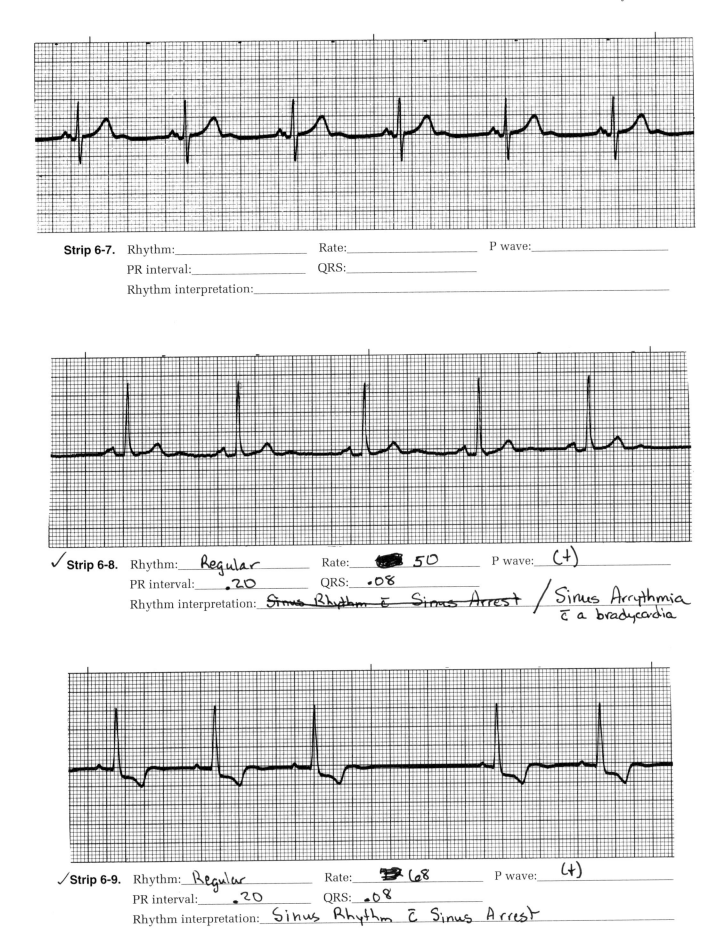

**Strip 6-7.** Rhythm:_____ Rate:_____ P wave:_____

PR interval:_____ QRS:_____

Rhythm interpretation:_____

✓**Strip 6-8.** Rhythm: Regular     Rate: ~~32~~ 50     P wave: (+)

PR interval: .20     QRS: .08

Rhythm interpretation: ~~Sinus Rhythm c̄ Sinus Arrest~~ / Sinus Arrythmia c̄ a bradycardia

✓**Strip 6-9.** Rhythm: Regular     Rate: ~~32~~ 68     P wave: (+)

PR interval: .20     QRS: .08

Rhythm interpretation: Sinus Rhythm c̄ Sinus Arrest

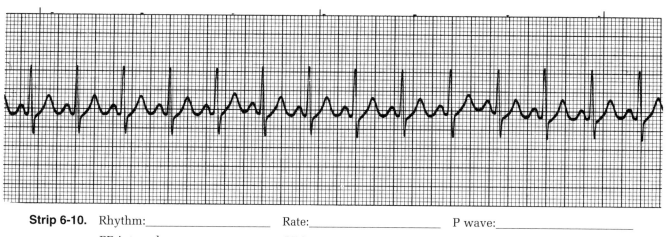

**Strip 6-10.** Rhythm:_____ Rate:_____ P wave:_____

PR interval:_____ QRS:_____

Rhythm interpretation:_____

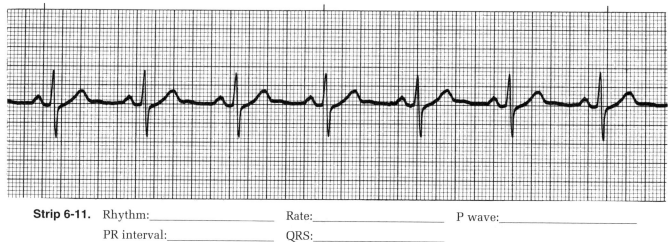

**Strip 6-11.** Rhythm:_____ Rate:_____ P wave:_____

PR interval:_____ QRS:_____

Rhythm interpretation:_____

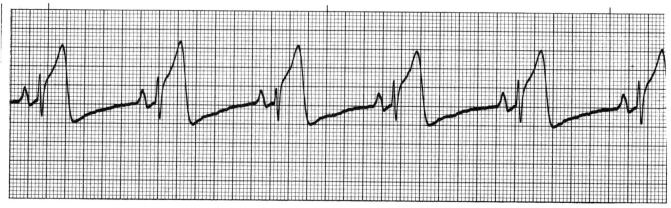

**Strip 6-12.** Rhythm:_____ Rate:_____ P wave:_____

PR interval:_____ QRS:_____

Rhythm interpretation:_____

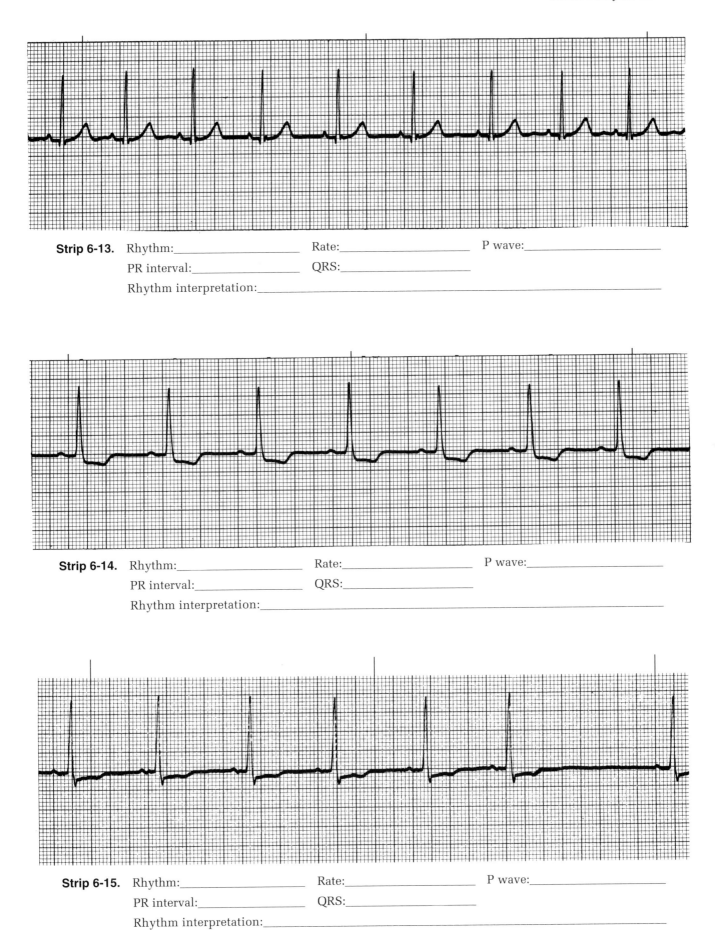

**Strip 6-13.** Rhythm:_____ Rate:_____ P wave:_____

PR interval:_____ QRS:_____

Rhythm interpretation:_____

**Strip 6-14.** Rhythm:_____ Rate:_____ P wave:_____

PR interval:_____ QRS:_____

Rhythm interpretation:_____

**Strip 6-15.** Rhythm:_____ Rate:_____ P wave:_____

PR interval:_____ QRS:_____

Rhythm interpretation:_____

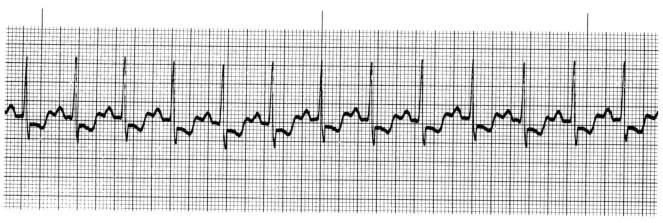

**Strip 6-16.** Rhythm:_____ Rate:_____ P wave:_____

PR interval:_____ QRS:_____

Rhythm interpretation:_____

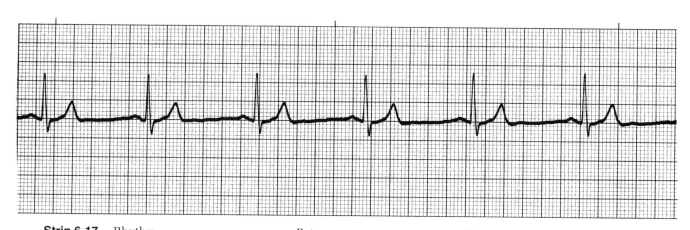

**Strip 6-17.** Rhythm:_____ Rate:_____ P wave:_____

PR interval:_____ QRS:_____

Rhythm interpretation:_____

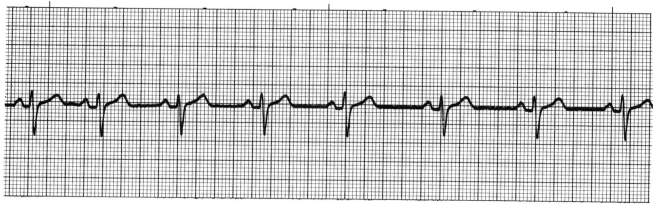

**Strip 6-18.** Rhythm:_____ Rate:_____ P wave:_____

PR interval:_____ QRS:_____

Rhythm interpretation:_____

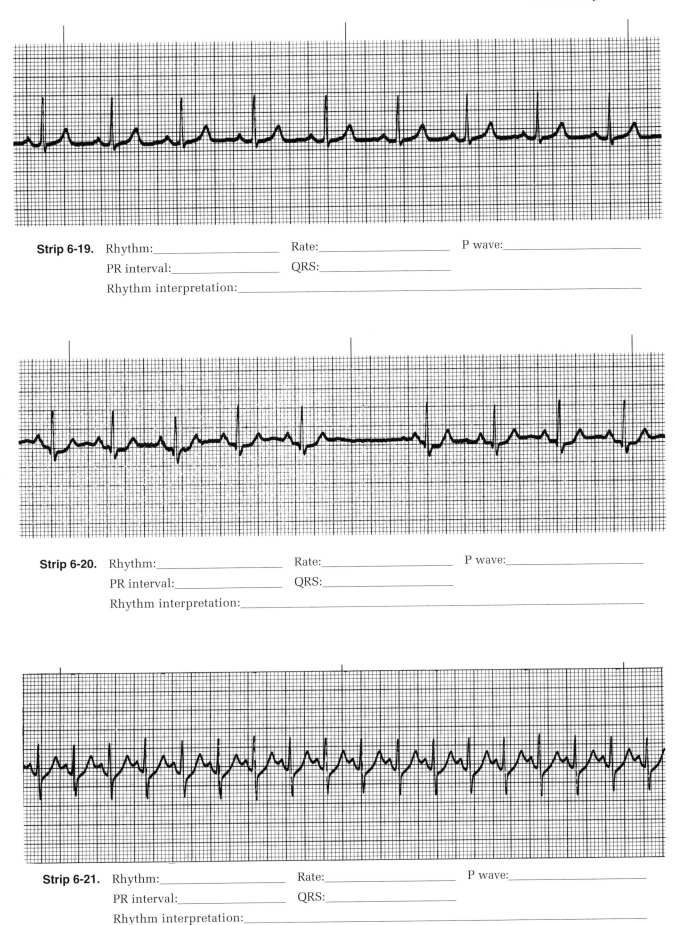

**Strip 6-19.** Rhythm:_____ Rate:_____ P wave:_____

PR interval:_____ QRS:_____

Rhythm interpretation:_____

**Strip 6-20.** Rhythm:_____ Rate:_____ P wave:_____

PR interval:_____ QRS:_____

Rhythm interpretation:_____

**Strip 6-21.** Rhythm:_____ Rate:_____ P wave:_____

PR interval:_____ QRS:_____

Rhythm interpretation:_____

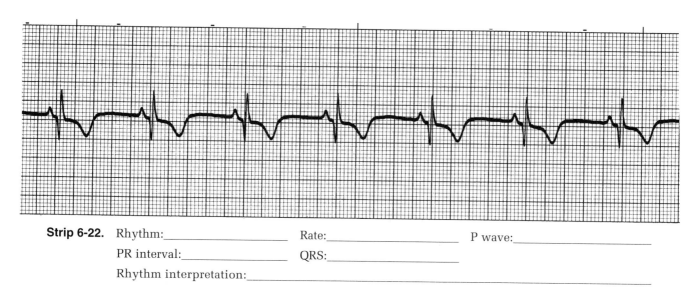

**Strip 6-22.** Rhythm:_____ Rate:_____ P wave:_____

PR interval:_____ QRS:_____

Rhythm interpretation:_____

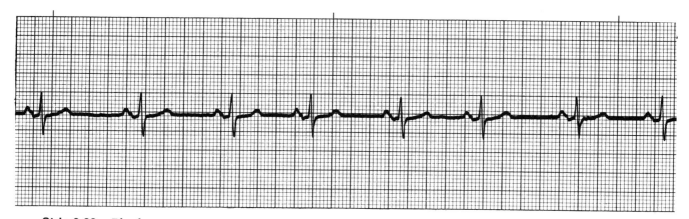

**Strip 6-23.** Rhythm:_____ Rate:_____ P wave:_____

PR interval:_____ QRS:_____

Rhythm interpretation:_____

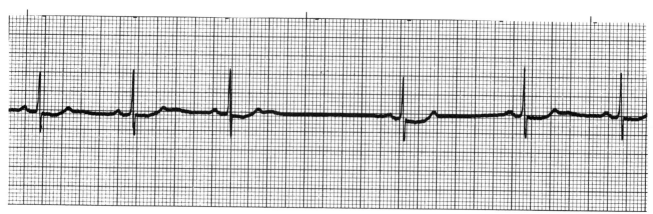

**Strip 6-24.** Rhythm:_____ Rate:_____ P wave:_____

PR interval:_____ QRS:_____

Rhythm interpretation:_____

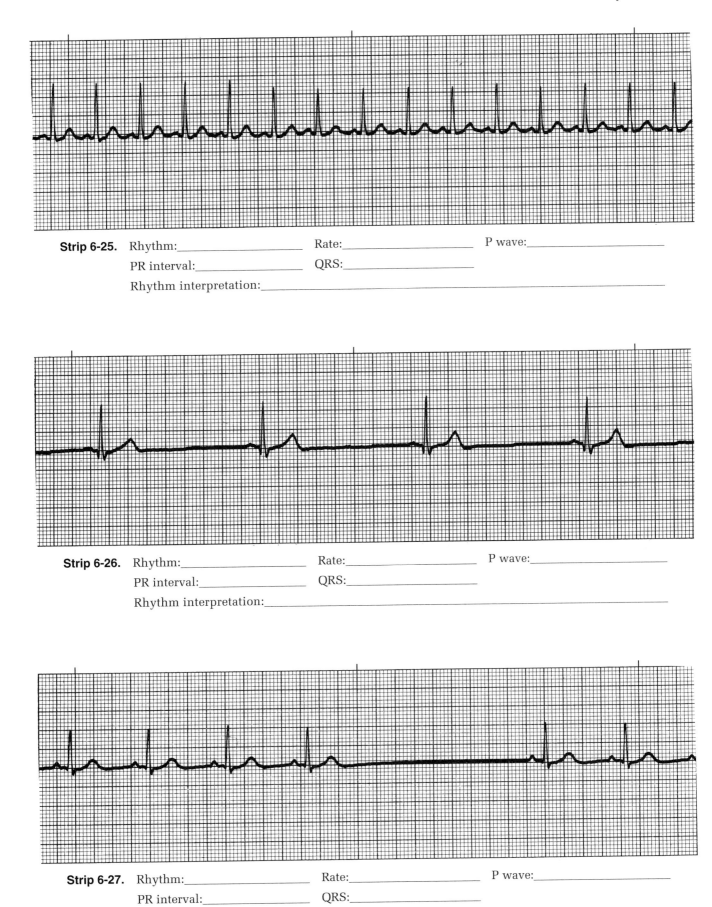

**Strip 6-25.** Rhythm:_____ Rate:_____ P wave:_____

PR interval:_____ QRS:_____

Rhythm interpretation:_____

**Strip 6-26.** Rhythm:_____ Rate:_____ P wave:_____

PR interval:_____ QRS:_____

Rhythm interpretation:_____

**Strip 6-27.** Rhythm:_____ Rate:_____ P wave:_____

PR interval:_____ QRS:_____

Rhythm interpretation:_____

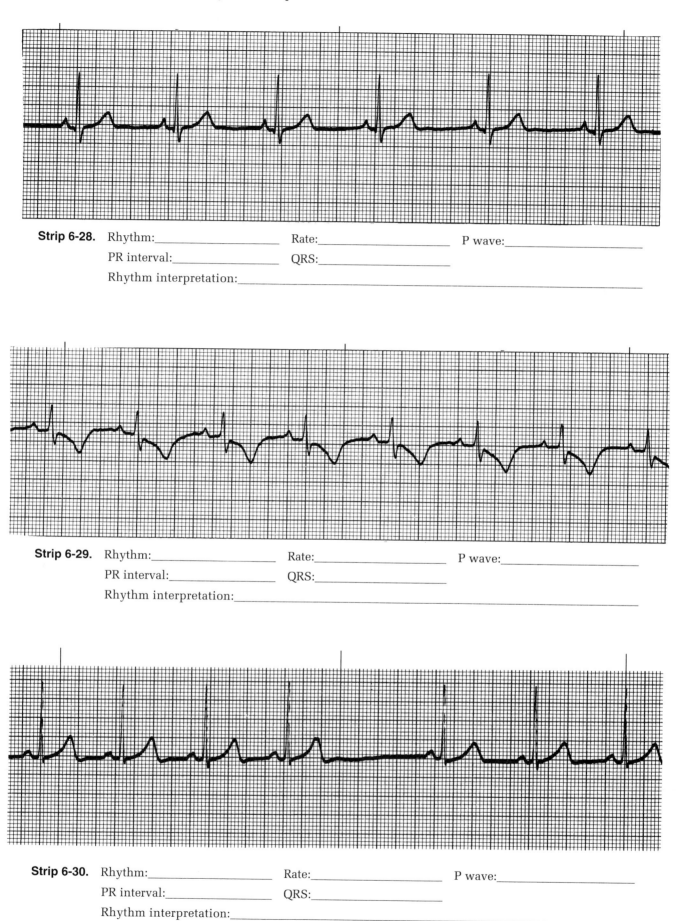

**Strip 6-28.** Rhythm:_____ Rate:_____ P wave:_____

PR interval:_____ QRS:_____

Rhythm interpretation:_____

**Strip 6-29.** Rhythm:_____ Rate:_____ P wave:_____

PR interval:_____ QRS:_____

Rhythm interpretation:_____

**Strip 6-30.** Rhythm:_____ Rate:_____ P wave:_____

PR interval:_____ QRS:_____

Rhythm interpretation:_____

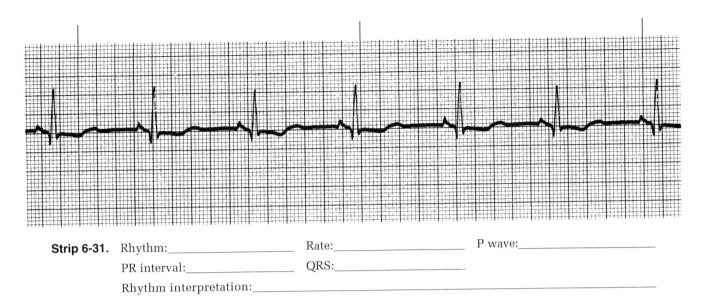

**Strip 6-31.** Rhythm:_____ Rate:_____ P wave:_____

PR interval:_____ QRS:_____

Rhythm interpretation:_____

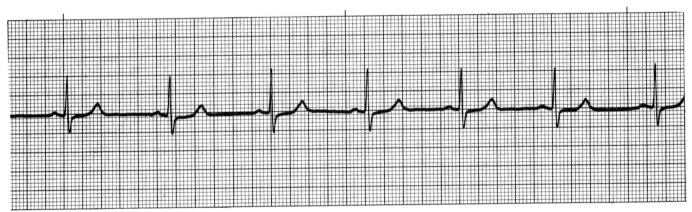

**Strip 6-32.** Rhythm:_____ Rate:_____ P wave:_____

PR interval:_____ QRS:_____

Rhythm interpretation:_____

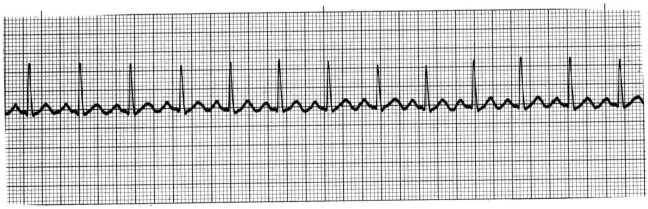

**Strip 6-33.** Rhythm:_____ Rate:_____ P wave:_____

PR interval:_____ QRS:_____

Rhythm interpretation:_____

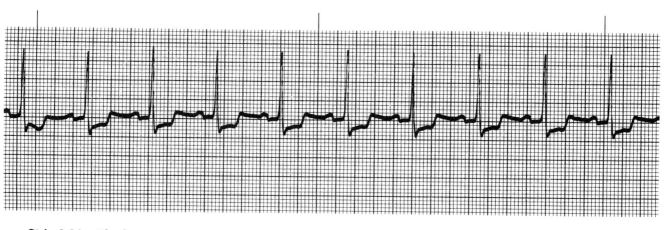

**Strip 6-34.**  Rhythm:_____  Rate:_____  P wave:_____

PR interval:_____  QRS:_____

Rhythm interpretation:_____

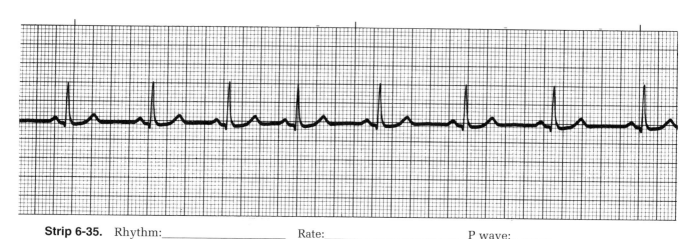

**Strip 6-35.**  Rhythm:_____  Rate:_____  P wave:_____

PR interval:_____  QRS:_____

Rhythm interpretation:_____

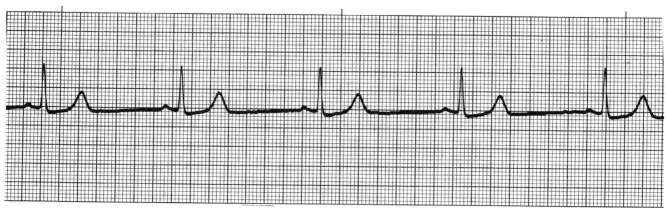

**Strip 6-36.**  Rhythm:_____  Rate:_____  P wave:_____

PR interval:_____  QRS:_____

Rhythm interpretation:_____

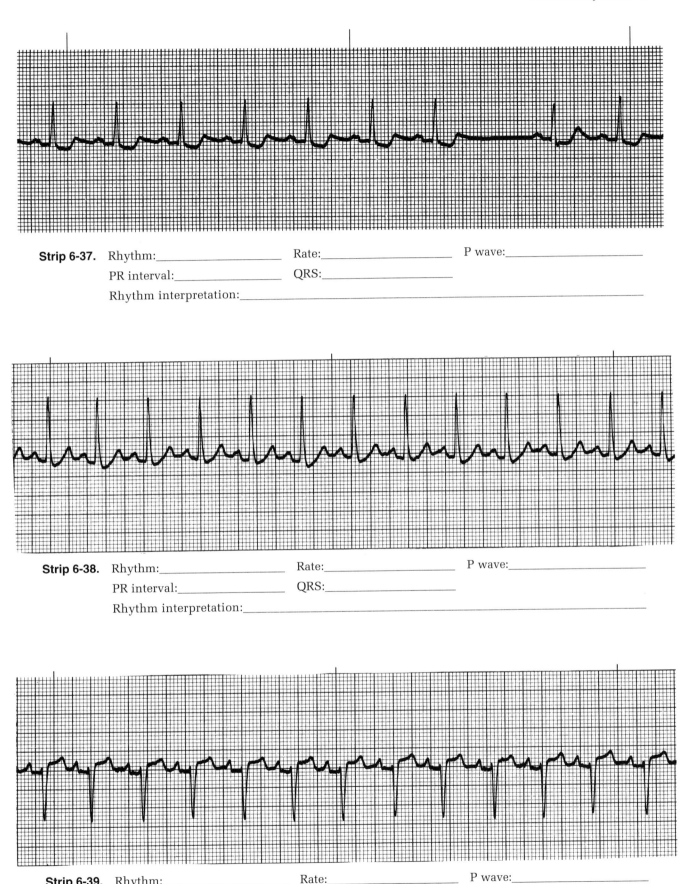

**Strip 6-37.** Rhythm:_____ Rate:_____ P wave:_____

PR interval:_____ QRS:_____

Rhythm interpretation:_____

**Strip 6-38.** Rhythm:_____ Rate:_____ P wave:_____

PR interval:_____ QRS:_____

Rhythm interpretation:_____

**Strip 6-39.** Rhythm:_____ Rate:_____ P wave:_____

PR interval:_____ QRS:_____

Rhythm interpretation:_____

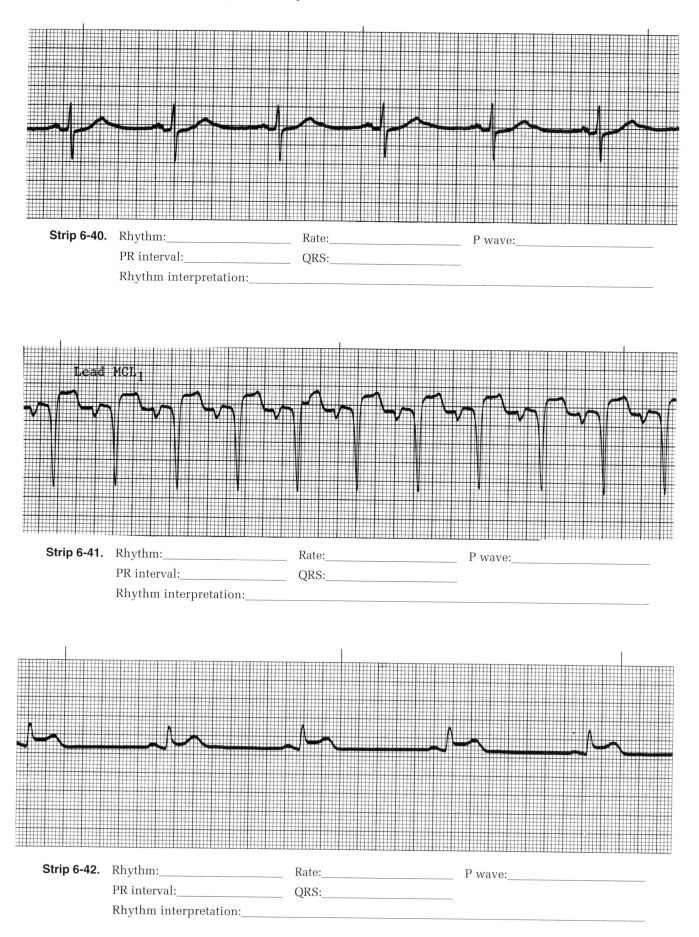

**Strip 6-40.** Rhythm:_____ Rate:_____ P wave:_____

PR interval:_____ QRS:_____

Rhythm interpretation:_____

**Strip 6-41.** Rhythm:_____ Rate:_____ P wave:_____

PR interval:_____ QRS:_____

Rhythm interpretation:_____

**Strip 6-42.** Rhythm:_____ Rate:_____ P wave:_____

PR interval:_____ QRS:_____

Rhythm interpretation:_____

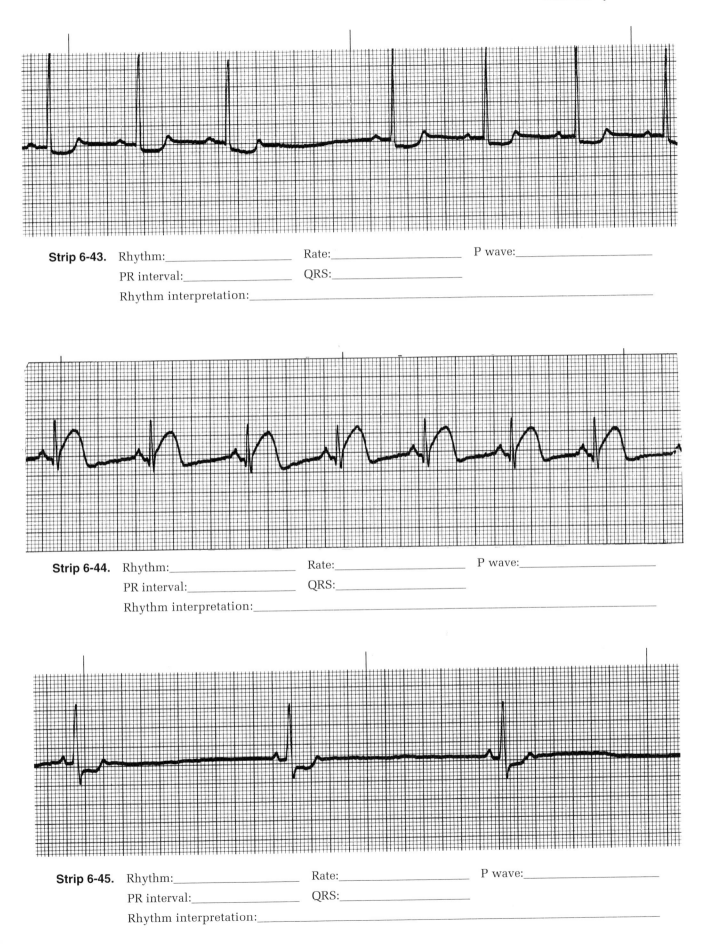

**Strip 6-43.** Rhythm:_____ Rate:_____ P wave:_____

PR interval:_____ QRS:_____

Rhythm interpretation:_____

**Strip 6-44.** Rhythm:_____ Rate:_____ P wave:_____

PR interval:_____ QRS:_____

Rhythm interpretation:_____

**Strip 6-45.** Rhythm:_____ Rate:_____ P wave:_____

PR interval:_____ QRS:_____

Rhythm interpretation:_____

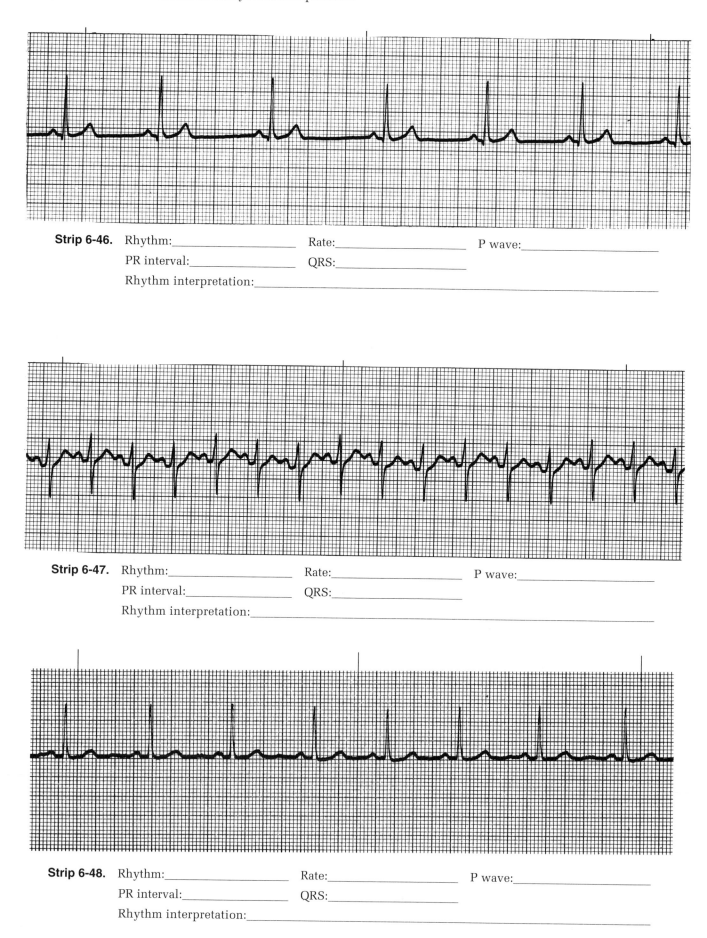

**Strip 6-46.** Rhythm:_____ Rate:_____ P wave:_____

PR interval:_____ QRS:_____

Rhythm interpretation:_____

**Strip 6-47.** Rhythm:_____ Rate:_____ P wave:_____

PR interval:_____ QRS:_____

Rhythm interpretation:_____

**Strip 6-48.** Rhythm:_____ Rate:_____ P wave:_____

PR interval:_____ QRS:_____

Rhythm interpretation:_____

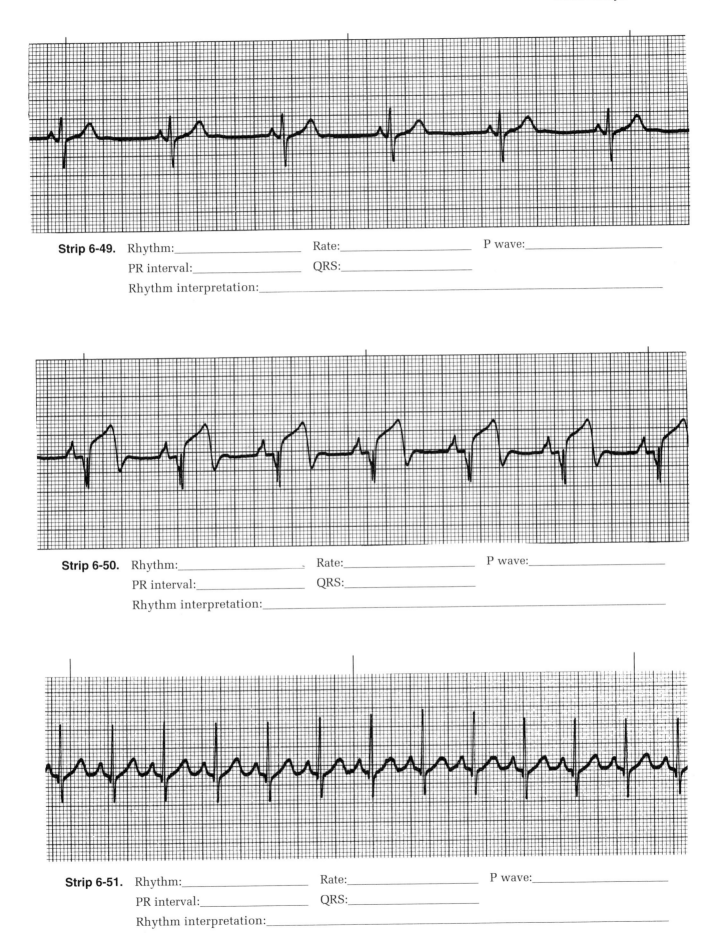

**Strip 6-49.** Rhythm:_____ Rate:_____ P wave:_____

PR interval:_____ QRS:_____

Rhythm interpretation:_____

**Strip 6-50.** Rhythm:_____ Rate:_____ P wave:_____

PR interval:_____ QRS:_____

Rhythm interpretation:_____

**Strip 6-51.** Rhythm:_____ Rate:_____ P wave:_____

PR interval:_____ QRS:_____

Rhythm interpretation:_____

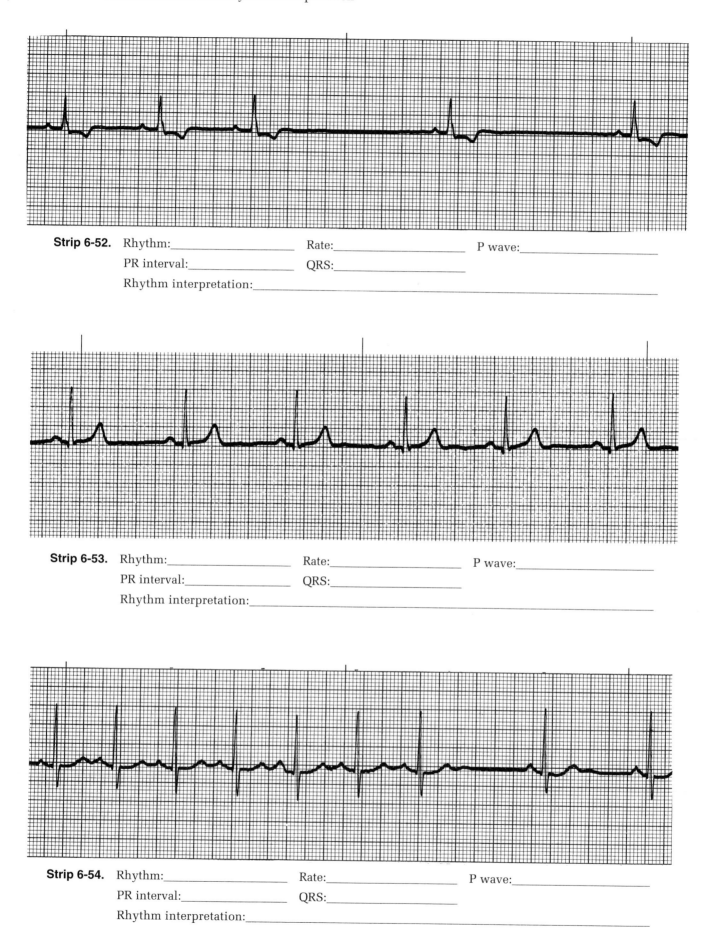

**Strip 6-52.** Rhythm:_____ Rate:_____ P wave:_____

PR interval:_____ QRS:_____

Rhythm interpretation:_____

**Strip 6-53.** Rhythm:_____ Rate:_____ P wave:_____

PR interval:_____ QRS:_____

Rhythm interpretation:_____

**Strip 6-54.** Rhythm:_____ Rate:_____ P wave:_____

PR interval:_____ QRS:_____

Rhythm interpretation:_____

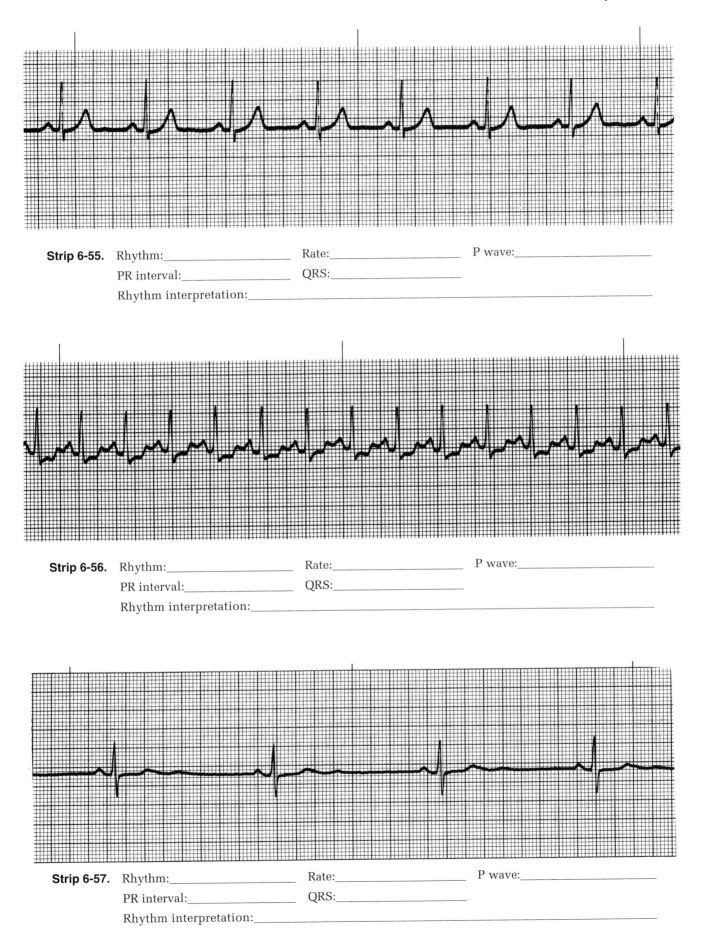

**Strip 6-55.** Rhythm:_____ Rate:_____ P wave:_____

PR interval:_____ QRS:_____

Rhythm interpretation:_____

**Strip 6-56.** Rhythm:_____ Rate:_____ P wave:_____

PR interval:_____ QRS:_____

Rhythm interpretation:_____

**Strip 6-57.** Rhythm:_____ Rate:_____ P wave:_____

PR interval:_____ QRS:_____

Rhythm interpretation:_____

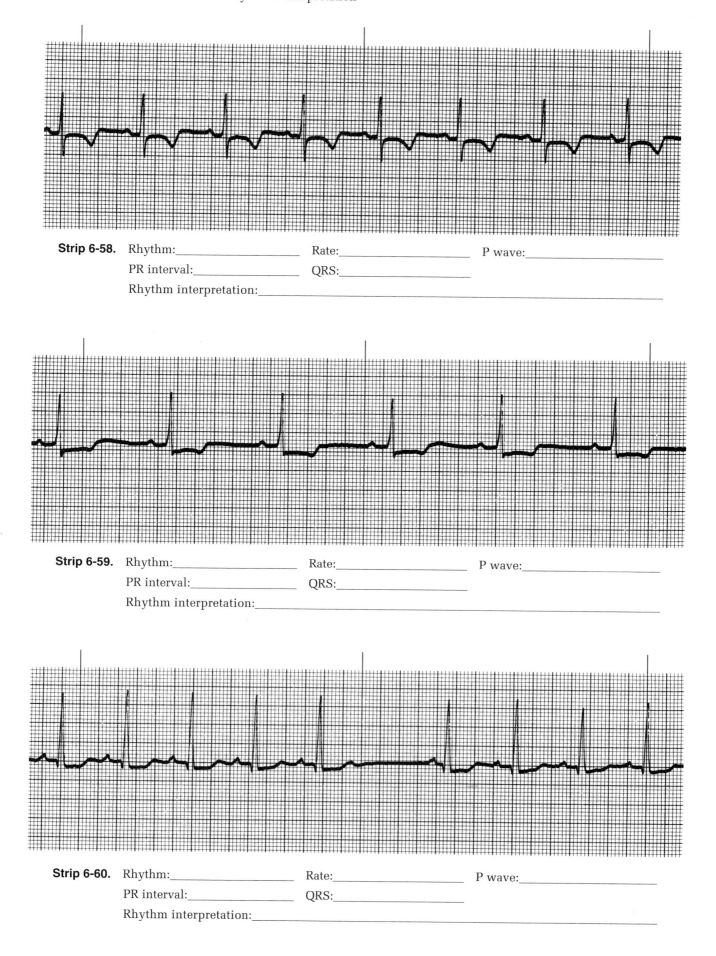

**Strip 6-58.** Rhythm:_____ Rate:_____ P wave:_____

PR interval:_____ QRS:_____

Rhythm interpretation:_____

**Strip 6-59.** Rhythm:_____ Rate:_____ P wave:_____

PR interval:_____ QRS:_____

Rhythm interpretation:_____

**Strip 6-60.** Rhythm:_____ Rate:_____ P wave:_____

PR interval:_____ QRS:_____

Rhythm interpretation:_____

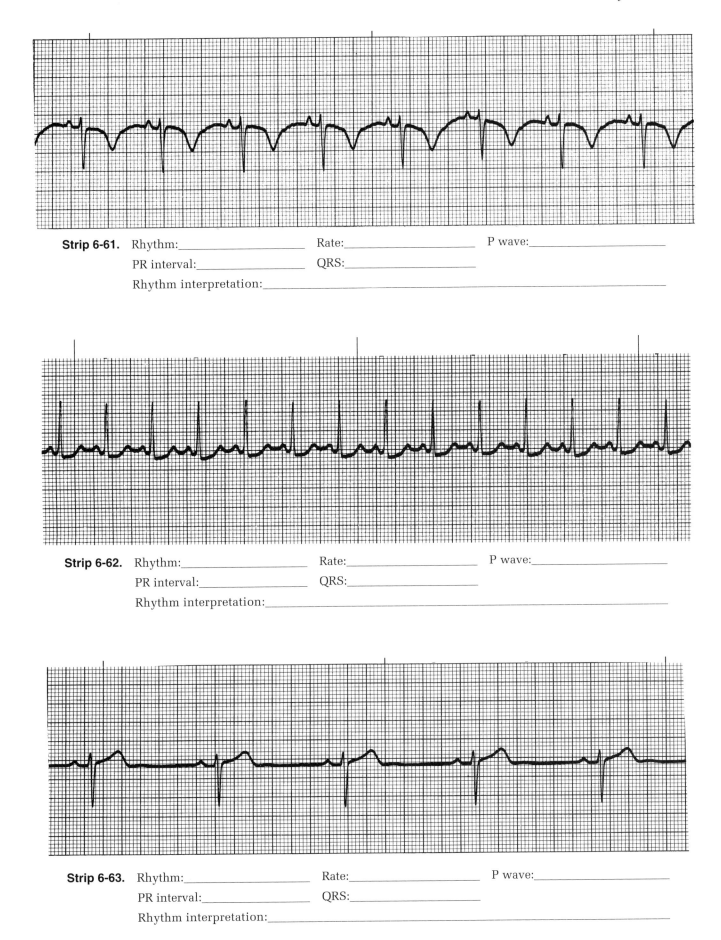

**Strip 6-61.** Rhythm:_____ Rate:_____ P wave:_____

PR interval:_____ QRS:_____

Rhythm interpretation:_____

**Strip 6-62.** Rhythm:_____ Rate:_____ P wave:_____

PR interval:_____ QRS:_____

Rhythm interpretation:_____

**Strip 6-63.** Rhythm:_____ Rate:_____ P wave:_____

PR interval:_____ QRS:_____

Rhythm interpretation:_____

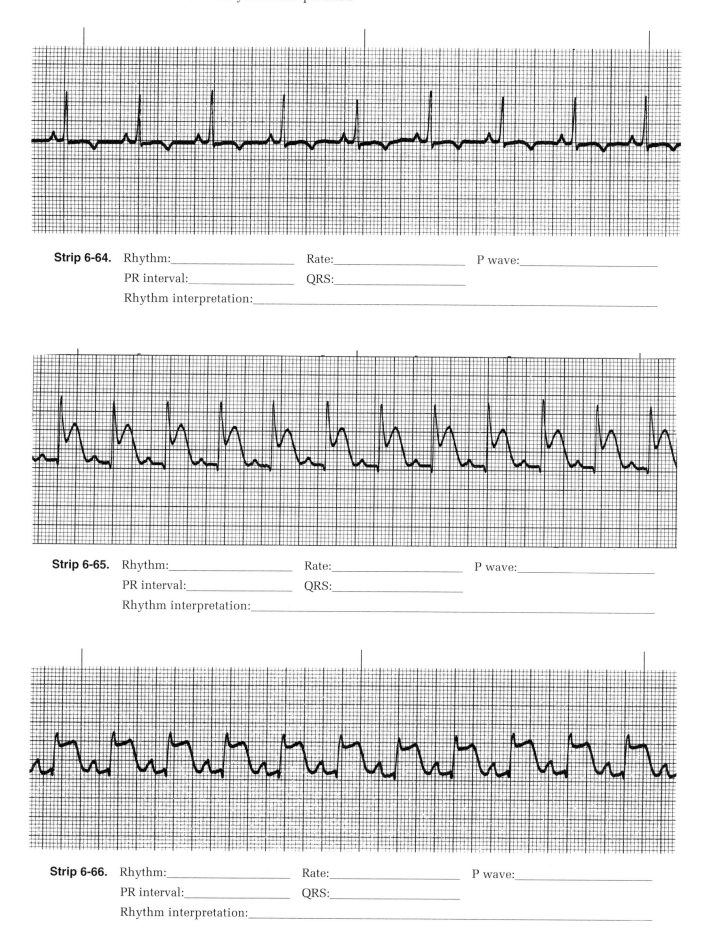

**Strip 6-64.** Rhythm:_____ Rate:_____ P wave:_____

PR interval:_____ QRS:_____

Rhythm interpretation:_____

**Strip 6-65.** Rhythm:_____ Rate:_____ P wave:_____

PR interval:_____ QRS:_____

Rhythm interpretation:_____

**Strip 6-66.** Rhythm:_____ Rate:_____ P wave:_____

PR interval:_____ QRS:_____

Rhythm interpretation:_____

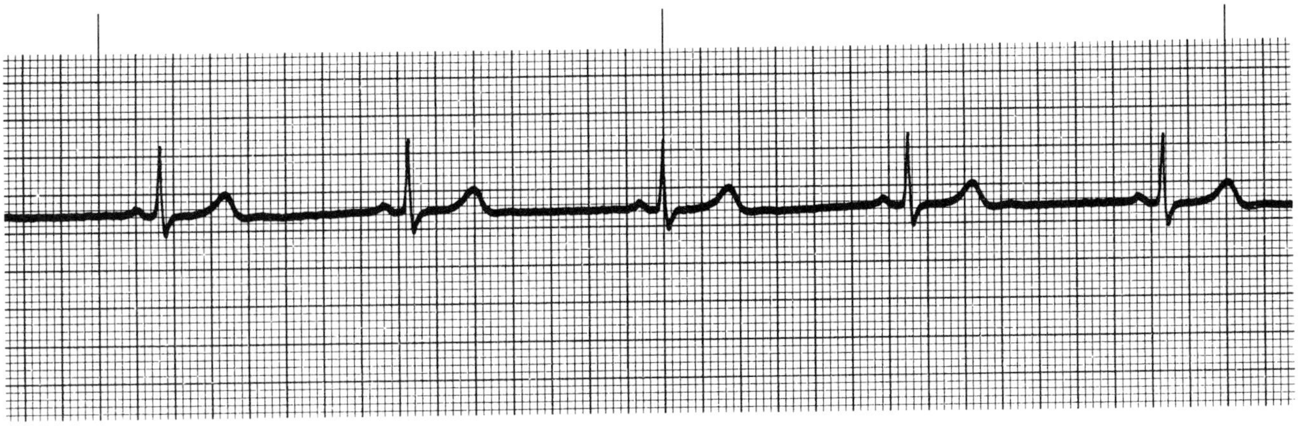

**Strip 6-67.** Rhythm:_____ Rate:_____ P wave:_____

PR interval:_____ QRS:_____

Rhythm interpretation:_____

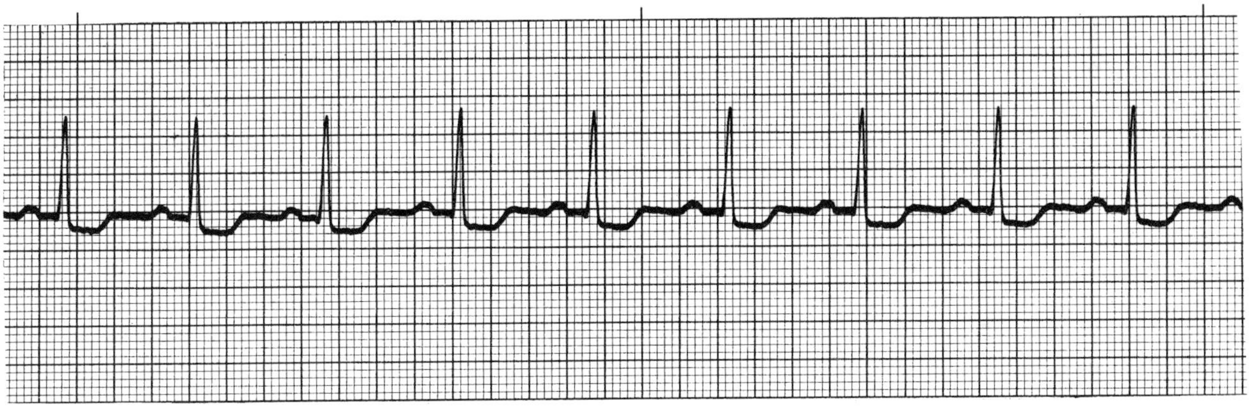

**Strip 6-68.** Rhythm:_____ Rate:_____ P wave:_____

PR interval:_____ QRS:_____

Rhythm interpretation:_____

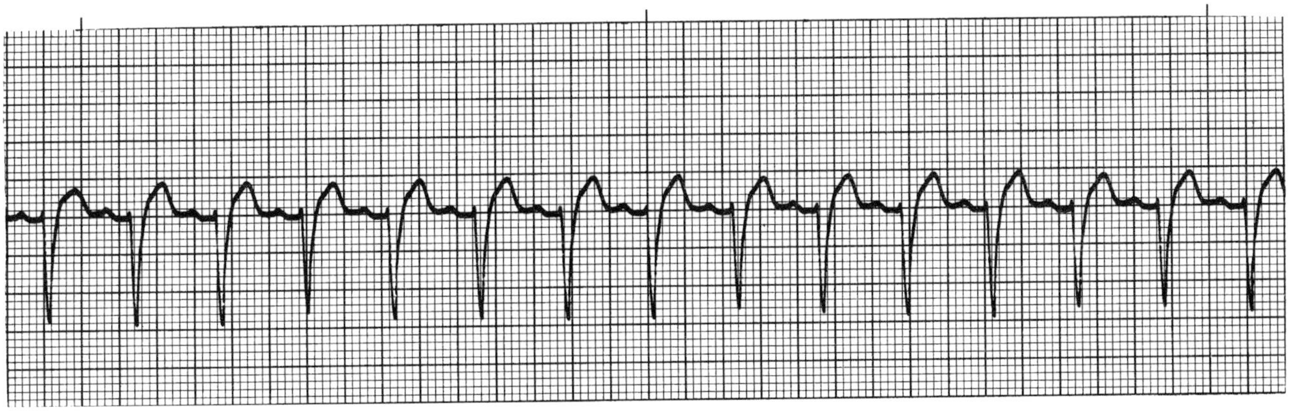

**Strip 6-69.** Rhythm:_____ Rate:_____ P wave:_____

PR interval:_____ QRS:_____

Rhythm interpretation:_____

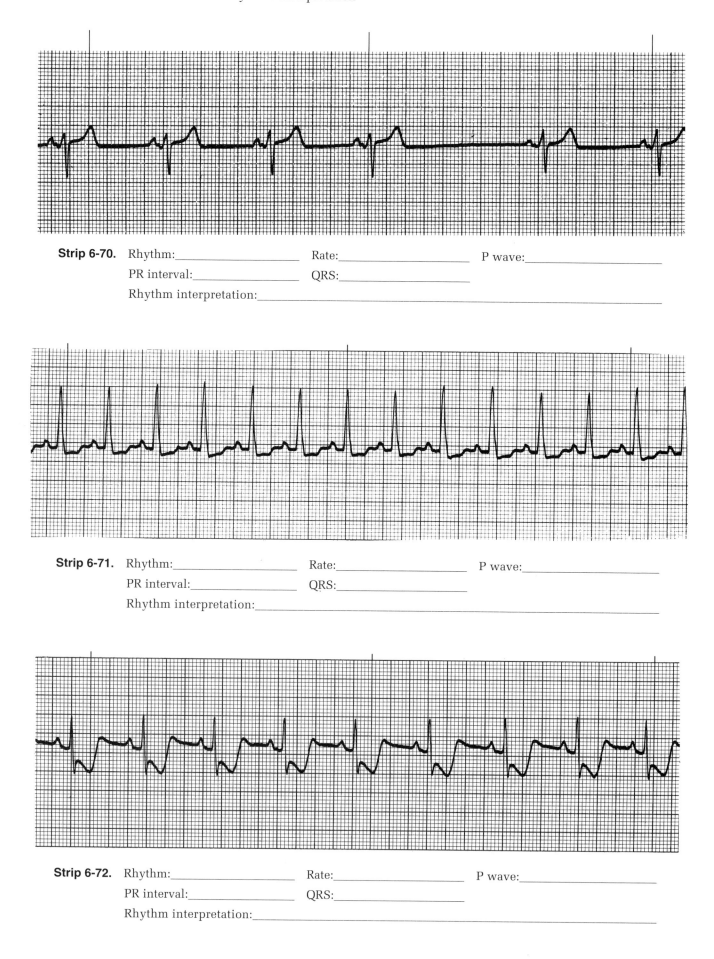

**Strip 6-70.** Rhythm:_____ Rate:_____ P wave:_____

PR interval:_____ QRS:_____

Rhythm interpretation:_____

**Strip 6-71.** Rhythm:_____ Rate:_____ P wave:_____

PR interval:_____ QRS:_____

Rhythm interpretation:_____

**Strip 6-72.** Rhythm:_____ Rate:_____ P wave:_____

PR interval:_____ QRS:_____

Rhythm interpretation:_____

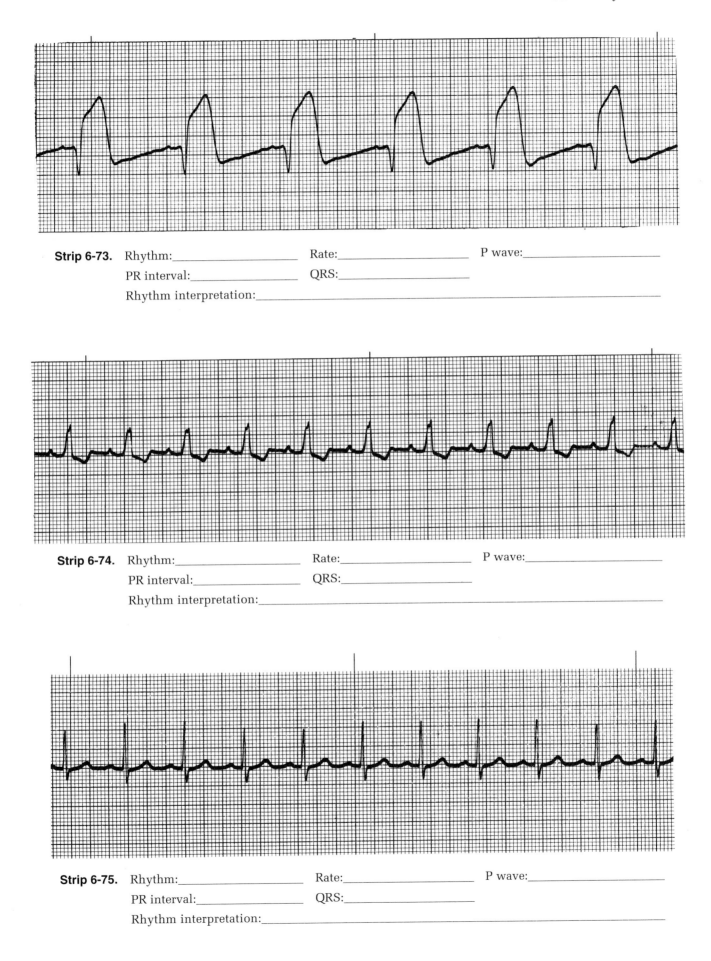

**Strip 6-73.** Rhythm:_____ Rate:_____ P wave:_____

PR interval:_____ QRS:_____

Rhythm interpretation:_____

**Strip 6-74.** Rhythm:_____ Rate:_____ P wave:_____

PR interval:_____ QRS:_____

Rhythm interpretation:_____

**Strip 6-75.** Rhythm:_____ Rate:_____ P wave:_____

PR interval:_____ QRS:_____

Rhythm interpretation:_____

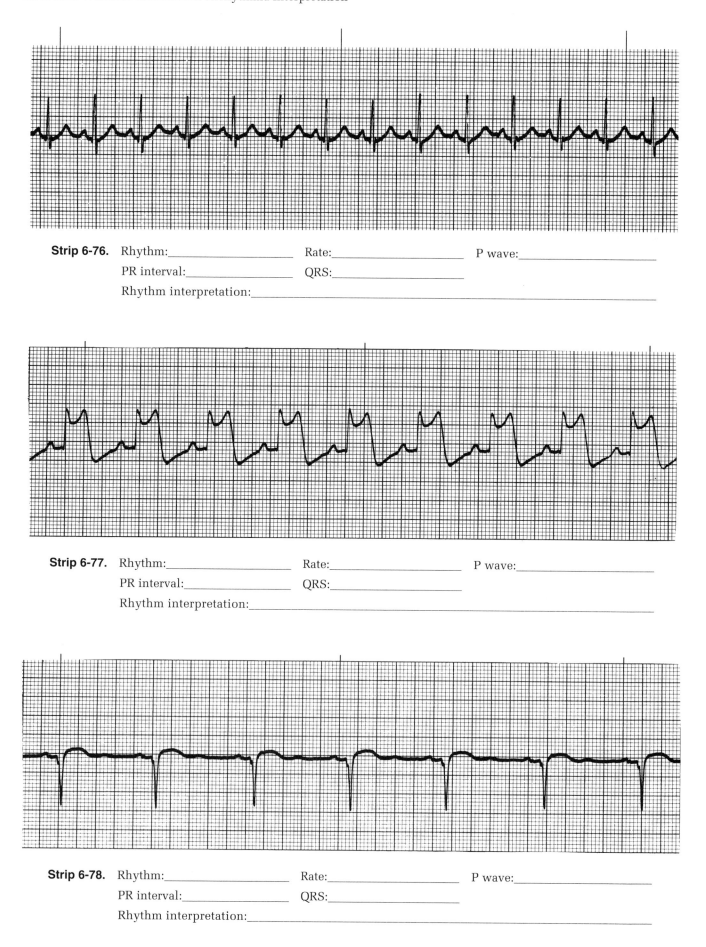

**Strip 6-76.** Rhythm:_____ Rate:_____ P wave:_____

PR interval:_____ QRS:_____

Rhythm interpretation:_____

**Strip 6-77.** Rhythm:_____ Rate:_____ P wave:_____

PR interval:_____ QRS:_____

Rhythm interpretation:_____

**Strip 6-78.** Rhythm:_____ Rate:_____ P wave:_____

PR interval:_____ QRS:_____

Rhythm interpretation:_____

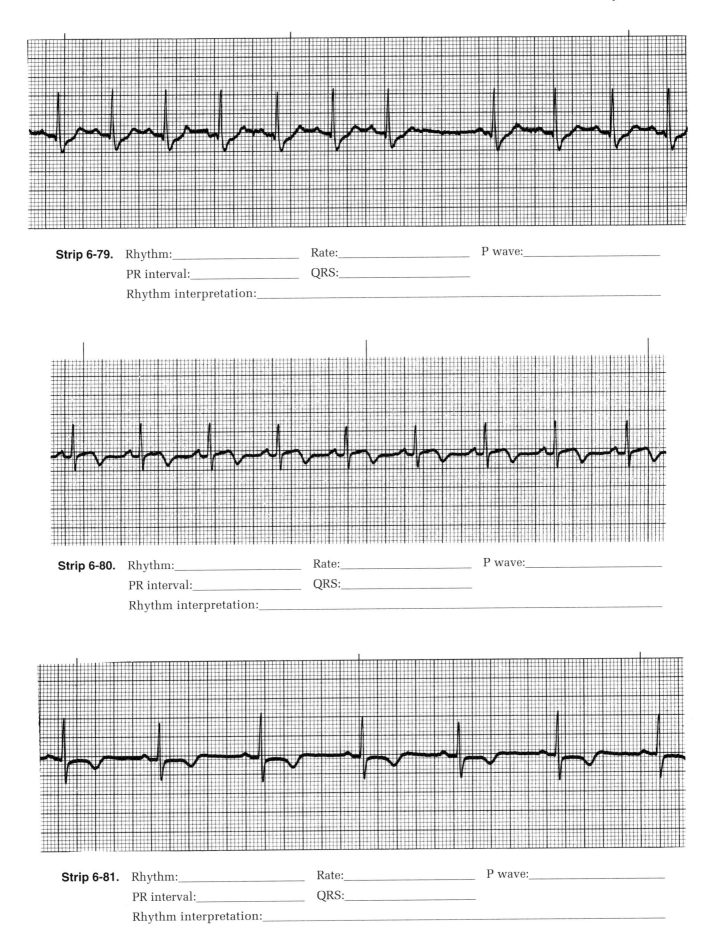

**Strip 6-79.** Rhythm:_____ Rate:_____ P wave:_____

PR interval:_____ QRS:_____

Rhythm interpretation:_____

**Strip 6-80.** Rhythm:_____ Rate:_____ P wave:_____

PR interval:_____ QRS:_____

Rhythm interpretation:_____

**Strip 6-81.** Rhythm:_____ Rate:_____ P wave:_____

PR interval:_____ QRS:_____

Rhythm interpretation:_____

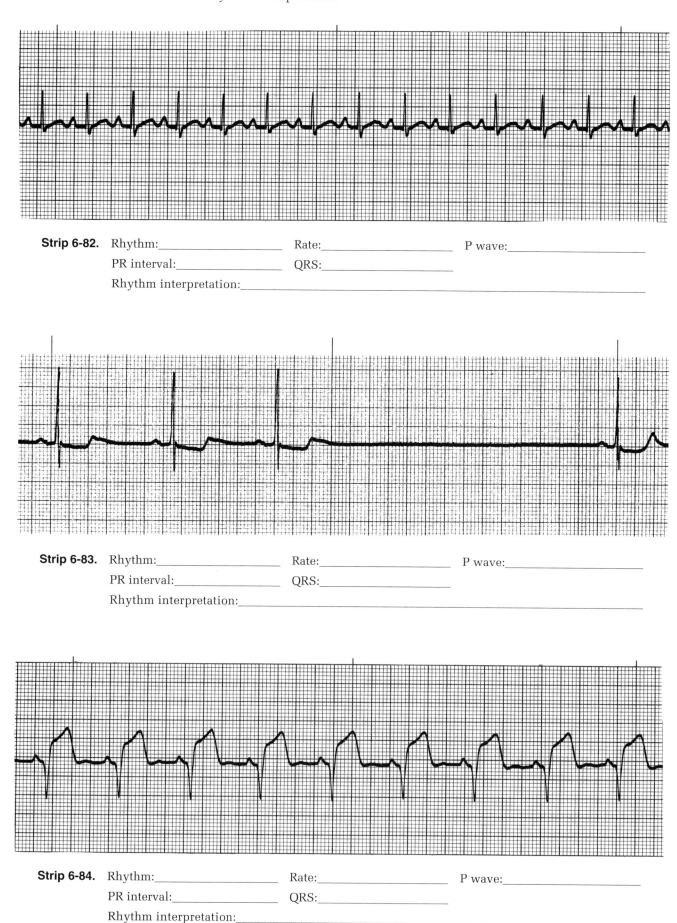

**Strip 6-82.** Rhythm:_____ Rate:_____ P wave:_____

PR interval:_____ QRS:_____

Rhythm interpretation:_____

**Strip 6-83.** Rhythm:_____ Rate:_____ P wave:_____

PR interval:_____ QRS:_____

Rhythm interpretation:_____

**Strip 6-84.** Rhythm:_____ Rate:_____ P wave:_____

PR interval:_____ QRS:_____

Rhythm interpretation:_____

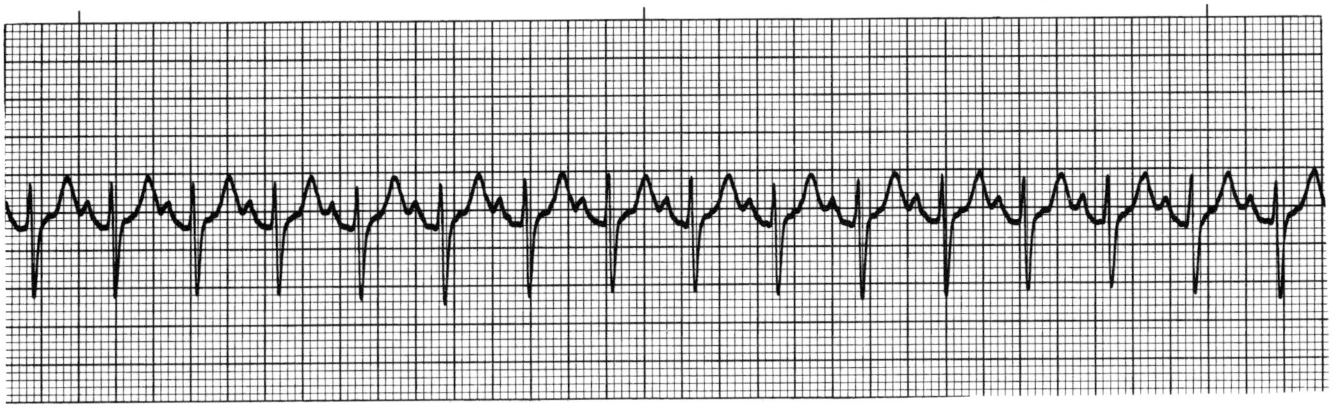

**Strip 6-85.** Rhythm:_____ Rate:_____ P wave:_____

PR interval:_____ QRS:_____

Rhythm interpretation:_____

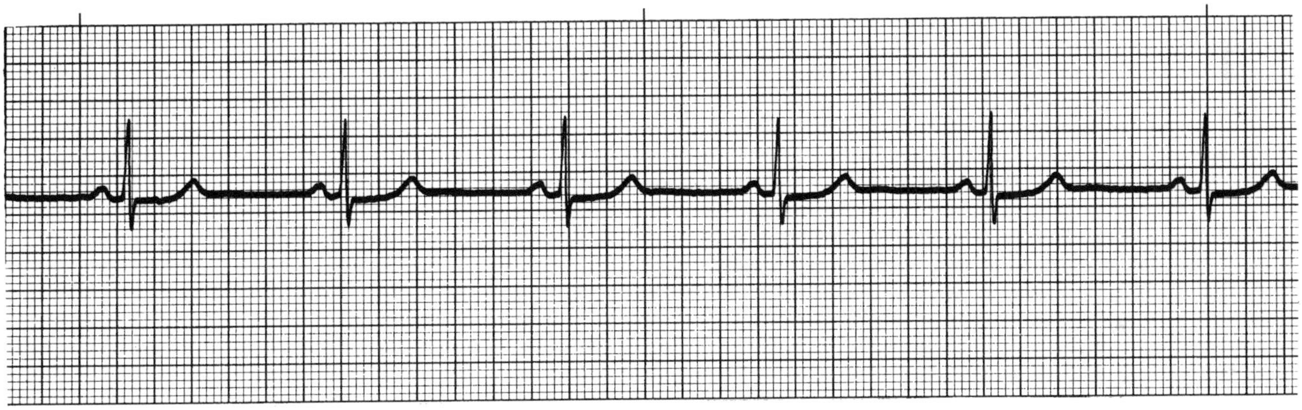

**Strip 6-86.** Rhythm:_____ Rate:_____ P wave:_____

PR interval:_____ QRS:_____

Rhythm interpretation:_____

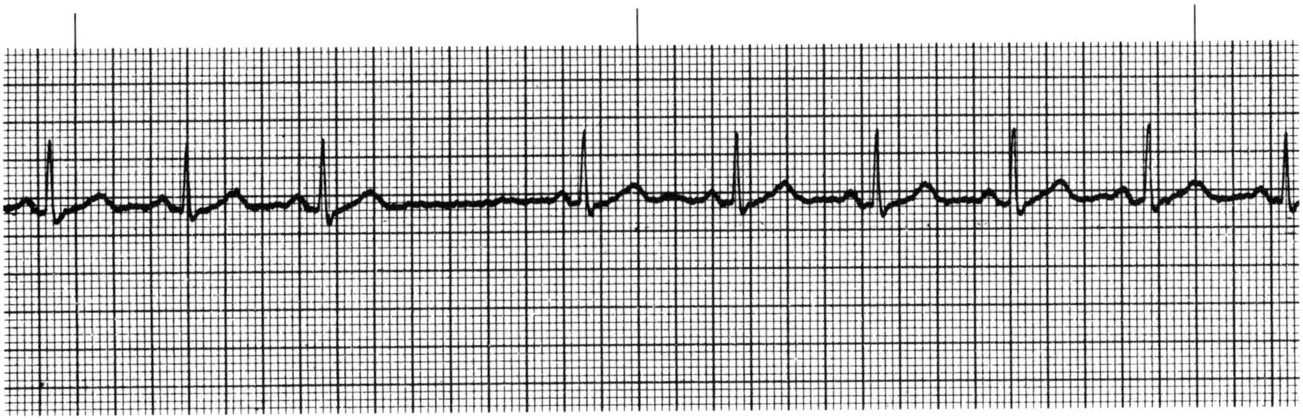

**Strip 6-87.** Rhythm:_____ Rate:_____ P wave:_____

PR interval:_____ QRS:_____

Rhythm interpretation:_____

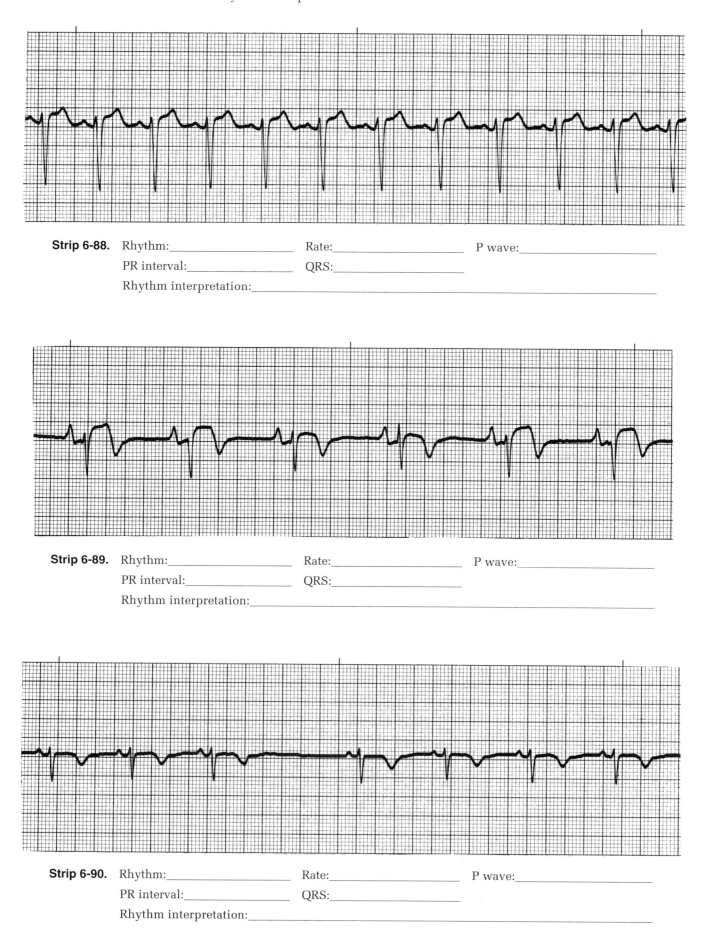

**Strip 6-88.** Rhythm:_____ Rate:_____ P wave:_____

PR interval:_____ QRS:_____

Rhythm interpretation:_____

**Strip 6-89.** Rhythm:_____ Rate:_____ P wave:_____

PR interval:_____ QRS:_____

Rhythm interpretation:_____

**Strip 6-90.** Rhythm:_____ Rate:_____ P wave:_____

PR interval:_____ QRS:_____

Rhythm interpretation:_____

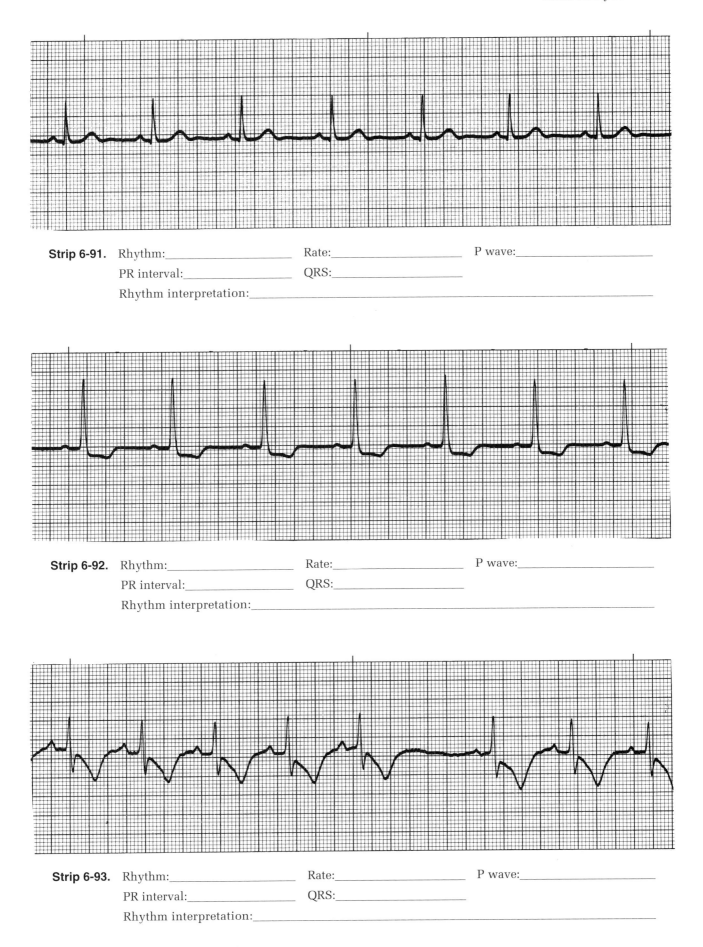

**Strip 6-91.** Rhythm:_____ Rate:_____ P wave:_____

PR interval:_____ QRS:_____

Rhythm interpretation:_____

**Strip 6-92.** Rhythm:_____ Rate:_____ P wave:_____

PR interval:_____ QRS:_____

Rhythm interpretation:_____

**Strip 6-93.** Rhythm:_____ Rate:_____ P wave:_____

PR interval:_____ QRS:_____

Rhythm interpretation:_____

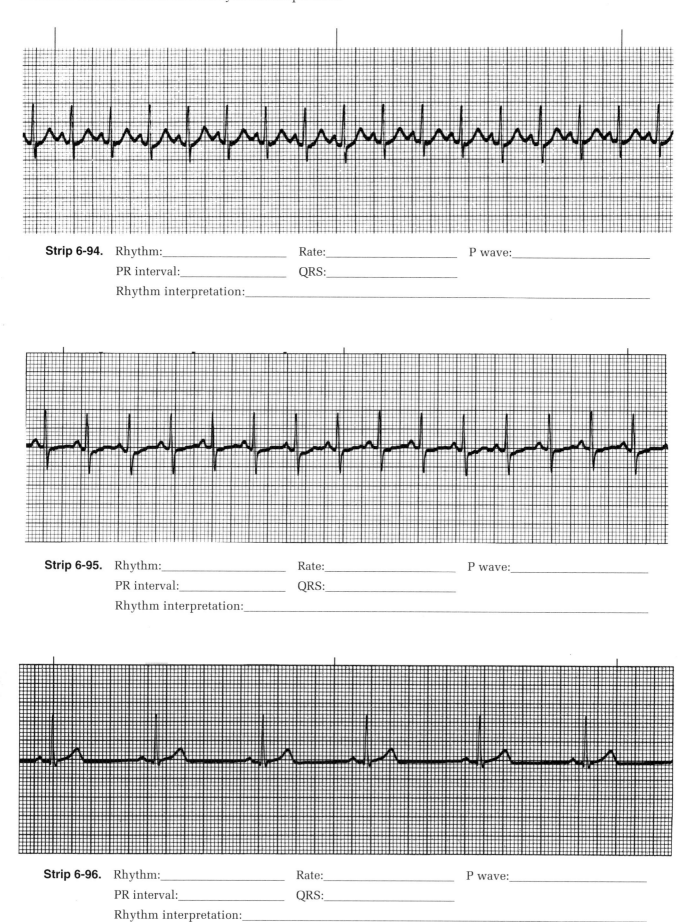

**Strip 6-94.** Rhythm:_____ Rate:_____ P wave:_____

PR interval:_____ QRS:_____

Rhythm interpretation:_____

**Strip 6-95.** Rhythm:_____ Rate:_____ P wave:_____

PR interval:_____ QRS:_____

Rhythm interpretation:_____

**Strip 6-96.** Rhythm:_____ Rate:_____ P wave:_____

PR interval:_____ QRS:_____

Rhythm interpretation:_____

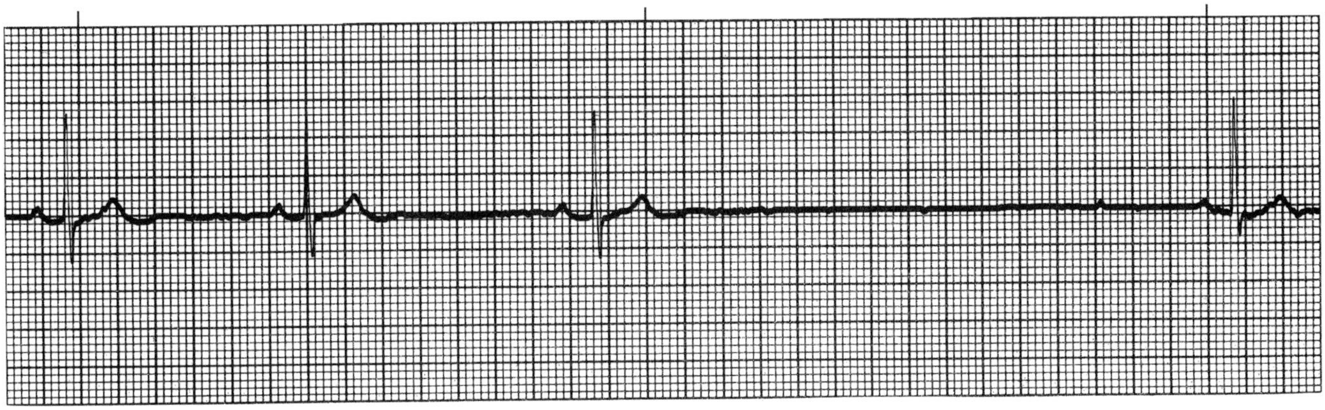

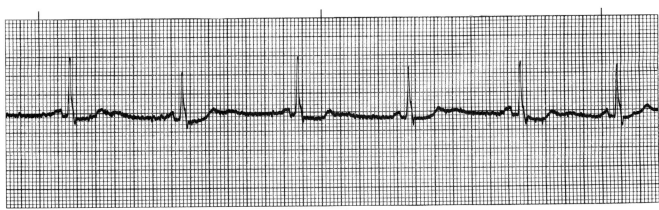

**Strip 6-97.** Rhythm:_____ Rate:_____ P wave:_____

PR interval:_____ QRS:_____

Rhythm interpretation:_____

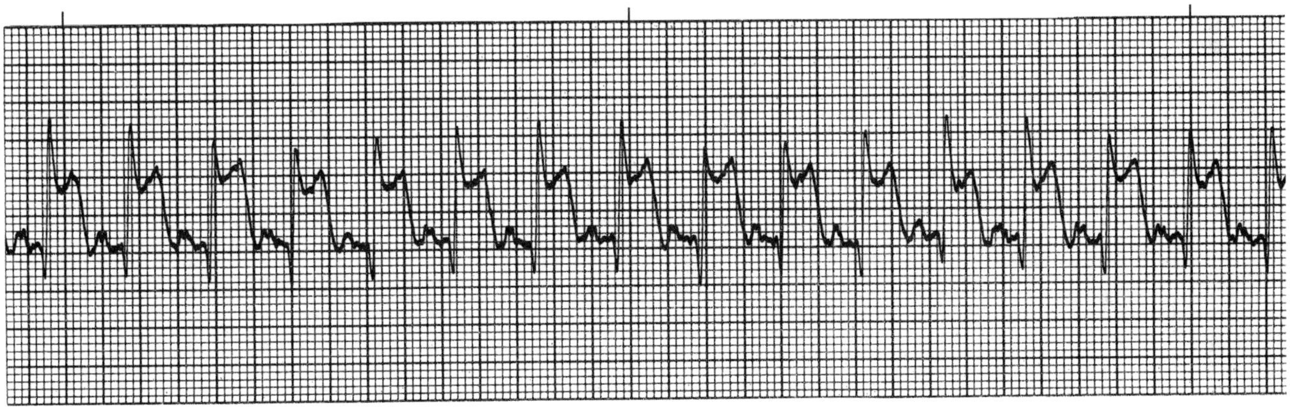

**Strip 6-98.** Rhythm:_____ Rate:_____ P wave:_____

PR interval:_____ QRS:_____

Rhythm interpretation:_____

**Strip 6-99.** Rhythm:_____ Rate:_____ P wave:_____

PR interval:_____ QRS:_____

Rhythm interpretation:_____

# 7

# ATRIAL ARRHYTHMIAS

Atrial arrhythmias (Figure 7-1) originate from ectopic sites in the atria. Because of the ectopic origin of the impulse, the P waves will be different in configuration (morphology) from the sinus P waves (Figure 7-2). In slower atrial rhythms (premature atrial beats, wandering atrial pacemaker), the P wave is often visible as a small, pointed, upright waveform, or it may be inverted if the impulse originates in the lower atrium near the AV junction. In faster atrial rhythms, the abnormal P wave is either superimposed on the preceding T wave (paroxysmal atrial tachycardia), appears in a sawtooth pattern (atrial flutter), or is seen as a wavy baseline (atrial fibrillation).

The electrophysiologic mechanisms most often responsible for atrial arrhythmias are altered automaticity and reentry. Normally, the automaticity of the sinus node exceeds that of all other parts of the conduction system, allowing it to control the heart rate and rhythm. A secondary pacemaking site, such as the atria, can initiate the cardiac rhythm either because it usurps control from the sinus node by accelerating its own automaticity or because the sinus node relinquishes its role by decreasing its automaticity. With reentry, an impulse can travel through an area of myocardium, depolarize it, and then reenter that same area to depolarize it again. Reentry produces a circular movement of the impulse, which continues as long as it encounters receptive cells. This type of impulse conduction often results in rapid heart rates.

When the atrial rate is extremely rapid, as seen in atrial flutter and atrial fibrillation, the AV node blocks some of the atrial impulses from being conducted to the ventricles, thus protecting the ventri-

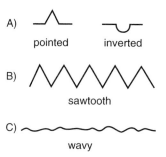

**Figure 7-2.** Atrial P waves.

cles from dangerously high rates. This results in a ventricular rate that is slower than the atrial rate (fewer QRS complexes than P waves). Younger patients and people without underlying heart disease may tolerate episodes of rapid heart rate with no serious problems. In patients with limited cardiac reserve, however, increased heart rates can have serious consequences. In atrial rhythms associated with rapid ventricular rates, cardiac output and coronary perfusion may be reduced secondary to decreased diastolic filling time in the ventricles. Treatment depends on the hemodynamic consequences of the arrhythmia.

## WANDERING ATRIAL PACEMAKER (WAP)

A wandering atrial pacemaker (Figure 7-3; Box 7-1) occurs when the pacemaker site shifts back and forth between the sinus node, other atrial sites, and sometimes the AV node. The P waves change their shape as the pacemaker "wanders" between the mul-

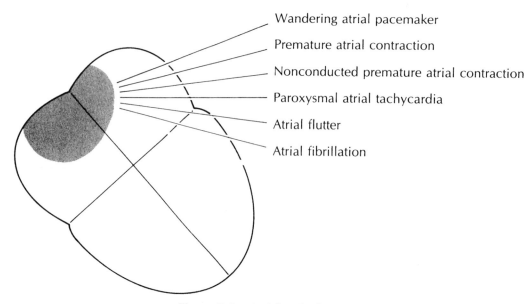

**Figure 7-1.** Atrial arrhythmias.

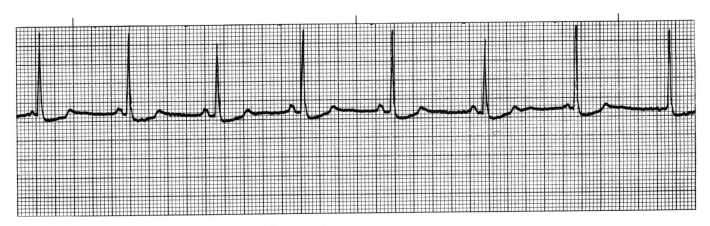

**Figure 7-3.** **Wandering Atrial Pacemaker**

| | |
|---|---|
| ***Rhythm:*** | Irregular |
| ***Rate:*** | 60 |
| ***P waves:*** | Vary in size, shape, across rhythm strip |
| ***PR interval:*** | 0.10–0.14 seconds |
| ***QRS:*** | 0.04–0.08 seconds |

tiple sites. Wandering atrial pacemaker is thought to result from multiple pacemaker sites competing with each other for control of the heart. The heart rate is usually normal, but can be slow. The rhythm may be regular or irregular. The PR interval may vary depending on the pacemaker site. The QRS is normal in duration. The distinguishing feature of this arrhythmia is the changing P wave configuration across the rhythm strip.

| **Box 7-1.** | **Wandering Atrial Pacemaker: Identifying ECG Features** |
|---|---|
| Rhythm: | Regular or irregular |
| Rate: | Usually normal (60–100) but may be slower |
| P waves: | Vary in size, shape, and direction across rhythm strip |
| PR: | May vary slightly depending on the changing pacemaker location |
| QRS: | Normal (0.10 seconds or less) |

WAP can be caused by increased vagal tone that slows the sinus pacemaker or by enhanced automaticity in atrial or junctional pacemaker cells, causing them to compete with the sinus node for control. WAP can be seen in chronic lung disease or valvular (especially mitral and tricuspid) heart disease. It may also be caused by the administration of digitalis. Occasionally, it develops in normal subjects, particularly during sleep.

Wandering atrial pacemaker is not a common arrhythmia, it is usually not clinically significant, and treatment is not indicated. If the heart rate is slow, medications should be reviewed and discontinued if necessary. Asking the patient to cough may decrease vagal tone and encourage the reappearance of a sinus rhythm.

## PREMATURE ATRIAL CONTRACTION (PAC)

A premature atrial contraction (Figures 7-4 through 7-10; Box 7-2) is an early beat that originates in an ectopic pacemaker in the atria and is usually caused by enhanced automaticity in the atrial tissue. It occurs in addition to the patient's underlying rhythm. PACs may originate from a single ectopic pacemaker site or from multiple sites in the atria. The early beat is characterized by an abnormal (occasionally normal appearing) P wave, a QRS complex that is identical or very similar to the QRS complex of the normally conducted beats, and is followed by a pause. An early ectopic atrial P wave followed by a QRS complex is considered a conducted PAC (the premature impulse is conducted to the ventricles).

The shape of the P wave depends on the location of the ectopic pacemaker site. If the ectopic focus is in the vicinity of the SA node, the P wave may closely resemble the sinus P wave (see Figure 7-4). Its sole distinguishing feature may be its prematurity. As a rule, however, the P wave is usually different from the sinus P waves. In Lead II, it is generally upright and often pointed (see Figure 7-8), or it may be inverted (see Figure 7-5) if the pacemaker site is near

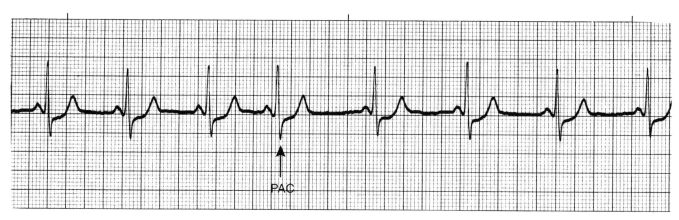

**Figure 7-4.   Normal Sinus Rhythm with Premature Atrial Contraction**

*Rhythm:*      Basic rhythm regular—irregular with PAC

*Rate:*        Basic rhythm rate 72—rate slows to 60 following PAC (temporary rate suppression is common following a pause in the basic rhythm—after several cardiac cycles the rate usually returns to the basic rhythm rate).

*P waves:*     Sinus P waves with basic rhythm; P wave associated with PAC is premature and closely resembles that of the sinus P waves in the underlying rhythm—this indicates the ectopic atrial pacemaker site is close to the SA node

*PR interval:* 0.12 seconds (basic rhythm and PAC)

*QRS:*         0.08 seconds (basic rhythm and PAC)

the AV junction. If the premature beat occurs very early, the abnormal P wave can be found hidden in the preceding T wave, causing a distortion of the T wave contour (see Figure 7-6).

| Box 7-2. | Premature Atrial Contraction (PAC): Identifying ECG Features |
|---|---|
| Rhythm: | Underlying rhythm usually regular; irregular with PACs |
| Rate: | Heart rate is that of underlying rhythm |
| P waves: | P wave associated with PAC is premature and abnormal in size, shape, or direction (in Lead II, the P wave is usually upright (often pointed), or it may be inverted); abnormal P wave often found hidden in preceding T wave, distorting the T wave contour. |
| PR: | Normal or prolonged—usually differs from that of underlying rhythm |
| QRS: | Normal (0.10 seconds or less) |

The PR intervals of the PACs may be normal in duration, but they usually differ from those of the underlying rhythm. Occasionally, the PR interval is prolonged if there is a delay in conduction (see Figure 7-7). The PR interval will not be measurable if the abnormal P wave is obscured in the preceding T wave.

The QRS of the PAC usually resembles that of the underlying rhythm because the conduction of the electrical impulse through the bundle branches is unchanged. If, however, the ectopic atrial impulse is discharged very early, the bundle branches may not have repolarized sufficiently to conduct the impulse normally. Abnormal (aberrant) conduction through the bundle branches results in a wide QRS complex. The term for such a PAC is *premature atrial contraction with aberrant ventricular conduction* (see Figure 7-7). This wide complex must be differentiated from a premature ventricular contraction (PVC), especially if the abnormal P wave associated with the PAC is obscured in the preceding T wave. PVCs are discussed in Chapter 9.

The pause associated with the PAC is usually noncompensatory (the measurement from the R wave before the PAC to the R wave after the PAC is less than two R-R intervals of the underlying rhythm; see Figure 7-8). This is because premature depolarization of the atria by the PAC results in subsequent premature depolarization of the sinus node, causing the sinus node to reset itself a little earlier than expected. Occasionally, the PAC will occur with a compensatory pause (a pause that equals two R-R intervals), but this is usually seen with the PVC. With the compensatory pause, the SA node is not depolarized by the PAC, its timing is not reset, and the underlying rhythm will appear at the time expected after the pause. Rarely, the PAC may occur with a pause that is longer than compensatory.

PACs may appear as a single beat, every other beat (bigeminal PACs; see Figure 7-9), every third

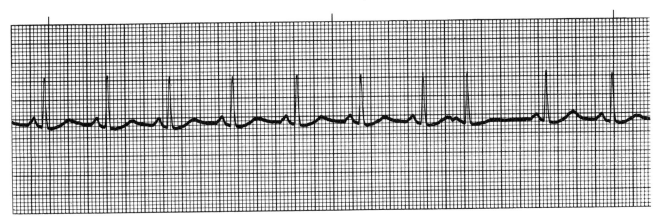

**Figure 7-5.** **Normal Sinus Rhythm with Premature Atrial Contraction**

*Rhythm:*     Basic rhythm regular, irregular with PAC

*Rate:*       Basic rhythm rate 88

*P waves:*    Sinus P waves with basic rhythm; premature, inverted P wave with PAC

*PR interval:* 0.14 to 0.16 seconds

*QRS:*        0.04 to 0.06 seconds

beat (trigeminal PACs), every fourth beat (quadrigeminal PACs), in pairs (also called couplets; see Figure 7-10), or in runs. When PACs occur in consecutive runs of three or more, atrial tachycardia is considered to be present. Frequent PACs may warn of or initiate more serious atrial arrhythmias such as paroxysmal atrial tachycardia, atrial flutter, or atrial fibrillation.

Premature atrial beats are very common. They can occur in people with a normal heart or in people with heart disease. In normal subjects, PACs are seen with emotional stress (which can increase sympathetic tone and catecholamine release) or ingestion of alcohol, caffeine, or nicotine. Other causes include electrolyte disturbances (low serum potassium or magnesium levels), hypoxia, myocardial ischemia, coronary artery disease, chronic lung disease, digitalis toxicity, hyperthyroidism, dilated or hypertrophied atria (commonly caused by mitral stenosis or atrial septal defect), and the administra-

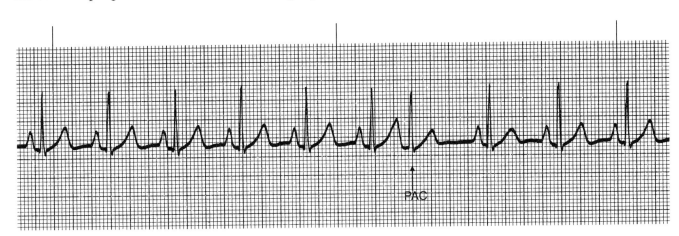

**Figure 7-6.** **Normal Sinus Rhythm with Premature Atrial Contraction**

*Rhythm:*     Basic rhythm regular, irregular with PAC

*Rate:*       Basic rhythm rate 84

*P waves:*    Sinus P waves with basic rhythm; premature, abnormal P wave with PAC. The P wave of the PAC is hidden in the preceding T wave distorting the T wave contour (T wave is taller and more pointed.)

*PR interval:* 0.12 to 0.14 seconds (basic rhythm)

*QRS:*        0.06 to 0.08 seconds

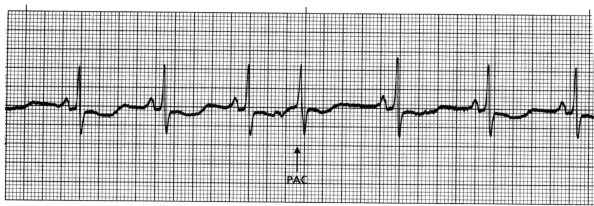

**Figure 7-7.** **Normal Sinus Rhythm with 1 PAC with Aberrant Ventricular Conduction**

*Rhythm:*      Basic rhythm regular, irregular with PAC

*Rate:*        Basic rhythm rate 68

*P waves:*     Sinus in basic rhythm; premature, abnormal P wave with PAC

*PR interval:* 0.16 to 0.18 seconds (basic rhythm)
              0.24 seconds (PAC)

*QRS:*         0.08 seconds
              0.12 seconds (PAC)

tion of sympathomimetic drugs (epinephrine, iso-proterenol, and theophylline). Because PACs may also result from stretch of the myocardium, they can be a warning signal in the development of congestive heart failure. PACs may also occur without apparent cause.

Infrequent PACs require no treatment. If treatment is needed, the best approach is to eliminate the cause (eg, caffeine, alcohol, tobacco, stress).

On some occasions, an ectopic atrial beat will occur late instead of early. These beats are called *atrial escape beats* (Figure 7-11). Atrial escape beats are

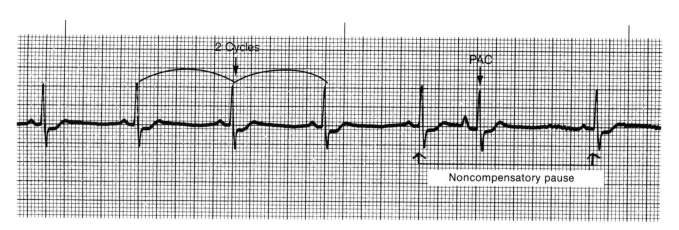

**Figure 7-8.** **Normal Sinus Rhythm with Premature Atrial Contraction**

*Rhythm:*      Basic rhythm regular, irregular with PAC

*Rate:*        Basic rhythm rate 60

*P waves:*     Sinus P waves with basic rhythm; premature, abnormal P wave with PAC

*PR interval:* 0.12 to 0.16 seconds (basic rhythm)

*QRS:*         0.08 seconds

*Comment:*     To determine the type of pause following premature beats, measure from the QRS preceding the premature beat to the QRS following the premature beat. If the measurement equals two RR intervals, the pause is compensatory. If the measurement is less than two RR intervals, the pause is noncompensatory. ST segment depression is present.

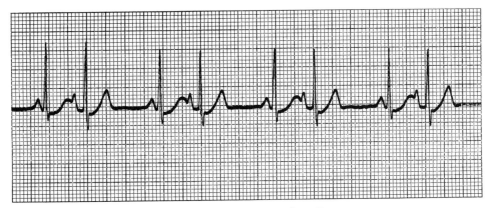

**Figure 7-9.** Bigeminal PACs.

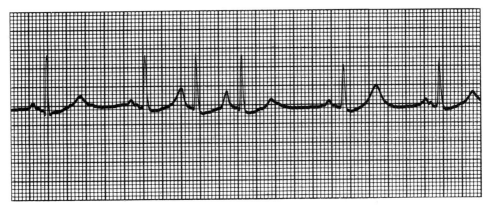

**Figure 7-10.** Paired PACs.

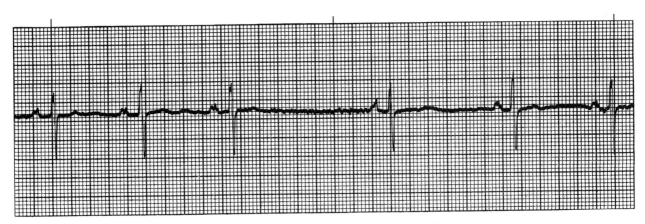

**Figure 7-11.** **Normal Sinus Rhythm with Sinus Arrest and Atrial Escape Beat**

*Rhythm:* Basic rhythm regular; irregular during pause

*Rate:* Basic rhythm rate 63—rate slows to 58 after pause due to temporary rate supression (common following pauses in the basic rhythm)

*P waves:* Sinus P waves; P waves are notched in basic rhythm which could be due to left atrial enlargement; peaked P wave with escape beat

*PR interval:* 0.18–0.20 seconds basic rhythm and escape beat

*QRS:* 0.08 seconds basic rhythm
0.06 seconds escape beat

more likely to occur as a result of increased vagal effect on the SA node rather than enhanced automaticity as is associated with the premature beat. Atrial escape beats may occur after a pause in the underlying rhythm (eg, sinus arrest, sinus block, nonconducted PAC, or type I second-degree AV block ). The morphologic characteristics of the late beat will be the same as the PAC. Escape beats require no treatment. It is important, however, to identify the cause of the initiating pause so appropriate intervention can be started if necessary.

## NONCONDUCTED PAC

A nonconducted PAC (Figures 7-12, 7-13, and 7-14; Box 7-3) results when an ectopic atrial focus occurs so early that it finds the AV node refractory and the impulse is not conducted to the ventricles. This results in an ectopic P wave not accompanied by a QRS complex, but followed by a pause (see Figure 7-12).

Like the conducted PAC, the P wave associated with the nonconducted PAC will be premature and abnormal in size, shape, or direction. Again, the P wave is often found hidden in the preceding T waves, distorting the T wave contour (see Figure 7-13), and the pause that follows is usually noncompensatory. The nonconducted PAC is the most com-

mon cause of unexpected pauses in a regular sinus rhythm.

| Box 7-3. | **Nonconducted PACs: Identifying ECG Features** |
|---|---|
| Rhythm: | Underlying rhythm usually regular; irregular with nonconducted PACs |
| Rate: | Heart rate is that of underlying rhythm |
| P waves: | P wave associated with the nonconducted PAC is premature, and abnormal in size, shape, or direction; often found hidden in preceding T wave, distorting the T wave contour |
| PR: | Absent with nonconducted PAC |
| QRS: | Absent with nonconducted PAC |

The nonconducted PAC can be confused with sinus arrest or block. All produce a sudden pause in the rhythm without QRS complexes. To differentiate between these rhythms, one must examine and compare T wave contours (see Figure 7-14). The early P wave of the nonconducted PAC will distort the preceding T wave. In sinus arrest or sinus block, there is no P wave produced and the T wave contour remains unchanged.

Nonconducted PACs have the same significance as conducted PACs and may be treated in the same manner.

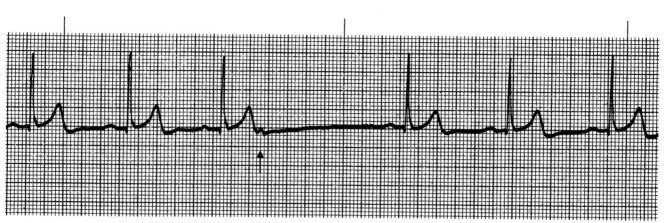

**Figure 7-12. Normal Sinus Rhythm with Nonconducted PAC**

*Rhythm:* Basic rhythm regular; irregular with nonconducted PAC

*Rate:* Basic rate 60; rate slows following nonconducted PAC; rate suppression can occur following a pause in the basic rhythm. After several cycles, the rate will return to the basic rhythm rate.

*P waves:* Sinus P waves with basic rhythm; premature, abnormal P wave with nonconducted PAC

*PR interval:* 0.20 seconds with basic rhythm

*QRS:* 0.06 to 0.08 seconds with basic rhythm

*Comment:* A U wave is present

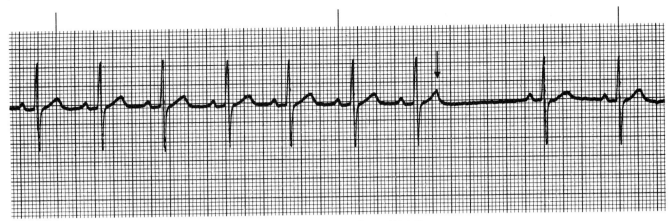

**Figure 7-13.** **Normal Sinus Rhythm with Nonconducted PAC**

*Rhythm:* Basic rhythm regular; irregular with nonconducted PACs

*Rate:* Basic rhythm rate 88

*P waves:* Sinus P waves with basic rhythm; P wave of nonconducted PAC is premature, abnormal, and hidden in the preceding T wave (T wave is taller and more pointed than those of underlying rhythm)

*PR interval:* 0.16 to 0.18 seconds (basic rhythm); not present with nonconducted PAC

*QRS:* 0.06 to 0.08 seconds (basic rhythm); not present with nonconducted PAC

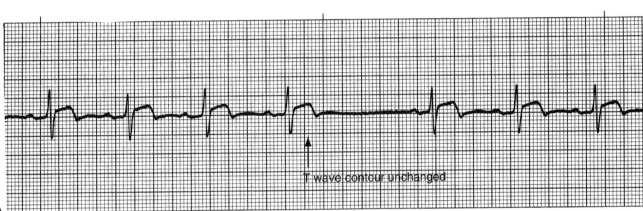

A

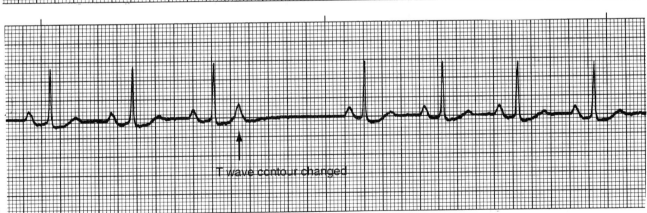

B

**Figure 7-14.** **Differentiation of Sinus Arrest or Block from the Nonconducted PAC**

*A Sinus Arrest or Block*
1. Sudden pause in the basic rhythm
2. No P wave present
3. T-wave contour occurring during pause remains unchanged

*B Nonconducted PAC*
1. Sudden pause in the basic rhythm
2. Abnormal, premature P wave present and often found hidden in T wave
3. T wave contour occurring during pause will be different from the contours of the basic rhythm

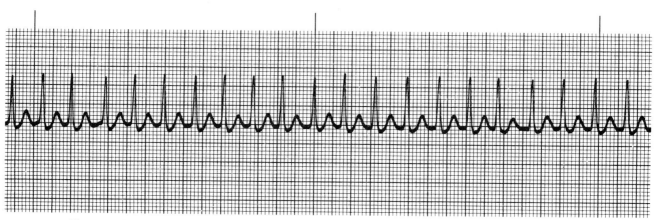

**Figure 7-15.** Paroxysmal Atrial Tachycardia

*Rhythm:* Regular

*Rate:* 188

*P waves:* Hidden

*PR interval:* Not measurable

*QRS:* 0.06 to 0.08 seconds

# PAROXYSMAL ATRIAL TACHYCARDIA (PAT)

Paroxysmal atrial tachycardia (Figures 7-15 and 7-16; Box 7-4) is an arrhythmia originating in an ectopic pacemaker site in the atria. This rhythm is most commonly caused by rapid firing of an ectopic atrial focus from accelerated automaticity or to a reentry circuit (usually involving the AV node) in which the impulse remains active and travels rapidly around the circuit pathway, repeatedly reactivating the myocardium. Atrial tachycardia commonly starts and ends abruptly, occurring in bursts or paroxysms (thus, the name "paroxysmal atrial tachycardia" or PAT). PAT is often initiated by a PAC. By definition, three or more consecutive PACs are considered to be atrial tachycardia (see Figure 7-16).

Atrial tachycardia is a regular tachycardia with an atrial rate between 140 and 250 per minute. The ventricular rate will be the same as the atrial rate un-

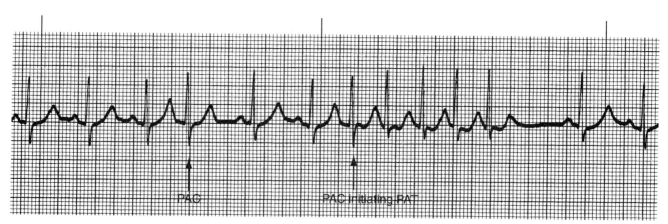

**Figure 7-16.** Normal Sinus Rhythm with PAC and Burst of PAT

*Rhythm:* Basic rhythm regular; irregular with PAC and burst of PAT

*Rate:* Basic rhythm rate 94; PAT rate (167)

*P waves:* Sinus P waves with basic rhythm; premature, pointed P waves with PAC and PAT (P waves are superimposed on preceding T waves)

*PR interval:* 0.16 seconds (basic rhythm)

*QRS:* 0.08 seconds

*Comment:* A run of three or more consecutive PACs is considered PAT

less AV block is involved. The P waves associated with atrial tachycardia are abnormal but may be difficult to identify because they are often hidden in the preceding T waves. The PR interval will not be measurable if the P waves are hidden. The QRS duration is normal.

| Box 7-4. | Atrial Tachycardia: Identifying ECG Features |
|---|---|
| Rhythm: | Regular |
| Rate: | Atrial: 140–250 |
| | Ventricular: 140–250 |
| P waves: | Abnormal (often pointed); usually hidden in preceding T wave |
| PR: | Not measurable |
| QRS: | Normal (0.10 seconds or less) |

In general, the causes of atrial tachycardia are similar to those of PACs. Atrial tachycardia has been associated with emotional stress, mitral valve disease, rheumatic heart disease, chronic obstructive pulmonary disease, digitalis toxicity, acute MI, and ingestion of alcohol, caffeine, or nicotine.

During an episode of PAT, many people can feel the rapid heart rate (palpitations), and this is a source of stress and anxiety. When the ventricular rate is very rapid, the ventricles are unable to fill completely during diastole, resulting in a significant reduction in cardiac output. In addition, a rapid heart rate increases myocardial oxygen requirements and cardiac workload. Treatment of atrial tachycardia is directed toward eliminating the cause and decreasing the ventricular rate.

Priorities of treatment depend on the patient's tolerance of the rhythm. If the patient is hemodynamically stable (systolic blood pressure of 90 mmHg or above; normal level of consciousness; skin warm and dry; free of chest pain, dyspnea, or signs of heart failure), try sedation first. In addition to relieving the anxiety that commonly accompanies tachyarrhythmias, sedation will often reduce sympathetic tone and might convert the arrhythmia to a sinus rhythm. If sedation does not convert the rhythm, vagal maneuvers should be tried next. Vagal maneuvers work by slowing the heart rate through increasing parasympathetic tone. The most common of these measures include carotid sinus massage and the Valsalva maneuver ("bearing down"). If vagal maneuvers fail, administer a 6-mg bolus of adenosine IV rapidly over 1 to 2 seconds, followed by a rapid 20-cc flush of saline or plain IV fluid. If the initial dose is ineffective after 1 to 2 minutes, administer a 12-mg bolus of adenosine IV rapidly over 1 to 2 seconds, followed by a rapid 20-cc flush of saline or plain IV fluid. If the second dose is ineffective after 1 to 2 minutes, repeat a 12-mg dose of adenosine in the same manner.

Additional treatment options for those patients who fail to respond to vagal maneuvers or adenosine include either a calcium channel blocker, a beta blocker, or digitalis, all of which increase block at the AV node and may slow ventricular response or terminate the arrhythmia. If the AV nodal agent is unsuccessful in terminating PAT, then electrical cardioversion is the next treatment of choice. Antiarrhythmics such as amiodarone and procainamide should be considered only when a AV nodal blocking agent and cardioversion are not successful. In patients with significantly impaired left ventricular function, drugs with negative inotropic properties should be avoided in favor of digitalis or amiodarone, or perhaps diltiazem, a negative inotropic drug that exhibits less depression of contractility when compared to similar agents. Amiodarone has the best balance between side effects and effectiveness in heart failure patients. Combined use of calcium channel blockers, beta blockers, and antiarrhythmic agents should be avoided because of the potential additive hypotensive, bradycardic, and proarrhythmic effects of these drugs in combination. Electrical cardioversion is the initial treatment of choice in patients who are hemodynamically unstable. Radiofrequency catheter ablation of the ectopic focus or reentry circuit may be necessary for recurrent PAT unresponsive to oral therapy.

## ATRIAL FLUTTER

Atrial flutter (Figures 7-17 and 7-18; Box 7-5) is an arrhythmia most commonly resulting from a rapidly firing ectopic site in the atria caused by accelerated automaticity or to a rapid reentry circuit in the atria. The atria are depolarized at rates of 250 to 400 times per minute. The atrial muscles respond to this rapid stimulation by producing wave deflections called *flutter waves* (F waves). The typical atrial flutter wave consists of an initial negative component followed by a positive component producing V-shaped waveforms with a sawtooth appearance. The sawtooth waves affect the whole baseline to such a degree that there is no isoelectric line between the F waves, and the T wave is completely or partially obscured by the flutter waves. Atrial flutter is primarily recognized by this sawtooth baseline. The QRS complexes are usually narrow as long as conduction in the ventricles is normal.

The AV node is bombarded by the rapid atrial impulses but will only conduct some of the impulses to the ventricles. The rest are not conducted. The AV node conducts the impulses in various ratios. For example, the AV node might allow every second im-

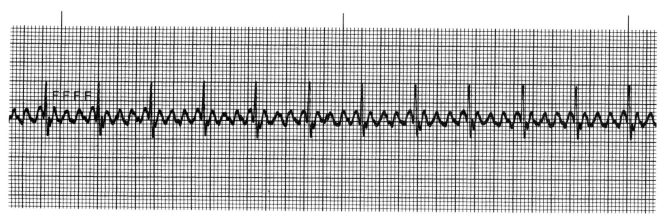

**Figure 7-17.** **Atrial Flutter with 4:1 AV Conduction**

*Rhythm:* Regular

*Rate:* Atrial: 428
Ventricular: 107
Note: If the ventricular rate is regular, multiply the number of flutter waves before each QRS × the ventricular rate to determine atrial rate.

*P waves:* Four flutter waves before each QRS (marked as F waves above)

*PR interval:* Not measurable

*QRS:* 0.06 to 0.08 seconds

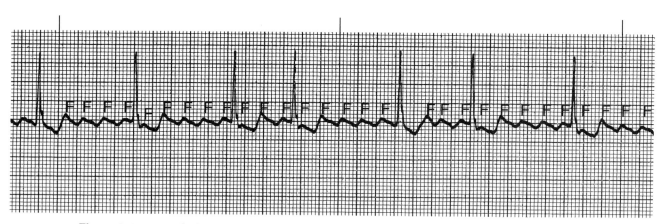

**Figure 7-18** **Atrial Flutter with Variable AV Conduction**

*Rhythm:* Irregular

*Rate:* Atrial: 280
Ventricular: 60
Note: If the ventricular rate is irregular, count the number of flutter waves in a 6-second strip and multiply × 10 to obtain atrial rate.

*P waves:* Flutter waves before each QRS (varying ratios)

*PR interval:* Not measurable

*QRS:* 0.06 to 0.08 seconds

pulse to travel through the AV junction to the ventricles, resulting in a 2:1 AV conduction ratio (a 2:1 conduction ratio indicates that, for every two flutter waves, only one is followed by a QRS). Even ratios (2:1, 4:1) are more common than odd ratios (3:1, 5:1). If the conduction ratio remains constant (eg, 2:1), the ventricular rhythm will be regular, and the rhythm is described as atrial flutter with 2:1 AV conduction. If the conduction ratio varies (from 4:1 to 2:1 to 6:1, and so forth), the ventricular rhythm will be irregular, and the rhythm is described as atrial flutter with variable AV conduction. In atrial flutter, the ventricular rate is slower than the atrial rate, with the rate depending on the number of impulses conducted through the AV node to the ventricles.

---

**Box 7-5.  Atrial Flutter: Identifying ECG Features**

Rhythm: Regular or irregular (depends on AV conduction ratios)

Rate: Atrial rate: 250–400

Ventricular rate: Varies with number of impulses conducted through AV node; will be less than the atrial rate

P waves: V-shaped waveforms with a sawtooth appearance called *flutter waves* (F waves)

PR: Not measurable

QRS: Normal (0.10 seconds or less)

---

Causes of atrial flutter include valvular heart disease, acute MI, hypertensive heart disease, cardiomyopathy, pulmonary disease, pulmonary emboli, congestive heart failure, pericarditis, and myocarditis. The arrhythmia can also occur after cardiac surgery.

Like PAT, the ventricular rate in atrial flutter may be rapid, increasing myocardial oxygen requirements and cardiac workload and decreasing cardiac output. In addition, the rapidly contracting atria do not contract strongly enough to empty all their contents. This results not only in a loss of the "atrial kick" but also in a stasis of blood, which may form clots in the atria (mural thrombi) leading to a risk of arterial or pulmonary emboli.

Priorities of treatment include controlling the ventricular rate, assessment of anticoagulation needs, and restoration of sinus rhythm. Pharmacologic rate control is the initial treatment for stable, rapid atrial flutter regardless of its duration. In patients with preserved left ventricular function, beta blockers, calcium channel blockers, or digitalis is the reasonable agent for rate control. In patients with congestive heart failure, digitalis, diltiazem, or amiodarone is recommended. Although amiodarone is ef-

fective for rate control, conversion to normal sinus rhythm (NSR) may occur. Therefore, in patients at risk for systemic emboli upon conversion to sinus rhythm (arrhythmia onset greater than 48 hours), amiodarone is recommended only when other medications for rate control have proved ineffective or are contraindicated, and the risk of possible pharmacologic cardioversion is believed to be justified. After rate control, electrical cardioversion is the treatment of choice to restore sinus rhythm in atrial flutter less than 48 hours old. If atrial flutter has been present for more than 48 hours, there is a risk of systemic embolization with conversion to sinus rhythm unless the patient has been adequately anticoagulated. In this situation, attempts to convert the rhythm with antiarrhythmics or cardioversion should be delayed. The patient should be treated with anticoagulants for 3 weeks, cardioverted, then placed on anticoagulants for an additional 4 weeks. Some physicians may prefer a more rapid approach of heparinization, cardiology consultation with the use of transesophageal echocardiography to exclude atrial thrombi, cardioversion within 24 hours, followed by anticoagulants for 4 more weeks. Hemodynamically unstable, rapid atrial flutter should be electrically cardioverted immediately regardless of the duration of the arrhythmia. For chronic or recurrent atrial flutter, radiofrequency catheter ablation of the reentry circuit is the treatment of choice.

## ATRIAL FIBRILLATION

Atrial fibrillation (Figures 7-19 through 7-22; Box 7-6) is an arrhythmia arising from multiple ectopic pacemakers or sites of rapid reentry circuits in the atria discharging impulses at a rate of 400 or more. These impulses are so rapid that they cause the atria to quiver instead of contract regularly, producing irregular, wavy deflections. These wavy deflections are called *fibrillatory waves* (f waves). If the waves are large, they are called *coarse* fibrillatory waves. If the waves are small, they are called *fine* fibrillatory waves. Sometimes, the f waves are so small (see Figure 7-21) that they appear to be almost a flat line between the QRS complexes. As in atrial flutter, the wavy deflections seen in atrial fibrillation affect the whole baseline. Flutter waves are sometimes seen mixed with the fibrillatory waves. This mixed rhythm is often called *fib-flutter*. The QRS complexes are usually narrow as long as conduction in the ventricles is normal.

As in atrial flutter, the AV node is being bombarded by these rapid atrial impulses but is refractory to most of the impulses and allows only a fraction to reach the ventricles. Characteristically, the

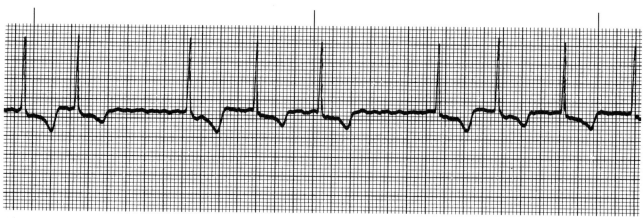

**Figure 7-19.   Atrial Fibrillation (Controlled rate)**

*Rhythm:*        Irregular

*Rate:*          Ventricular rate 70

*P waves:*       Fibrillatory waves present

*PR interval:*   Not measurable

*QRS:*           0.04 to 0.06 seconds

*Comment:*       ST segment depression and T wave inversion are present.

ventricular rate is grossly irregular because the AV junction is being stimulated in an apparently random fashion by the rapidly fibrillating atria. The ventricular rate is slower than the atrial rate and will depend on the number of impulses conducted through the AV node to the ventricles. When the ventricular rate is less than 100 per minute, the rhythm is called *controlled atrial fibrillation*. When the ventricular rate is greater than 100 per minute, the rhythm is called *uncontrolled atrial fibrillation*, or *atrial fibrillation with a rapid ventricular response*. Atrial fibrillation is recognized primarily by the wavy baseline and the grossly irregular ventricular rhythm (unless the ventricular rate is very rapid, in which case the rhythm becomes more regular).

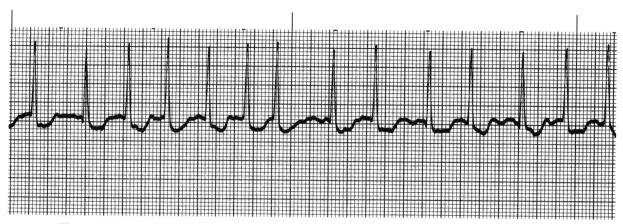

**Figure 7-20.   Atrial Fibrillation (Uncontrolled rate)**

*Rhythm:*        Irregular

*Rate:*          Ventricular rate 130

*P waves:*       Fibrillatory waves present

*PR interval:*   Not measurable

*QRS:*           0.06 to 0.08 seconds

*Comment:*       ST segment depression is present.

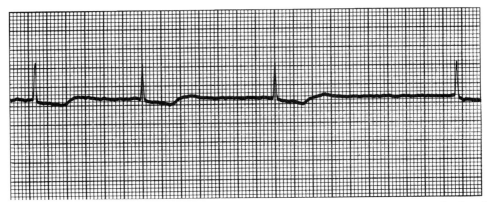

**Figure 7-21.** Atrial fibrillation with f waves so small they appear to be almost a flat line between QRS complexes.

Atrial fibrillation is the most common rhythm seen next to sinus rhythm. Atrial fibrillation can occur in normal people or in those with heart disease. In normal people, the rhythm is usually temporary, lasting only a few hours or days and may be associated with emotional stress or with excessive ingestion of alcohol or caffeine, or it may occur without any apparent cause. This type of atrial fibrillation often spontaneously reverts to sinus rhythm or is easily converted with pharmacologic therapy alone. In other people, the rhythm is chronic and may persist indefinitely. Chronic atrial fibrillation is associated with valvular heart disease (especially mitral valve stenosis and mitral regurgitation), hypertension, coronary heart disease, cardiomyopathy, myocarditis, pericarditis, heart failure, hyperthyroidism, pulmonary disease, and congenital heart disease (especially atrial septal defect). Atrial fibrillation is also common after cardiac surgery.

The clinical consequences of atrial fibrillation are similar to atrial flutter. The ventricular rate may be rapid, increasing myocardial oxygen demands and cardiac workload and decreasing cardiac output. With atrial fibrillation, normal atrial depolarization is lost and the atria fibrillate (quiver) instead of contracting synchronously. In this circumstance, the normal "atrial kick" is lost, further compromising cardiac output. Decreased cardiac output will be especially marked in patients with underlying cardiac impairment and in the elderly, who appear to depend more on atrial contraction for filling of the ventricles. Decreased cardiac output in atrial fibrillation is related to the rapid ventricular rate as well as to the loss of the "atrial kick."

**Box 7-6. Atrial Fibrillation: Identifying ECG Features**

| | |
|---|---|
| Rhythm: | Grossly irregular (unless the ventricular rate is very rapid, in which case the rhythm becomes more regular) |
| Rate: | Atrial rate: 400 or more—not measurable on surface ECG |
| | Ventricular rate: Varies with number of impulses conducted through AV node to ventricles |
| P waves: | Irregular wavy deflections called *fibrillatory waves* (f waves) |
| PR: | Not measurable |
| QRS: | Normal (0.10 seconds or less) |

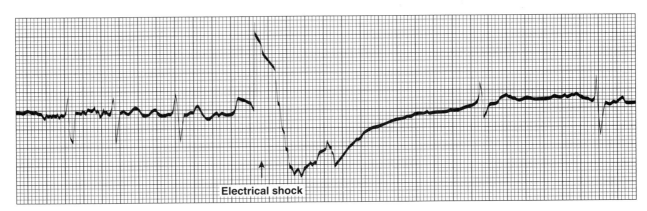

**Figure 7-22.** Cardioversion of atrial fibrillation to NSR.

The noncontracting atria also tend to pool blood in the atrial chamber, increasing the potential for thrombus formation. These clots (mural thrombi) may dislodge into the pulmonary circulation and cause pulmonary emboli or enter the arterial circulation causing a cerebrovascular accident, or an occlusion of the blood supply to the legs, intestines, or kidneys.

Treatment of atrial fibrillation includes controlling the heart rate, providing anticoagulation as a prophylaxis for thromboembolism, and returning the atria to a sinus rhythm. The treatment protocols for atrial fibrillation are the same as atrial flutter. Rate control should be achieved first, using pharmacologic agents (beta blockers, calcium channel blockers, or digitalis for patients with preserved left ventricular function and digitalis, diltiazem, or amiodarone for patients with congestive heart failure). As with atrial flutter, amiodarone should be reserved for use within the first 48 hours of arrhythmia onset because of the possibility of pharmacologic conversion to NSR and subsequent risk of systemic emboli. After rate control, electrical cardioversion is recommended for atrial fibrillation less than 48 hours old. If atrial fibrillation has been present for greater than 48 hours, the patient must be adequately anticoagulated (refer to anticoagulation protocols for atrial flutter) before attempts to restore sinus rhythm using electrical cardioversion or antiarrhythmics. Hemodynamically unstable atrial fibrillation should be electrically cardioverted immediately, regardless of the duration of the arrhythmia. Patients with chronic atrial fibrillation (present for months or years) may not convert to sinus rhythm with any therapy. Treatment of these patients should be directed at controlling the ventricular rate and providing anticoagulation. Figure 7-22 is an example of atrial fibrillation converting to sinus rhythm after electrical shock (cardioversion).

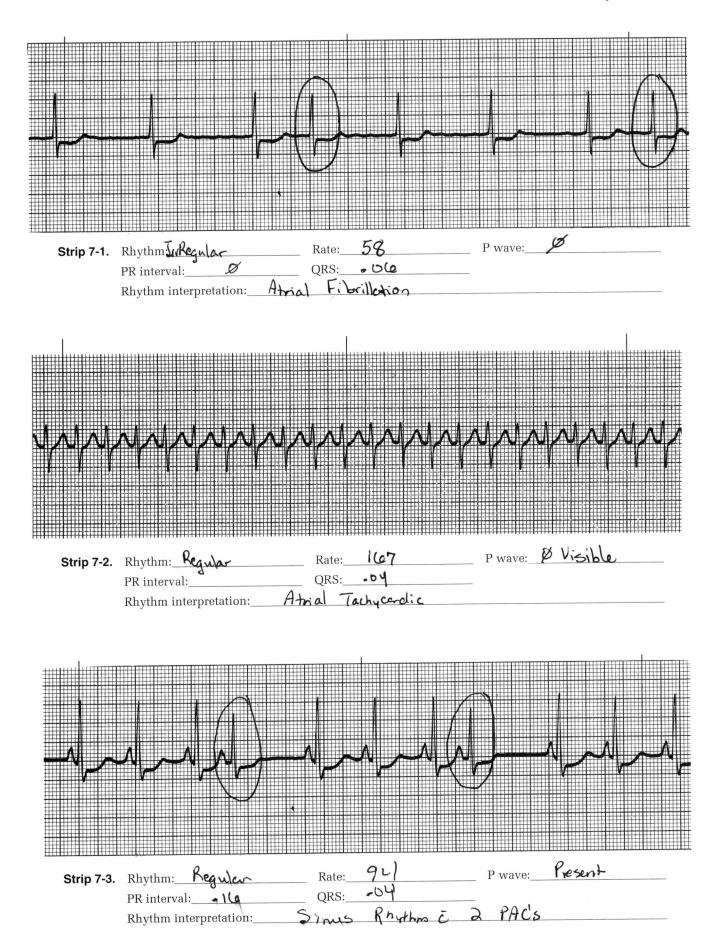

**Strip 7-1.** Rhythm: Irregular     Rate: 58     P wave: Ø
PR interval: Ø     QRS: .06
Rhythm interpretation: Atrial Fibrillation

**Strip 7-2.** Rhythm: Regular     Rate: 167     P wave: Ø Visible
PR interval:     QRS: .04
Rhythm interpretation: Atrial Tachycardia

**Strip 7-3.** Rhythm: Regular     Rate: 92     P wave: Present
PR interval: .16     QRS: .04
Rhythm interpretation: Sinus Rhythm c̄ 2 PAC's

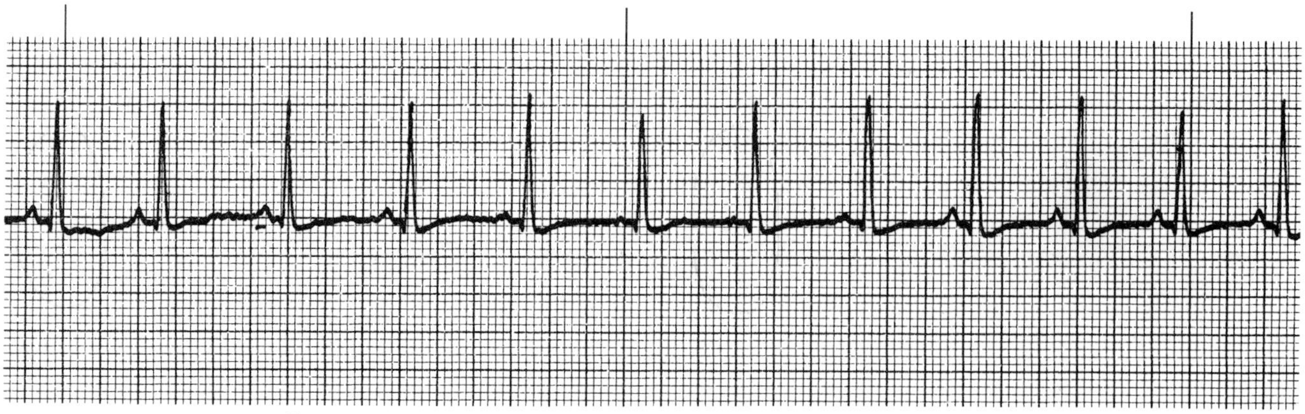

**Strip 7-4.** Rhythm: _Irregular_  Rate: _100_  P wave: _Present_
PR interval: _.16_  QRS: _.08_
Rhythm interpretation: _Wandering Atrial Pacemaker_

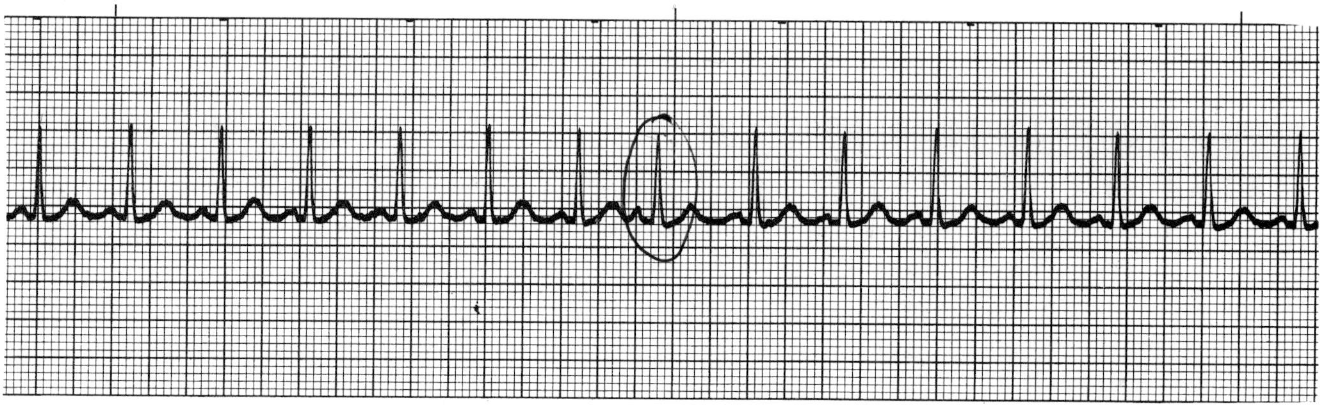

**Strip 7-5.** Rhythm: _Regular_  Rate: _125_  P wave: _Present_
PR interval: _.16_  QRS: _.04_
Rhythm interpretation: _Sinus Tachycardia c̄ 1 PAC_

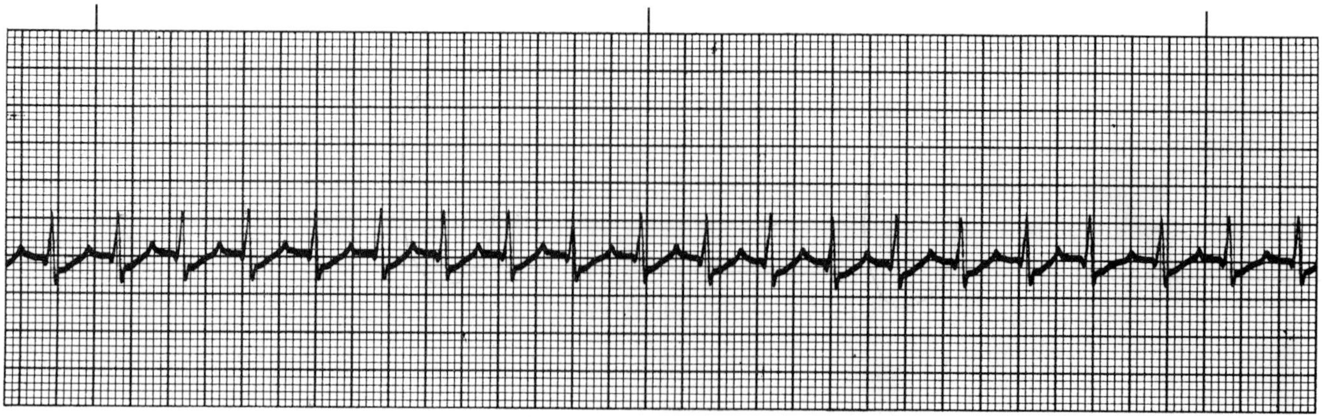

**Strip 7-6.** Rhythm: _Regular_  Rate: _150_  P wave: _____
PR interval: _____  QRS: _.06_
Rhythm interpretation: _Supraventricular Tachycardia_

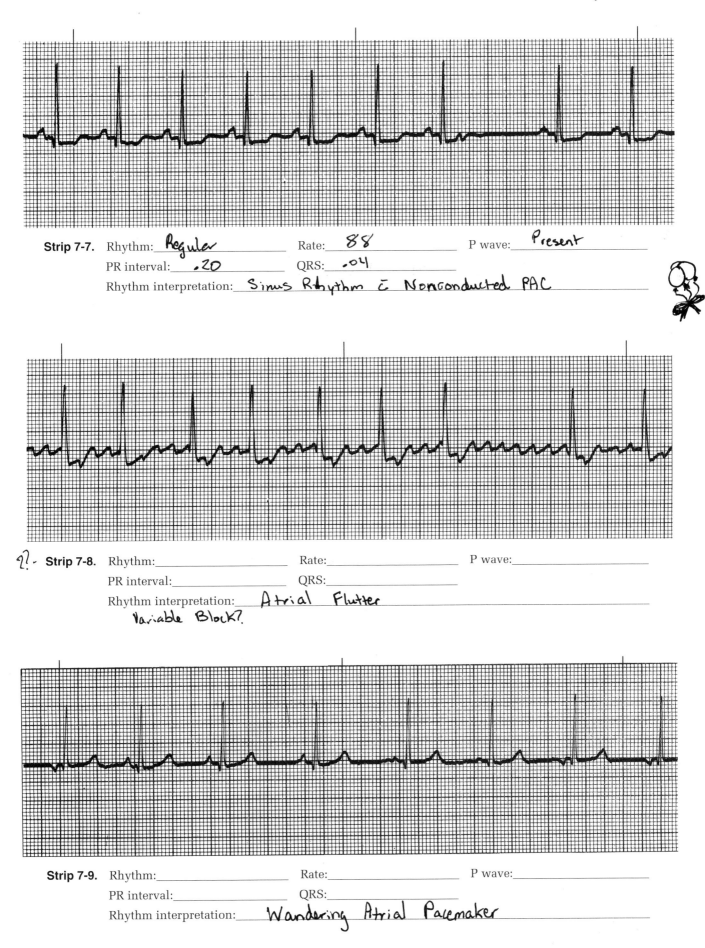

**Strip 7-7.** Rhythm: _Regular_     Rate: _88_     P wave: _Present_

PR interval: _.20_     QRS: _.04_

Rhythm interpretation: _Sinus Rhythm c̄ Nonconducted PAC_

?? - **Strip 7-8.** Rhythm: _____     Rate: _____     P wave: _____

PR interval: _____     QRS: _____

Rhythm interpretation: _Atrial Flutter_

_Variable Block?_

**Strip 7-9.** Rhythm: _____     Rate: _____     P wave: _____

PR interval: _____     QRS: _____

Rhythm interpretation: _Wandering Atrial Pacemaker_

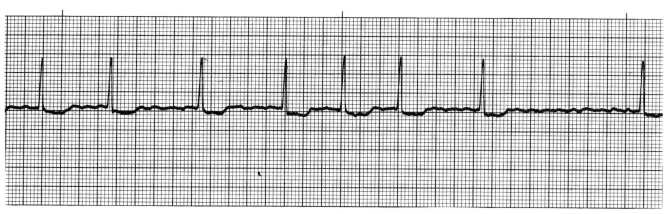

*Stop Here* ⭐

**Strip 7-10.** Rhythm:_____ Rate:_____ P wave:_____

PR interval:_____ QRS:_____

Rhythm interpretation:_____ Atrial Fibrillation _____

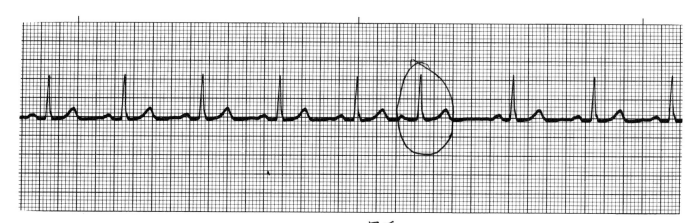

**Strip 7-11.** Rhythm:_____ Rate:_____ 75 _____ P wave:_____

PR interval:_____ QRS:_____

Rhythm interpretation:_____

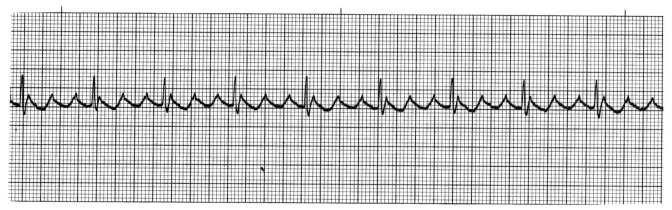

**Strip 7-12.** Rhythm:_____ Rate:_____ P wave:_____

PR interval:_____ QRS:_____

Rhythm interpretation:_____

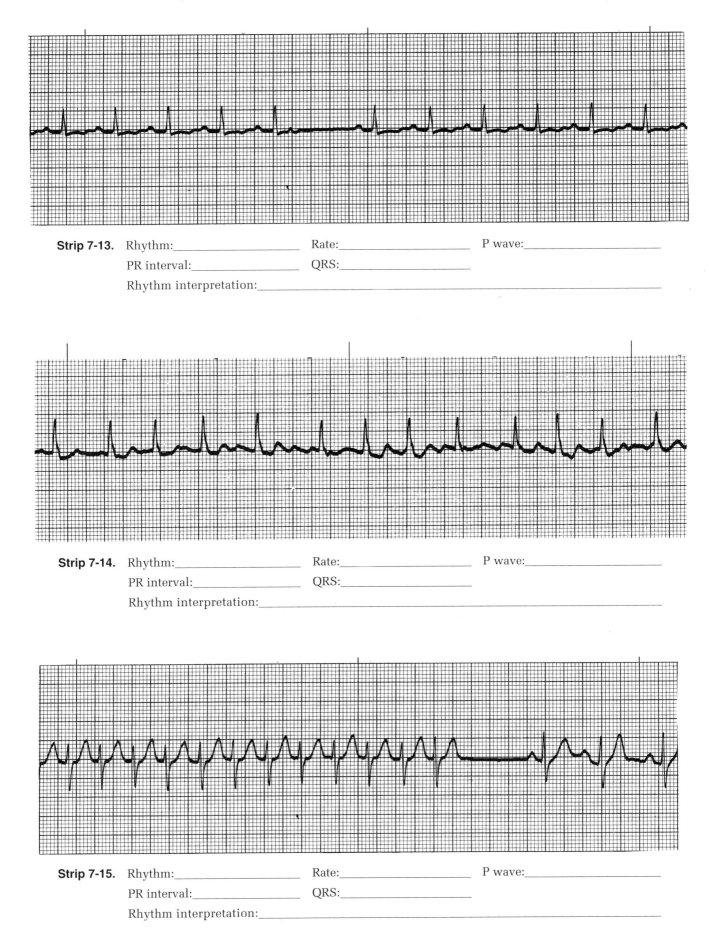

**Strip 7-13.** Rhythm:_____ Rate:_____ P wave:_____

PR interval:_____ QRS:_____

Rhythm interpretation:_____

**Strip 7-14.** Rhythm:_____ Rate:_____ P wave:_____

PR interval:_____ QRS:_____

Rhythm interpretation:_____

**Strip 7-15.** Rhythm:_____ Rate:_____ P wave:_____

PR interval:_____ QRS:_____

Rhythm interpretation:_____

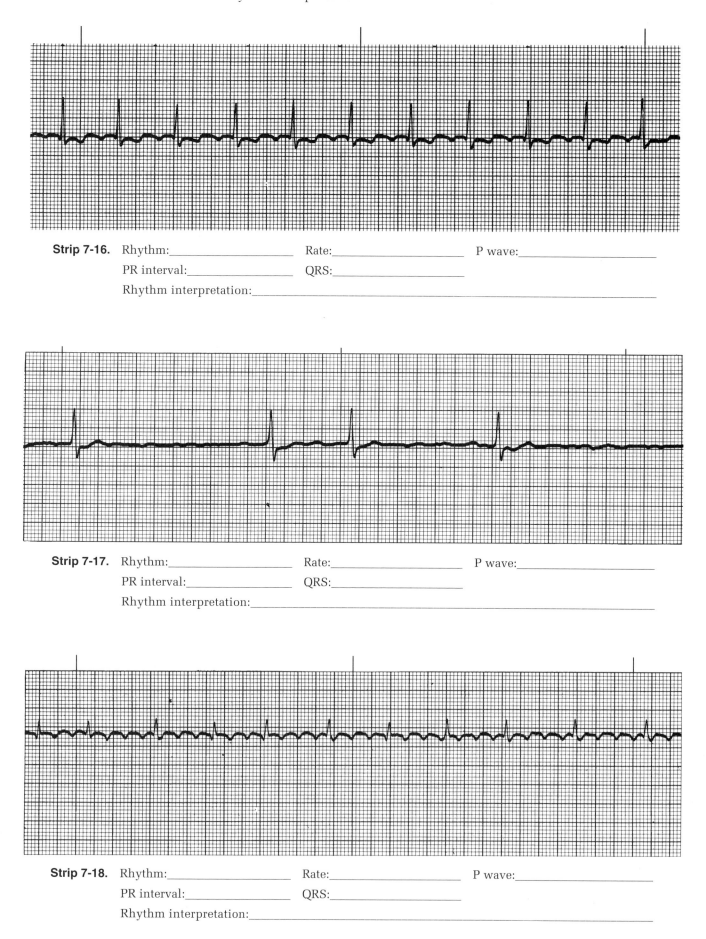

**Strip 7-16.** Rhythm:_____ Rate:_____ P wave:_____

PR interval:_____ QRS:_____

Rhythm interpretation:_____

**Strip 7-17.** Rhythm:_____ Rate:_____ P wave:_____

PR interval:_____ QRS:_____

Rhythm interpretation:_____

**Strip 7-18.** Rhythm:_____ Rate:_____ P wave:_____

PR interval:_____ QRS:_____

Rhythm interpretarion:_____

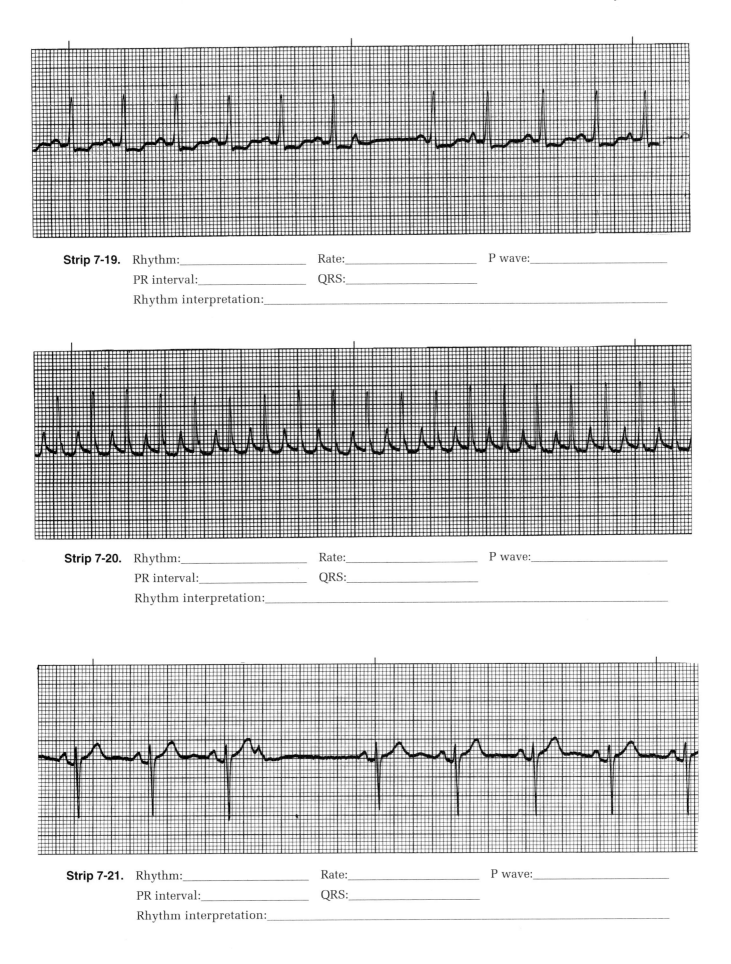

**Strip 7-19.** Rhythm:_____ Rate:_____ P wave:_____

PR interval:_____ QRS:_____

Rhythm interpretation:_____

**Strip 7-20.** Rhythm:_____ Rate:_____ P wave:_____

PR interval:_____ QRS:_____

Rhythm interpretation:_____

**Strip 7-21.** Rhythm:_____ Rate:_____ P wave:_____

PR interval:_____ QRS:_____

Rhythm interpretation:_____

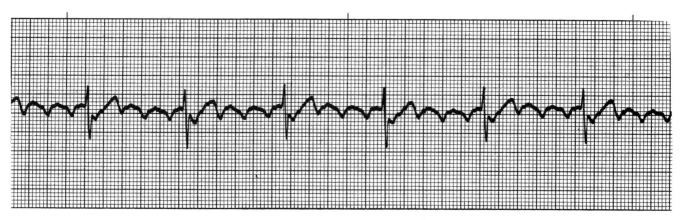

**Strip 7-22.** Cardioversion of atrial fibrillation to NSR.

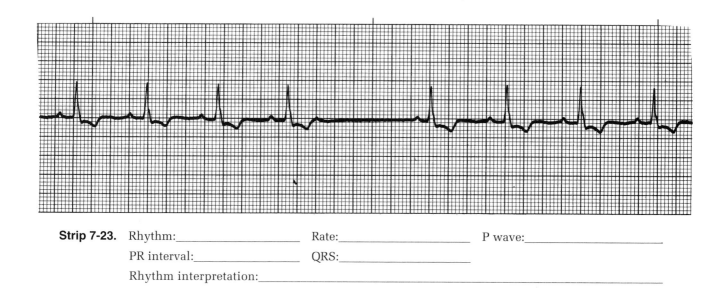

**Strip 7-23.** Rhythm:_____ Rate:_____ P wave:_____

PR interval:_____ QRS:_____

Rhythm interpretation:_____

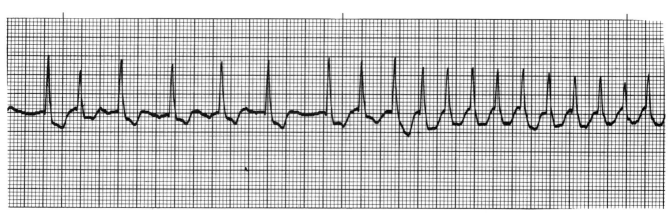

**Strip 7-24.** Rhythm:_____ Rate:_____ P wave:_____

PR interval:_____ QRS:_____

Rhythm interpretion:_____

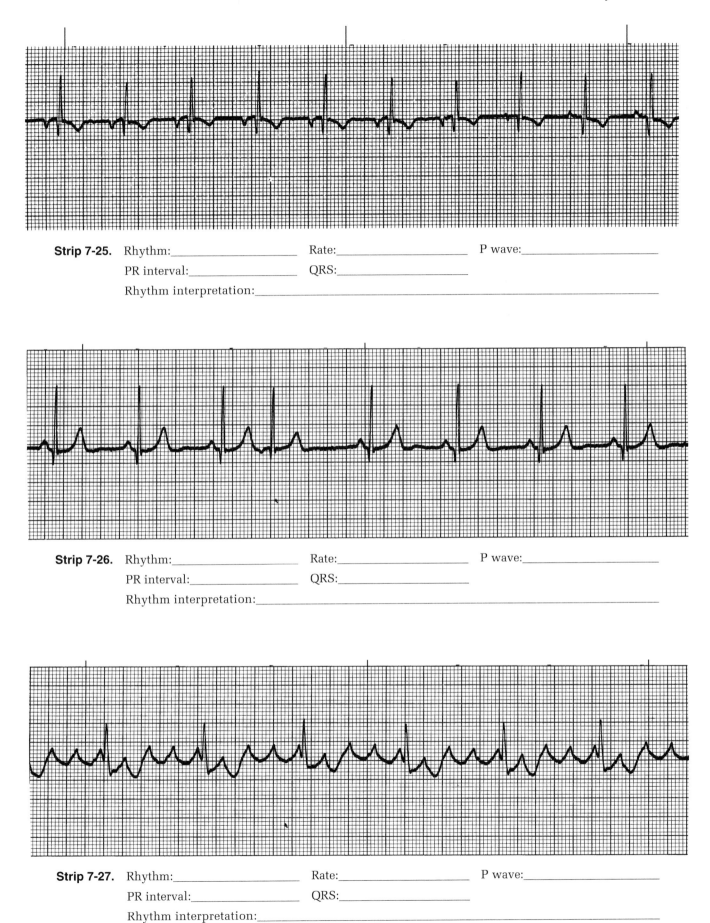

**Strip 7-25.** Rhythm:_____ Rate:_____ P wave:_____

PR interval:_____ QRS:_____

Rhythm interpretation:_____

**Strip 7-26.** Rhythm:_____ Rate:_____ P wave:_____

PR interval:_____ QRS:_____

Rhythm interpretation:_____

**Strip 7-27.** Rhythm:_____ Rate:_____ P wave:_____

PR interval:_____ QRS:_____

Rhythm interpretation:_____

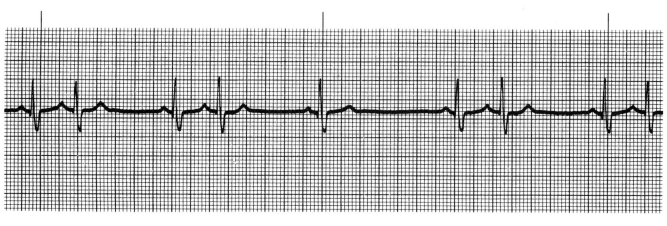

**Strip 7-28.** Rhythm:_____ Rate:_____ P wave:_____

PR interval:_____ QRS:_____

Rhythm interpretation:_____

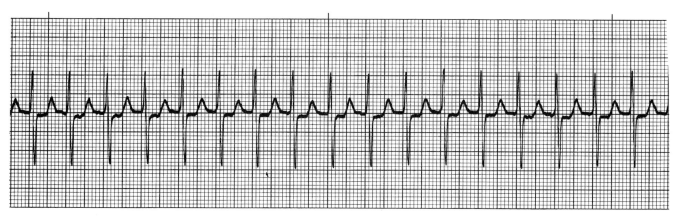

**Strip 7-29.** Rhythm:_____ Rate:_____ P wave:_____

PR interval:_____ QRS:_____

Rhythm interpretation:_____

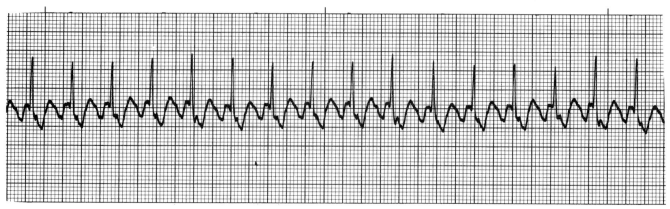

**Strip 7-30.** Rhythm:_____ Rate:_____ P wave:_____

PR interval:_____ QRS:_____

Rhythm interpretation:_____

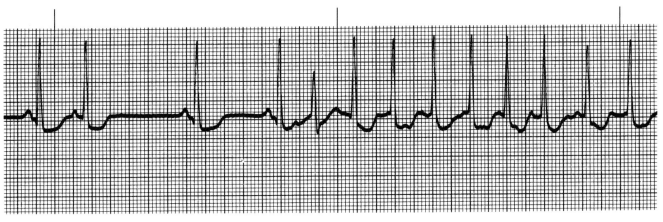

**Strip 7-31.** Rhythm:_____ Rate:_____ P wave:_____

PR interval:_____ QRS:_____

Rhythm interpretation:_____

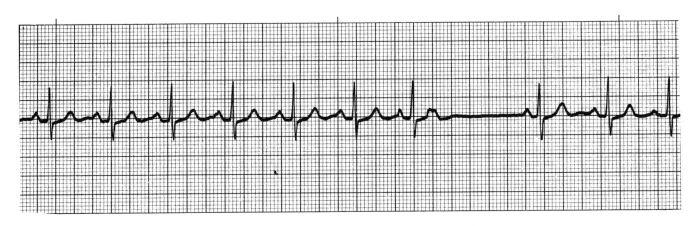

**Strip 7-32.** Rhythm:_____ Rate:_____ P wave:_____

PR interval:_____ QRS:_____

Rhythm interpretation:_____

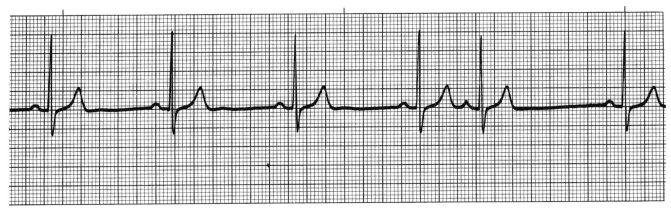

**Strip 7-33.** Rhythm:_____ Rate:_____ P wave:_____

PR interval:_____ QRS:_____

Rhythm interpretation:_____

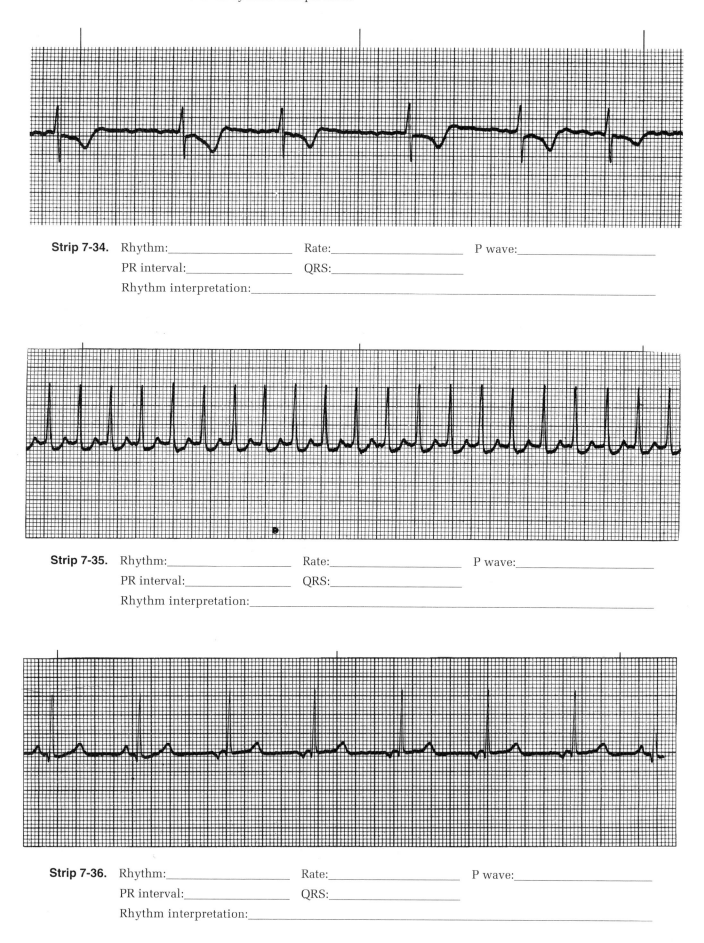

**Strip 7-34.** Rhythm:_____ Rate:_____ P wave:_____

PR interval:_____ QRS:_____

Rhythm interpretation:_____

**Strip 7-35.** Rhythm:_____ Rate:_____ P wave:_____

PR interval:_____ QRS:_____

Rhythm interpretation:_____

**Strip 7-36.** Rhythm:_____ Rate:_____ P wave:_____

PR interval:_____ QRS:_____

Rhythm interpretation:_____

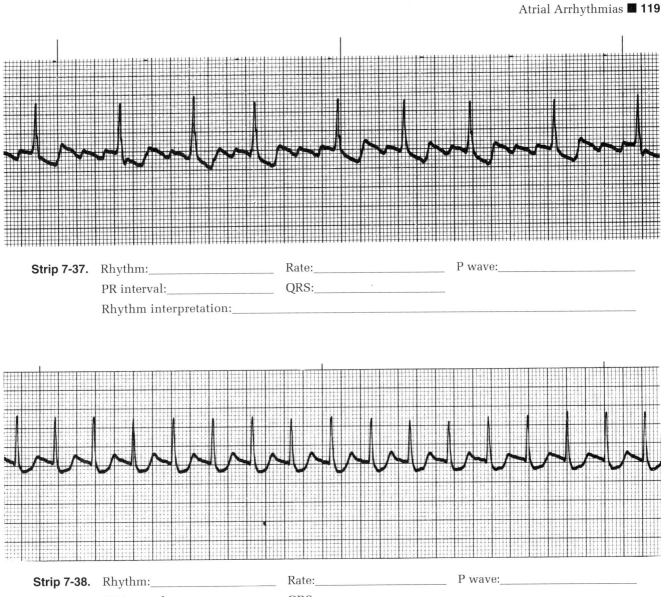

**Strip 7-37.** Rhythm:_____ Rate:_____ P wave:_____

PR interval:_____ QRS:_____

Rhythm interpretation:_____

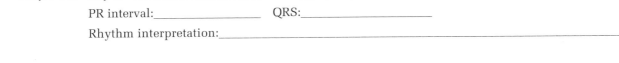

**Strip 7-38.** Rhythm:_____ Rate:_____ P wave:_____

PR interval:_____ QRS:_____

Rhythm interpretation:_____

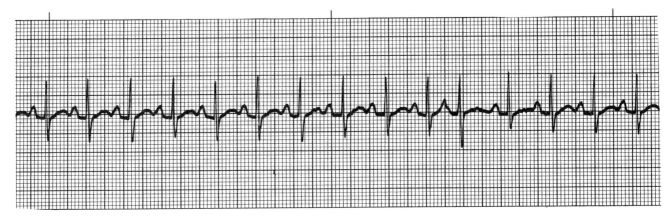

**Strip 7-39.** Rhythm:_____ Rate:_____ P wave:_____

PR interval:_____ QRS:_____

Rhythm interpretation:_____

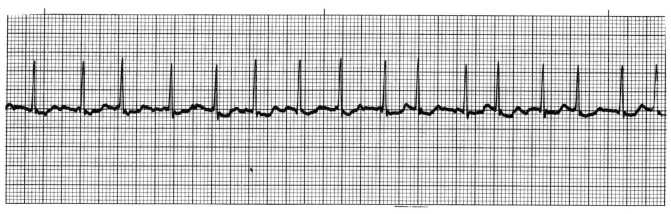

**Strip 7-40.** Rhythm:_____ Rate:_____ P wave:_____

PR interval:_____ QRS:_____

Rhythm interpretation:_____

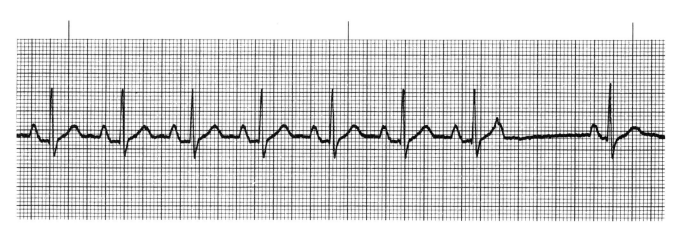

**Strip 7-41.** Rhythm:_____ Rate:_____ P wave:_____

PR interval:_____ QRS:_____

Rhythm interpretation:_____

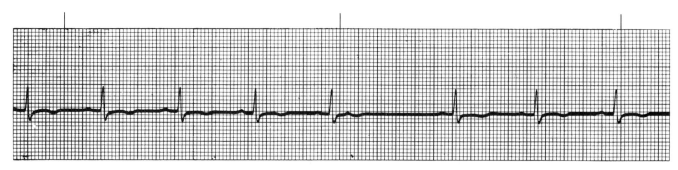

**Strip 7-42.** Rhythm:_____ Rate:_____ P wave:_____

PR interval:_____ QRS:_____

Rhythm interpretion:_____

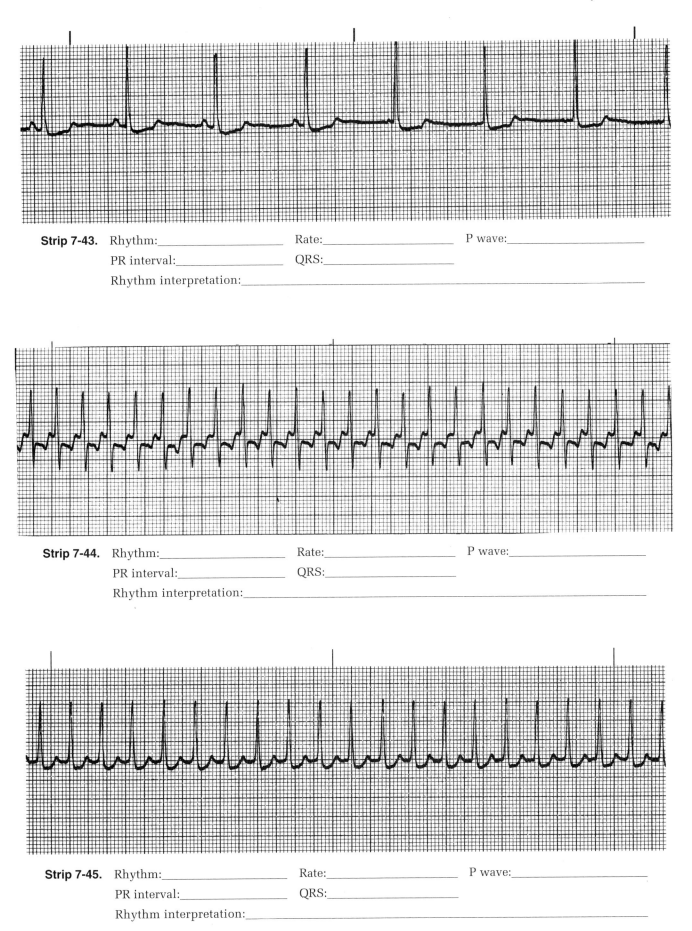

**Strip 7-43.** Rhythm:_____ Rate:_____ P wave:_____

PR interval:_____ QRS:_____

Rhythm interpretation:_____

**Strip 7-44.** Rhythm:_____ Rate:_____ P wave:_____

PR interval:_____ QRS:_____

Rhythm interpretation:_____

**Strip 7-45.** Rhythm:_____ Rate:_____ P wave:_____

PR interval:_____ QRS:_____

Rhythm interpretation:_____

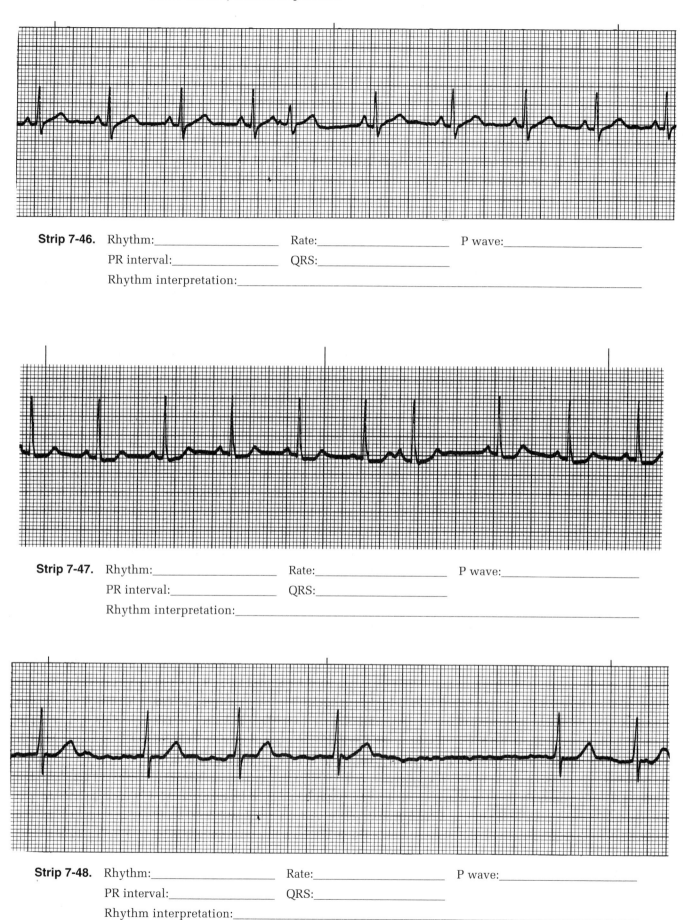

**Strip 7-46.** Rhythm:_____ Rate:_____ P wave:_____

PR interval:_____ QRS:_____

Rhythm interpretation:_____

**Strip 7-47.** Rhythm:_____ Rate:_____ P wave:_____

PR interval:_____ QRS:_____

Rhythm interpretation:_____

**Strip 7-48.** Rhythm:_____ Rate:_____ P wave:_____

PR interval:_____ QRS:_____

Rhythm interpretation:_____

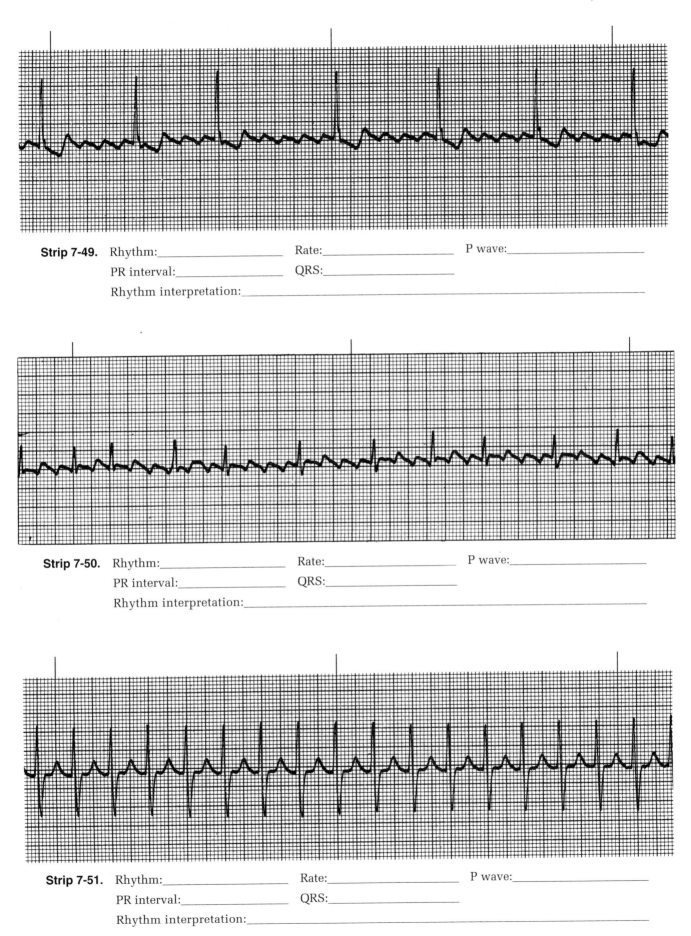

**Strip 7-49.** Rhythm:_____ Rate:_____ P wave:_____

PR interval:_____ QRS:_____

Rhythm interpretation:_____

**Strip 7-50.** Rhythm:_____ Rate:_____ P wave:_____

PR interval:_____ QRS:_____

Rhythm interpretation:_____

**Strip 7-51.** Rhythm:_____ Rate:_____ P wave:_____

PR interval:_____ QRS:_____

Rhythm interpretation:_____

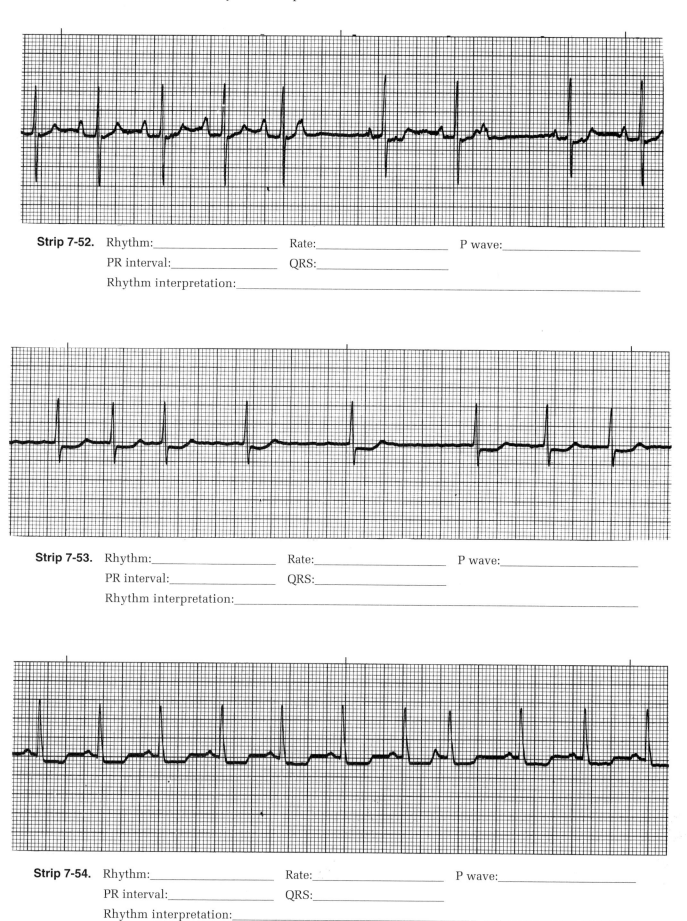

**Strip 7-52.** Rhythm:_____ Rate:_____ P wave:_____

PR interval:_____ QRS:_____

Rhythm interpretation:_____

**Strip 7-53.** Rhythm:_____ Rate:_____ P wave:_____

PR interval:_____ QRS:_____

Rhythm interpretation:_____

**Strip 7-54.** Rhythm:_____ Rate:_____ P wave:_____

PR interval:_____ QRS:_____

Rhythm interpretation:_____

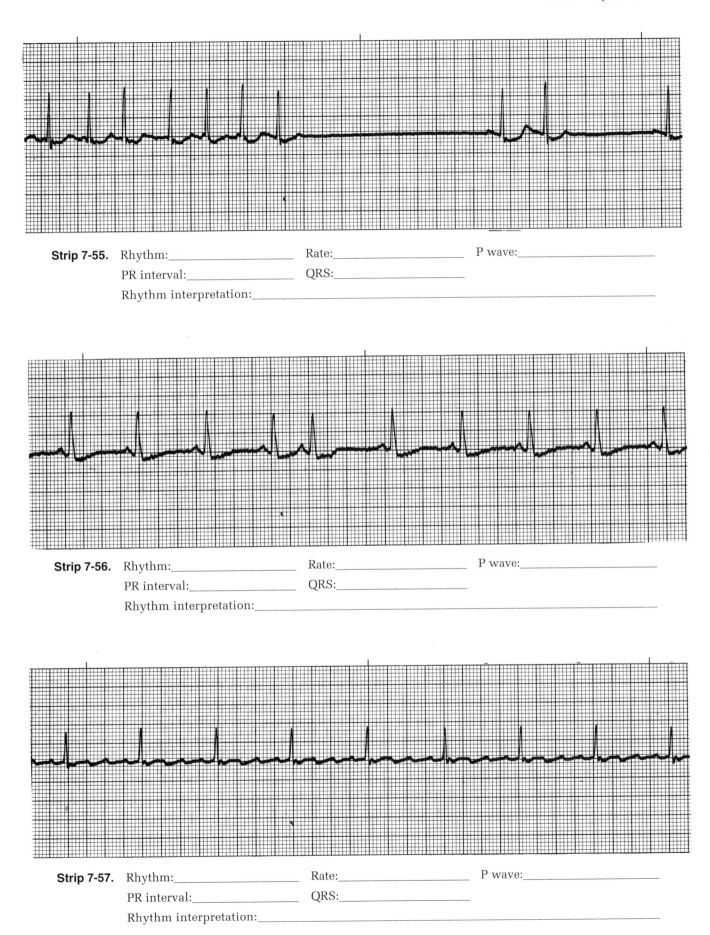

**Strip 7-55.** Rhythm:_____ Rate:_____ P wave:_____

PR interval:_____ QRS:_____

Rhythm interpretation:_____

**Strip 7-56.** Rhythm:_____ Rate:_____ P wave:_____

PR interval:_____ QRS:_____

Rhythm interpretation:_____

**Strip 7-57.** Rhythm:_____ Rate:_____ P wave:_____

PR interval:_____ QRS:_____

Rhythm interpretation:_____

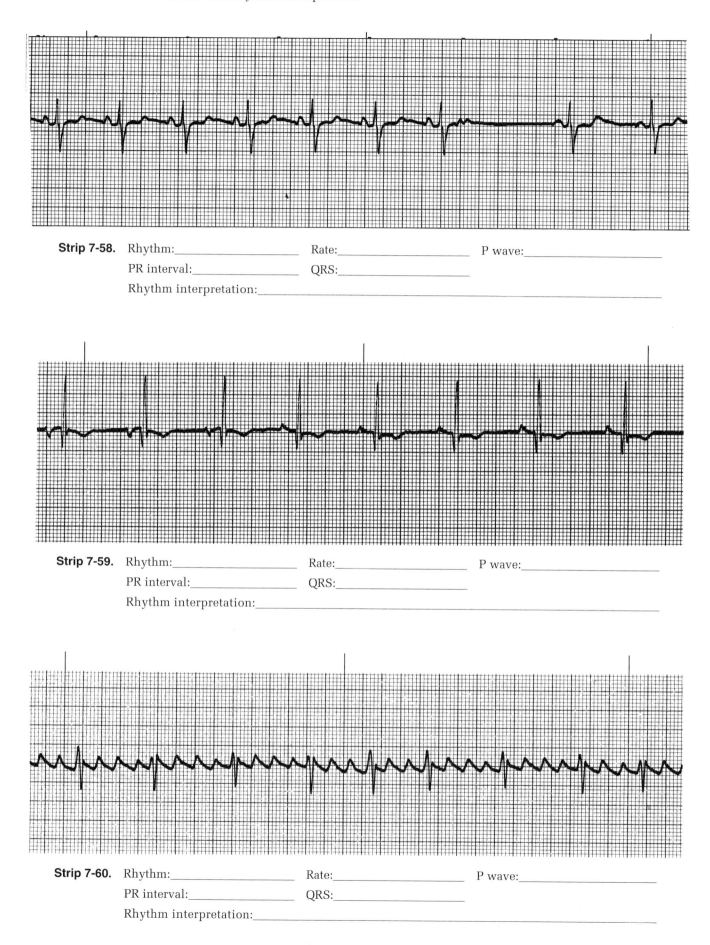

**Strip 7-58.** Rhythm:_____ Rate:_____ P wave:_____

PR interval:_____ QRS:_____

Rhythm interpretation:_____

**Strip 7-59.** Rhythm:_____ Rate:_____ P wave:_____

PR interval:_____ QRS:_____

Rhythm interpretation:_____

**Strip 7-60.** Rhythm:_____ Rate:_____ P wave:_____

PR interval:_____ QRS:_____

Rhythm interpretation:_____

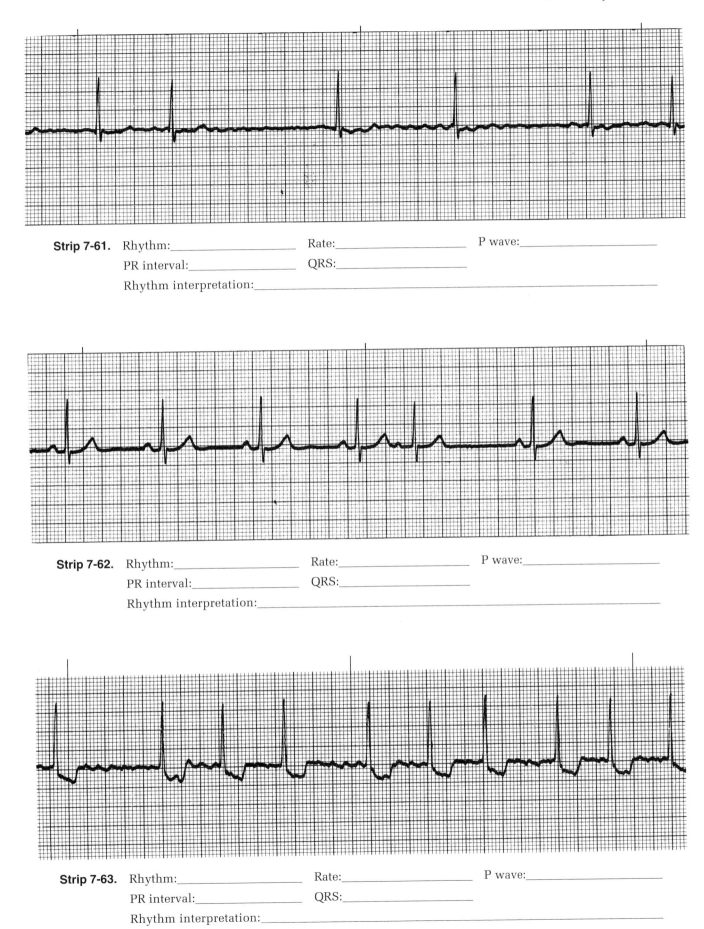

**Strip 7-61.** Rhythm:_____ Rate:_____ P wave:_____

PR interval:_____ QRS:_____

Rhythm interpretation:_____

**Strip 7-62.** Rhythm:_____ Rate:_____ P wave:_____

PR interval:_____ QRS:_____

Rhythm interpretation:_____

**Strip 7-63.** Rhythm:_____ Rate:_____ P wave:_____

PR interval:_____ QRS:_____

Rhythm interpretation:_____

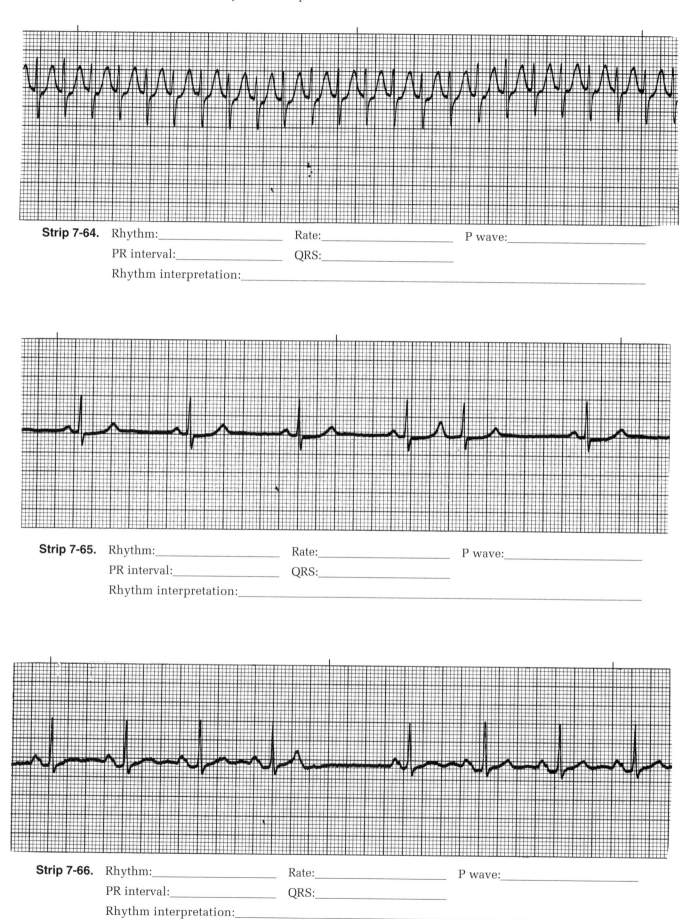

**Strip 7-64.** Rhythm:_____ Rate:_____ P wave:_____

PR interval:_____ QRS:_____

Rhythm interpretation:_____

**Strip 7-65.** Rhythm:_____ Rate:_____ P wave:_____

PR interval:_____ QRS:_____

Rhythm interpretation:_____

**Strip 7-66.** Rhythm:_____ Rate:_____ P wave:_____

PR interval:_____ QRS:_____

Rhythm interpretation:_____

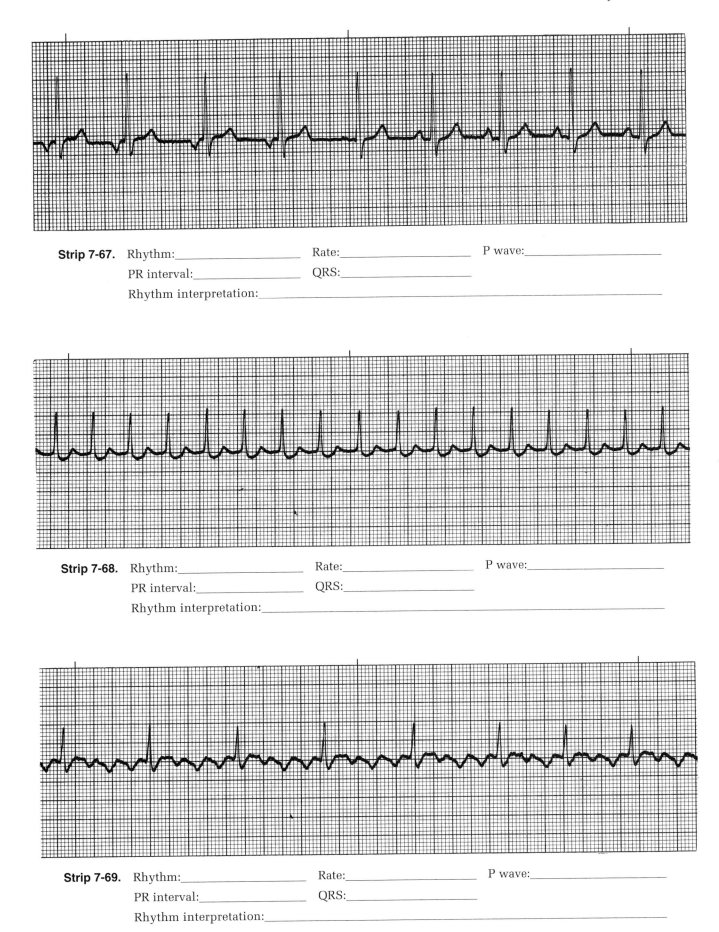

**Strip 7-67.** Rhythm:_____ Rate:_____ P wave:_____

PR interval:_____ QRS:_____

Rhythm interpretation:_____

**Strip 7-68.** Rhythm:_____ Rate:_____ P wave:_____

PR interval:_____ QRS:_____

Rhythm interpretation:_____

**Strip 7-69.** Rhythm:_____ Rate:_____ P wave:_____

PR interval:_____ QRS:_____

Rhythm interpretation:_____

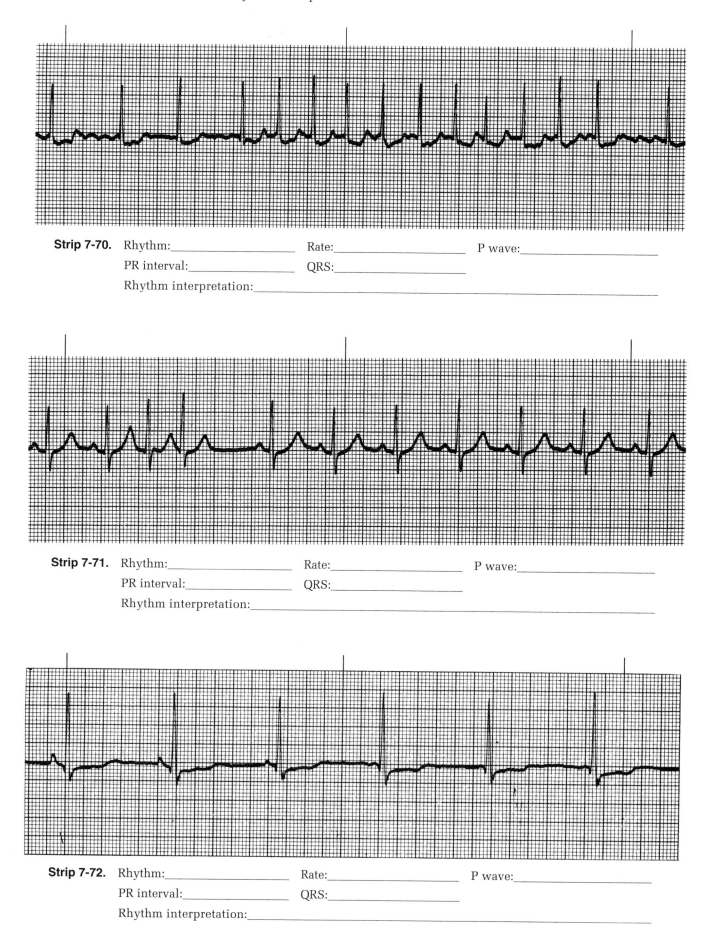

**Strip 7-70.** Rhythm:_____ Rate:_____ P wave:_____

PR interval:_____ QRS:_____

Rhythm interpretation:_____

**Strip 7-71.** Rhythm:_____ Rate:_____ P wave:_____

PR interval:_____ QRS:_____

Rhythm interpretation:_____

**Strip 7-72.** Rhythm:_____ Rate:_____ P wave:_____

PR interval:_____ QRS:_____

Rhythm interpretation:_____

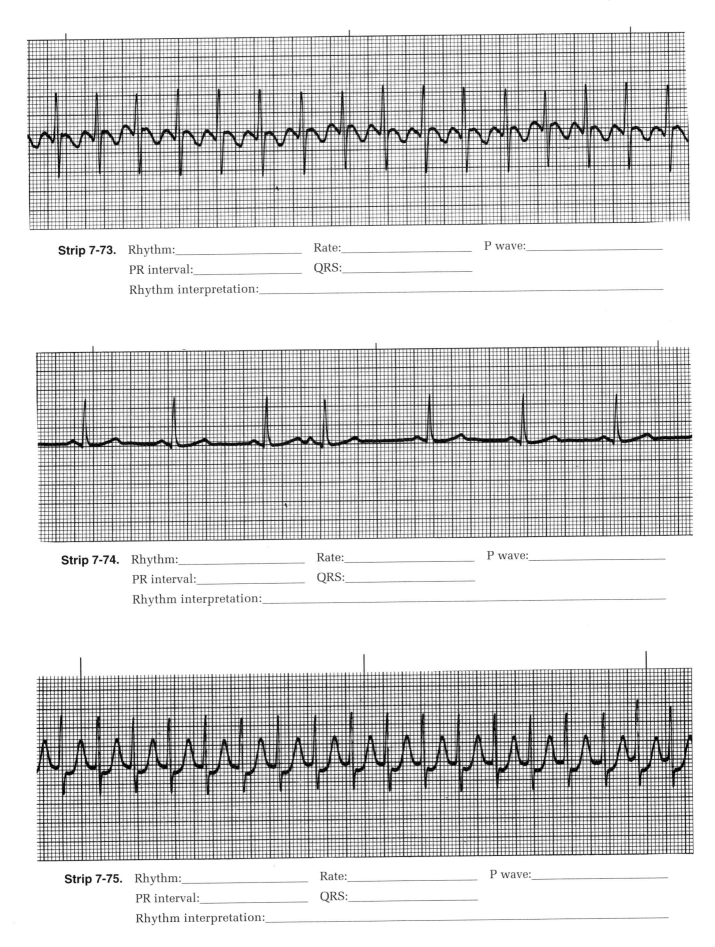

**Strip 7-73.**  Rhythm:_____  Rate:_____  P wave:_____

PR interval:_____  QRS:_____

Rhythm interpretation:_____

**Strip 7-74.**  Rhythm:_____  Rate:_____  P wave:_____

PR interval:_____  QRS:_____

Rhythm interpretation:_____

**Strip 7-75.**  Rhythm:_____  Rate:_____  P wave:_____

PR interval:_____  QRS:_____

Rhythm interpretation:_____

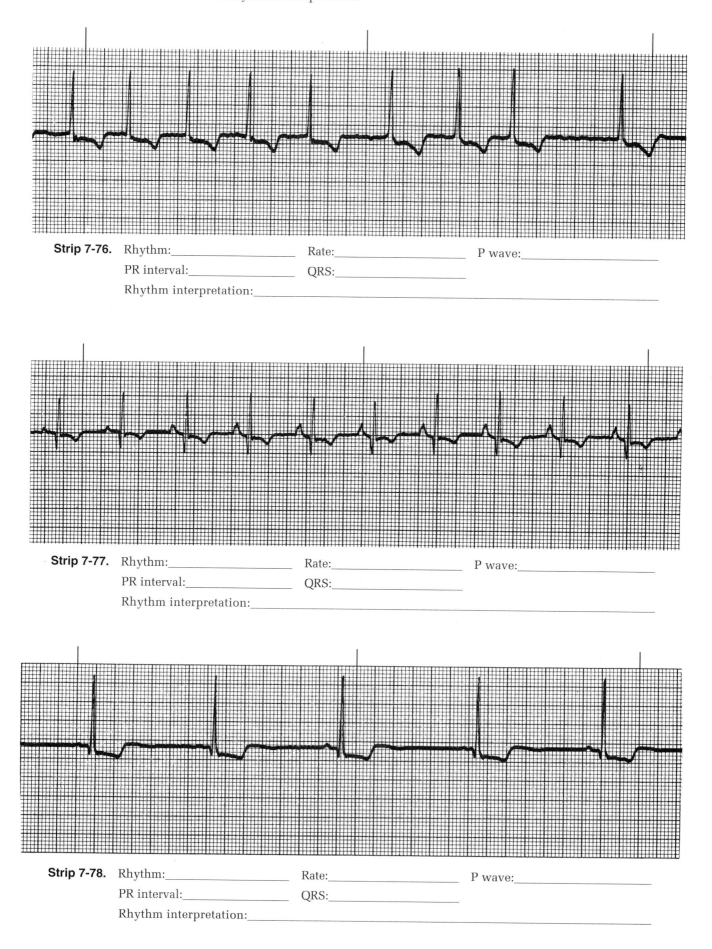

**Strip 7-76.** Rhythm:_____ Rate:_____ P wave:_____

PR interval:_____ QRS:_____

Rhythm interpretation:_____

**Strip 7-77.** Rhythm:_____ Rate:_____ P wave:_____

PR interval:_____ QRS:_____

Rhythm interpretation:_____

**Strip 7-78.** Rhythm:_____ Rate:_____ P wave:_____

PR interval:_____ QRS:_____

Rhythm interpretation:_____

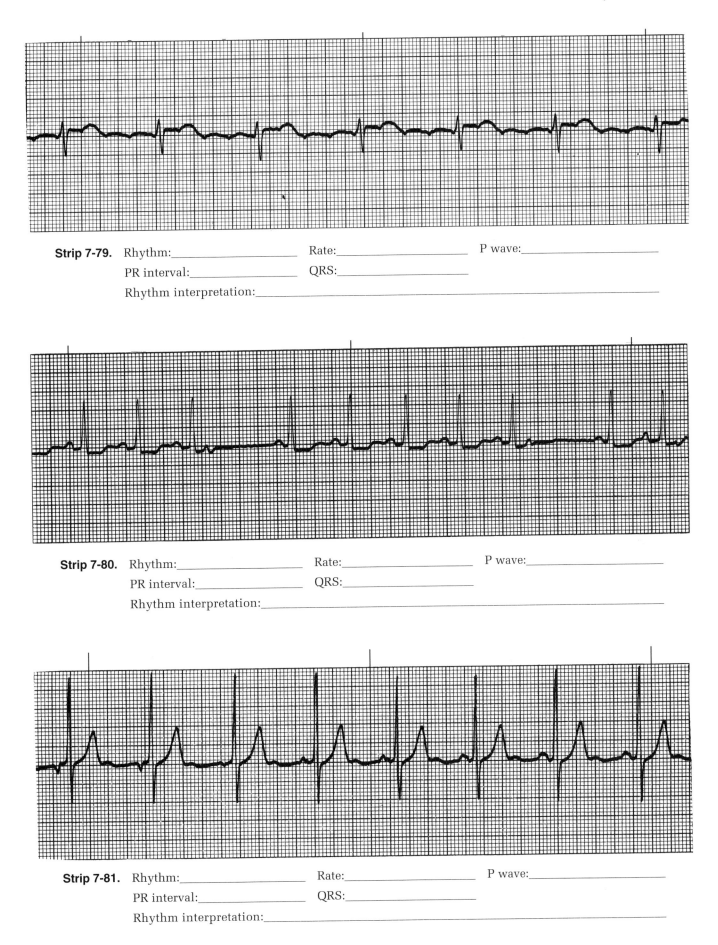

**Strip 7-79.** Rhythm:_____ Rate:_____ P wave:_____

PR interval:_____ QRS:_____

Rhythm interpretation:_____

**Strip 7-80.** Rhythm:_____ Rate:_____ P wave:_____

PR interval:_____ QRS:_____

Rhythm interpretation:_____

**Strip 7-81.** Rhythm:_____ Rate:_____ P wave:_____

PR interval:_____ QRS:_____

Rhythm interpretation:_____

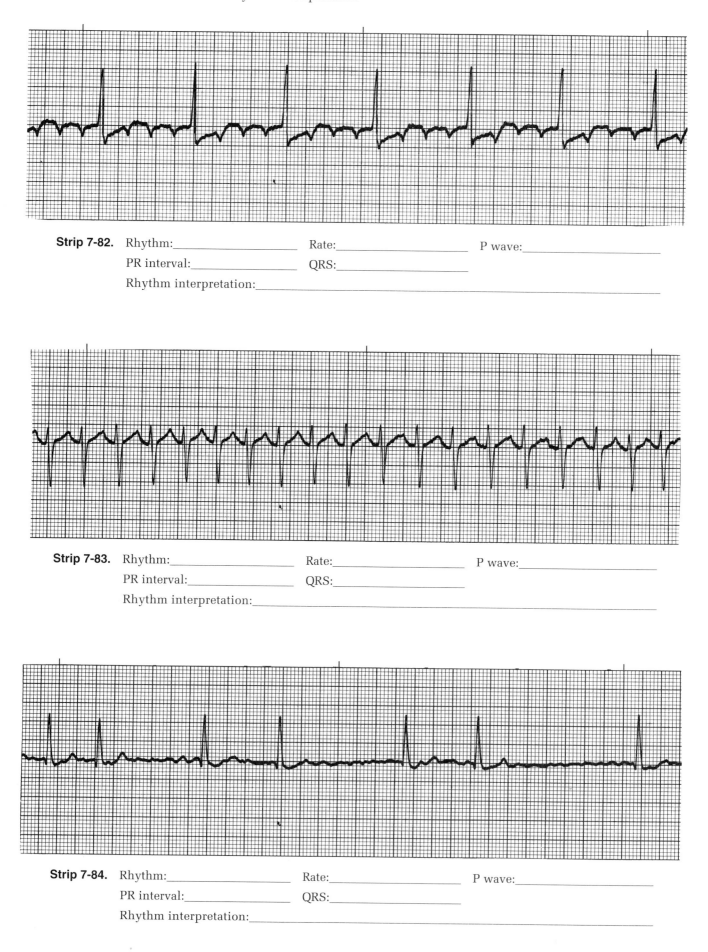

**Strip 7-82.** Rhythm:_____ Rate:_____ P wave:_____

PR interval:_____ QRS:_____

Rhythm interpretation:_____

**Strip 7-83.** Rhythm:_____ Rate:_____ P wave:_____

PR interval:_____ QRS:_____

Rhythm interpretation:_____

**Strip 7-84.** Rhythm:_____ Rate:_____ P wave:_____

PR interval:_____ QRS:_____

Rhythm interpretation:_____

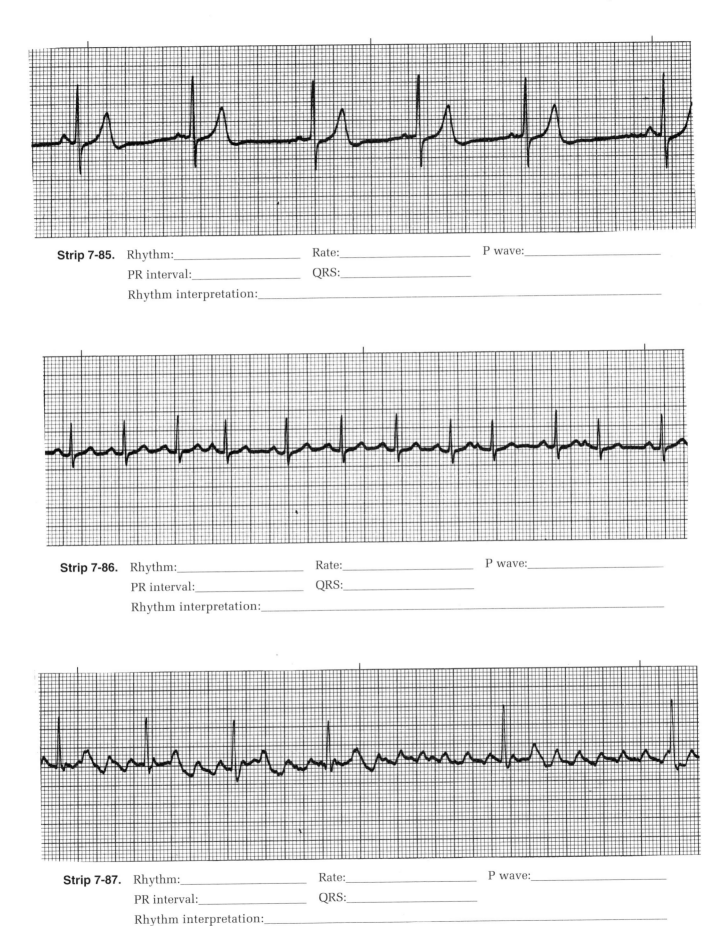

**Strip 7-85.** Rhythm:_____ Rate:_____ P wave:_____

PR interval:_____ QRS:_____

Rhythm interpretation:_____

**Strip 7-86.** Rhythm:_____ Rate:_____ P wave:_____

PR interval:_____ QRS:_____

Rhythm interpretation:_____

**Strip 7-87.** Rhythm:_____ Rate:_____ P wave:_____

PR interval:_____ QRS:_____

Rhythm interpretation:_____

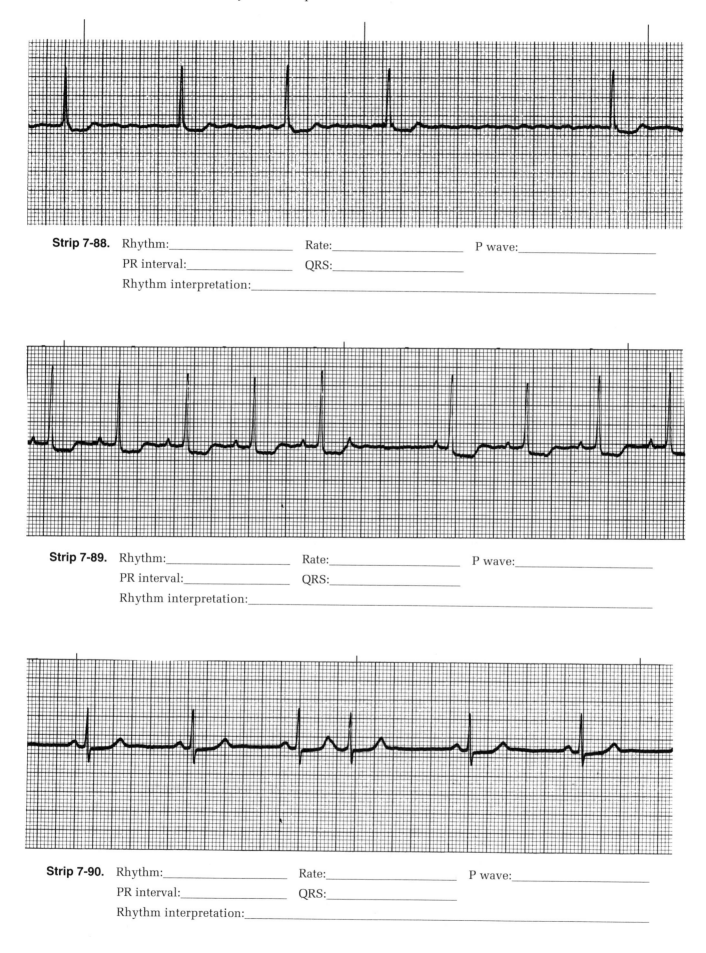

**Strip 7-88.** Rhythm:_____ Rate:_____ P wave:_____

PR interval:_____ QRS:_____

Rhythm interpretation:_____

**Strip 7-89.** Rhythm:_____ Rate:_____ P wave:_____

PR interval:_____ QRS:_____

Rhythm interpretation:_____

**Strip 7-90.** Rhythm:_____ Rate:_____ P wave:_____

PR interval:_____ QRS:_____

Rhythm interpretation:_____

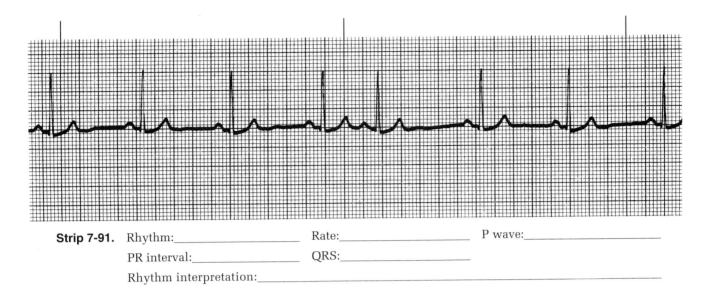

**Strip 7-91.** Rhythm:_____ Rate:_____ P wave:_____

PR interval:_____ QRS:_____

Rhythm interpretation:_____

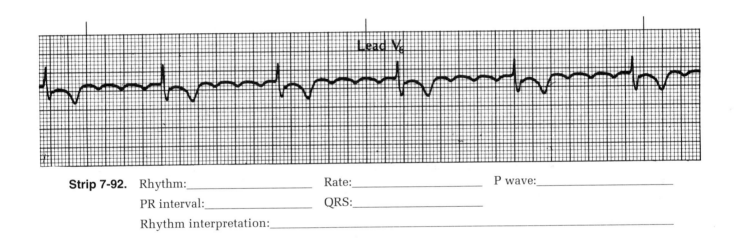

**Strip 7-92.** Rhythm:_____ Rate:_____ P wave:_____

PR interval:_____ QRS:_____

Rhythm interpretation:_____

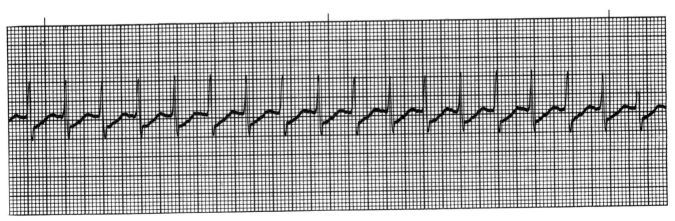

**Strip 7-93.** Rhythm:_____ Rate:_____ P wave:_____

PR interval:_____ QRS:_____

Rhythm interpretation:_____

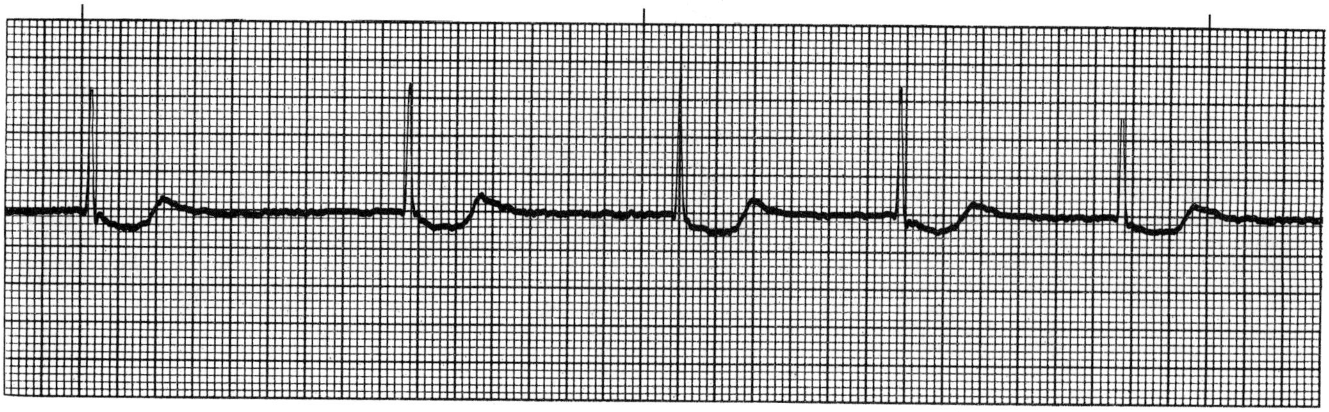

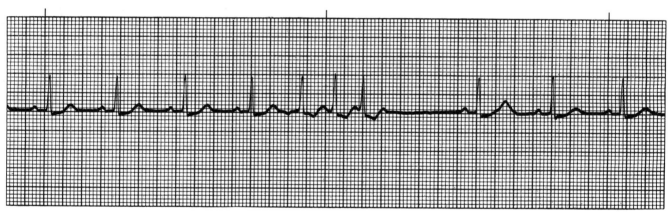

**Strip 7-94.** Rhythm:_____ Rate:_____ P wave:_____

PR interval:_____ QRS:_____

Rhythm interpretation:_____

**Strip 7-95.** Rhythm:_____ Rate:_____ P wave:_____

PR interval:_____ QRS:_____

Rhythm interpretation:_____

# 8

# AV JUNCTIONAL ARRHYTHMIAS AND AV BLOCKS

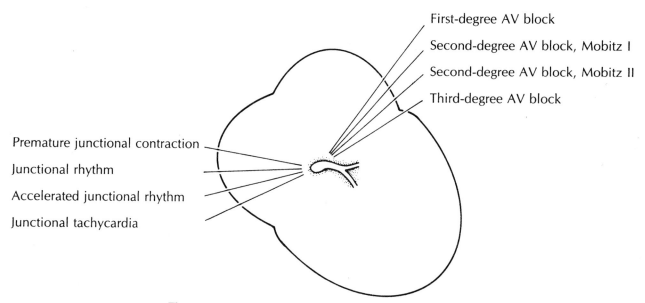

**Figure 8-1.** AV junctional arrhythmias and AV blocks.

AV junctional arrhythmias (Figure 8-1) originate from the area in and around the AV node. The AV node contains specialized pacemaker cells and can serve as a secondary pacemaker site if the SA node fails to function properly as the primary pacemaker. The inherent firing rate of the junctional pacemaker cells is 40 to 60 per minute. A rhythm occurring at this rate is called a *junctional rhythm.* On some occasions, enhanced automaticity of the junctional pacemaker cells may accelerate the rate beyond its inherent firing rate. Three arrhythmias may result from this increased activity: premature junctional contractions, accelerated junctional rhythm, and junctional tachycardia.

When the AV node is functioning as the pacemaker of the heart, the electrical impulse leaves the AV junction and is conducted backward (retrograde) to depolarize the atria, and forward (antegrade) to depolarize the ventricles. The location of the P wave relative to the QRS depends on the speed of antegrade and retrograde conduction:

**1.** If the electrical impulse from the AV junction depolarizes the atria first and then depolarizes the ventricles, the P wave will be in front of the QRS complex.

**2.** If the electrical impulse from the AV junction depolarizes the ventricles first and then depolarizes the atria, the P wave will be after the QRS complex.

**3.** If the electrical impulse from the AV junction depolarizes both the atria and the ventricles simultaneously, the P wave will be hidden in the QRS complex.

Retrograde stimulation of the atria is just opposite the direction of atrial depolarization when normal sinus rhythm is present, and will produce negative P waves (instead of upright) in Lead II. The PR interval will be short (0.10 seconds or less). The ventricles will be depolarized normally, resulting in a narrow QRS. Identifying features of AV junctional rhythms are shown in Figure 8-2.

**Figure 8-2.** Identifying features of junctional rhythms.
1. P waves inverted in Lead II
2. P waves will occur in one of three patterns:
   a. immediately before the QRS
   b. immediately after the QRS
   c. hidden within the QRS complex
3. PR interval will be short (0.10 seconds or less)
4. QRS will be normal (0.10 seconds or less)

Lead II      Lead II      Lead II

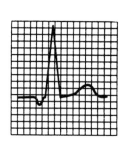
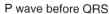
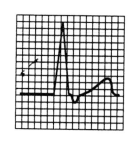
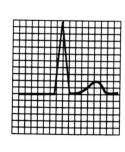

P wave before QRS      P wave after QRS      P wave hidden in QRS

Lead II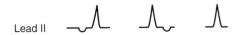

**Figure 8-3.** Premature junctional contractions will appear as a single beat in any of the above three patterns.

# PREMATURE JUNCTIONAL CONTRACTIONS (PJC)

A premature junctional contraction (PJC) (Figures 8-3 through 8-7; Box 8-1) is an early beat that originates in an ectopic pacemaker site in the AV junction and is usually caused by enhanced automaticity of the junctional tissue. Like the PAC, the premature junctional beat is characterized by an abnormal P wave, a QRS complex that is identical or very similar to the QRS complex of the normally conducted beats, and is followed by a pause that is usually noncompensatory. Some differences do exist, however. Because atrial depolarization occurs in a retrograde fashion with the PJC, the P wave associated with the premature beat will be negative (inverted) in Lead II and will occur immediately before the QRS, immediately after the QRS, or will be hidden within the QRS complex. The PR interval will be short (0.10 seconds or less). Inverted P waves in Lead II may also occur with PACs arising from the lower atria, but the associated PR interval will not be short. If difficulty is encountered in differentiating PJCs from PACs, keep the following in mind—PACs are much more common than PJCs. As a result, narrow complex premature beats should probably not be interpreted as PJCs unless P waves are definitely absent or the P wave is inverted in Lead II with a short PR interval.

**Box 8-1. Premature Junctional Contraction: Identifying ECG Features**

| | |
|---|---|
| Rhythm: | Underlying rhythm usually regular; irregular with PJC |
| Rate: | Rate is that of underlying rhythm |
| P waves: | P wave associated with the PJC will be inverted in Lead II and will occur immediately before the QRS, immediately after the QRS, or will be hidden within the QRS complex |
| PR: | Short (0.10 seconds or less) |
| QRS: | Normal (0.10 seconds or less) |

PJCs occur in addition to the underlying rhythm. They occur in the same patterns as PACs: as a single beat; in pairs (Figure 8-7); in bigeminal, trigeminal, or quadrigeminal patterns. A series of three or more consecutive junctional beats is considered a rhythm (ie, junctional rhythm, accelerated junctional rhythm, or junctional tachycardia). Differentiation of the rhythm will depend on the heart rate.

Causes of premature junctional contractions include excessive vagal tone, emotional stress, ingestion of caffeine or alcohol, heart failure, myocardial ischemia, pericarditis, valvular heart disease, coronary artery disease, chronic lung disease, hyperthyroidism, hypokalemia, and digitalis toxicity. PJCs may also occur without apparent cause.

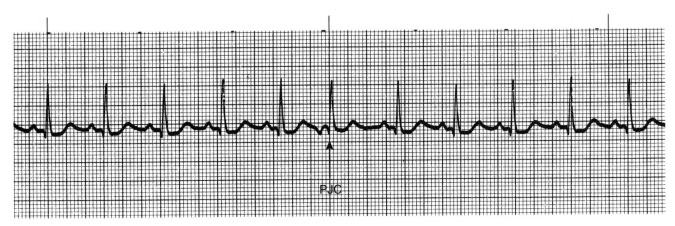

**Figure 8-4.** **Normal Sinus Rhythm with One PJC**

| | |
|---|---|
| *Rhythm:* | Basic rhythm regular; irregular with PJC |
| *Rate:* | Basic rhythm rate 94 |
| *P waves:* | Sinus P waves with basic rhythm; inverted P wave with PJC |
| *PR:* | 0.14 to 0.16 seconds (basic rhythm) 0.08 seconds (PJC) |
| *QRS:* | 0.08 seconds |
| *Comment:* | ST segment depression is present. |

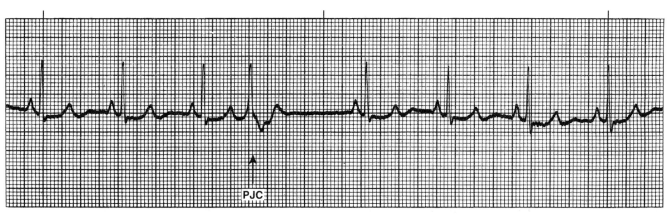

**Figure 8-5.** **Normal Sinus Rhythm with One PJC**

*Rhythm:* Basic rhythm regular; irregular with PJC

*Rate:* Basic rhythm rate 72

*P waves:* Sinus P waves with basic rhythm; inverted P wave after PJC (4th QRS complex)

*PR interval:* 0.14–0.16 seconds (basic rhythm); 0.06–0.08 seconds PJC

*QRS:* 0.06–0.08 seconds (basic rhythm); 0.08 seconds PJC

*Comment:* A U wave is present.

Isolated PJCs are not treated. If PJCs increase in frequency, the best approach is to eliminate the cause, if possible. Frequent PJCs may warn of or initiate more serious junctional arrhythmias.

Occasionally, an ectopic junctional beat will occur late instead of early. These are called *junctional escape beats* (Figure 8-8). Escape beats are more likely to occur as a result of increased vagal effect on the SA node rather than to enhanced automaticity, as is associated with the premature beat. Junctional escape beats are common after a pause in the underlying rhythm (eg, sinus arrest or block, nonconducted PACs, type I second-degree AV block). The morphologic characteristics of the late beat are the same as

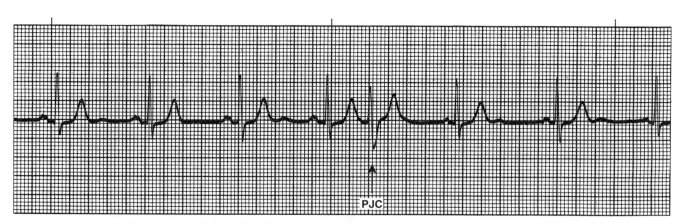

**Figure 8-6.** **Normal Sinus Rhythm with One PJC**

*Rhythm:* Basic rhythm regular; irregular with PJC

*Rate:* Basic rhythm rate 63; rate slows to 56 following PJC due to rate suppression (common following a pause in the basic rhythm).

*P waves:* Sinus P waves with basic rhythm; P wave associated with PJC is hidden in the QRS complex

*PR interval:* 0.16–0.18 seconds (basic rhythm)

*QRS:* 0.06–0.08 seconds (basic rhythm); 0.10 seconds PJC

*Comment:* A U wave is present.

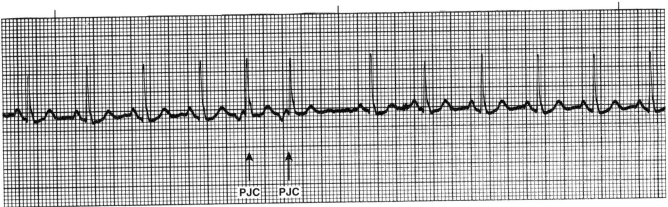

**Figure 8-7.** **Normal Sinus Rhythm with Paired PJCs**

*Rhythm:*    Basic rhythm regular; irregular following paired PJCs

*Rate:*    Basic rhythm rate 100

*P waves:*    Sinus P waves with basic rhythm; inverted P waves with PJCs

*PR interval:* 0.12–0.14 seconds basic rhythm; 0.008 seconds with PJCs

*QRS:*    0.06–0.08 seconds (basic rhythm and PJCs)

the PJC. Escape beats require no treatment. It is important, however, to identify the cause of the initiating pause so appropriate intervention can be started, if necessary.

## JUNCTIONAL RHYTHM

Junctional rhythm (Figures 8-9 through 8-12; Box 8-2) is an arrhythmia originating in the AV junction with a rate between 40 and 60 beats per minute. This rhythm is often referred to as *junctional escape rhythm* because it usually only appears secondary to depression of the higher pacing center of the heart, the SA node. Junctional rhythm is the normal response of the AV junction when the rate of the dominant pacemaker (usually the SA node) becomes less than the rate of the AV node or when the electrical impulses from the SA node fail to reach the AV node as in sinus arrest, sinus block, or third-degree AV block. When an electrical

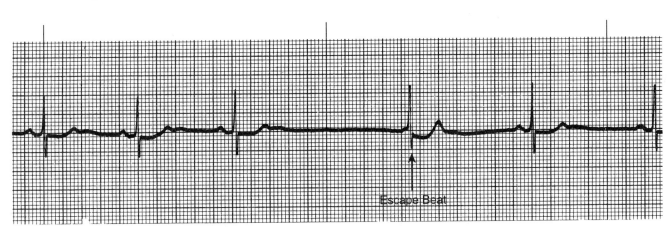

**Figure 8-8.** **Normal Sinus Rhythm with Sinus Arrest and Junctional Escape Beat**

*Rhythm:*    Basic rhythm regular; irregular with escape beat

*Rate:*    Basic rhythm 60; rate slows to 45 after escape beat. Rate suppression can occur following any pause in the basic rhythm. After several cycles the rate will return to the basic rate.

*P waves:*    Sinus P waves with basic rhythm; hidden P wave with escape beat

*PR:*    0.16 seconds

*QRS:*    0.06 seconds

*Comment:*    ST segment depression and a U wave are present.

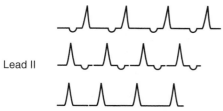

Lead II

**Figure 8-9.** Junctional rhythm will appear as a continuous rhythm at a rate of 40–60 beats per minute in either of the above three patterns.

impulse fails to reach the AV junction within 1 to 1½ seconds, the escape pacemaker in the AV junction begins to generate electrical impulses at its inherent firing rate of 40 to 60 per minute. The result could be a junctional escape beat or junctional escape rhythm.

---

**Box 8-2. Junctional Rhythm: Identifying ECG Features**

| | |
|---|---|
| Rhythm: | Regular |
| Rate: | 40–60 |
| P waves: | Inverted in Lead II and occurs immediately before the QRS, immediately after the QRS, or is hidden within the QRS complex |
| PR: | Short (0.10 seconds or less) |
| QRS: | Normal (0.10 seconds or less) |

---

Retrograde stimulation of the atria by the AV node impulse produces a rhythm with the following characteristics:

**1.** Negative P waves in Lead II that occur immediately before the QRS, immediately after the QRS, or are hidden within the QRS

**2.** A short PR interval of 0.10 seconds or less

**3.** A QRS complex that is identical or very similar to the normally conducted beats

Junctional rhythm is a continuous rhythm, usually transient in nature, with the same ECG characteristics as accelerated junctional rhythm and junctional tachycardia. This rhythm is differentiated from the other junctional rhythms by the heart rate (40 to 60).

Junctional rhythm can be seen in a number of clinical settings. It may be caused by drug effects (digitalis, beta blockers, calcium channel blockers), damage to the AV node secondary to acute inferior wall myocardial infarction (MI), electrolyte disturbances, heart failure, valvular heart disease, cardiomyopathy, and myocarditis.

The slow rate and loss of normal atrial depolarization (atrial kick) associated with junctional rhythm may cause a decrease in cardiac output. Treatment for symptomatic junctional rhythm includes increasing the heart rate (atropine, transcutaneous pacing, or transvenous pacing) and reversing the consequences of reduced cardiac output. Treatment should also be directed at identifying and correcting the underlying cause of the rhythm, if possible. All medications should be reviewed and discontinued, if indicated.

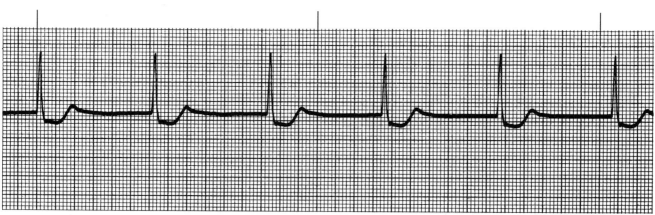

**Figure 8-10.  Junctional Rhythm**

| | |
|---|---|
| *Rhythm:* | Regular |
| *Rate:* | 50 |
| *P waves:* | Hidden in QRS complexes |
| *PR:* | Not measurable |
| *QRS:* | 0.06 to 0.08 seconds |
| *Comment:* | ST segment depression is present. |

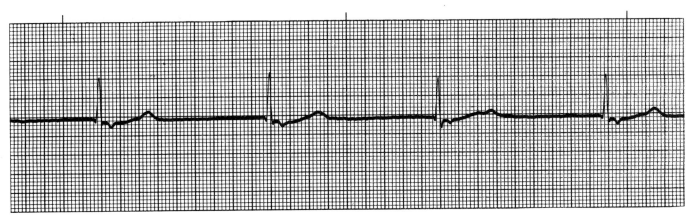

**Figure 8-11.  Junctional Rhythm**

| | |
|---|---|
| *Rhythm:* | Regular |
| *Rate:* | 33 |
| *P waves:* | Inverted after QRS |
| *PR:* | 0.08–0.10 seconds |
| *QRS:* | 0.08 to 0.10 seconds |

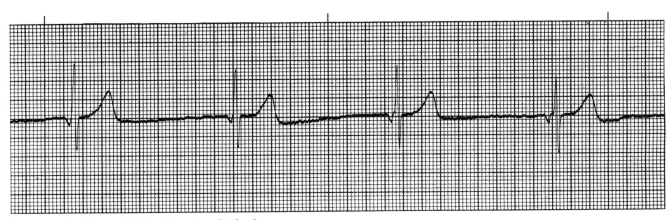

**Figure 8-12.  Junctional Rhythm**

| | |
|---|---|
| *Rhythm:* | Regular |
| *Rate:* | 35 |
| *P waves:* | Inverted before the QRS |
| *PR:* | 0.06–0.08 seconds |
| *QRS:* | 0.06 to 0.08 seconds |

## ACCELERATED JUNCTIONAL RHYTHM

Accelerated junctional rhythm (Figures 8-13 through 8-15; Box 8-3) is an arrhythmia originating in the AV junction with a rate between 60 and 100. The term *accelerated* denotes a rhythm that occurs at a rate that exceeds the inherent junctional escape rate of 40 to 60 but is not fast enough to be junctional tachycardia. This rhythm is usually caused by enhanced automaticity of the AV junctional tissue.

**Box 8-3.  Accelerated Junctional Rhythm: Identifying ECG Features**

| | |
|---|---|
| Rhythm: | Regular |
| Rate: | 60–100 |
| P waves: | Inverted in Lead II and occurs immediately before the QRS, immediately after the QRS, or is hidden within the QRS complex |
| PR: | Short (0.10 seconds or less) |
| QRS: | Normal (0.10 seconds or less) |

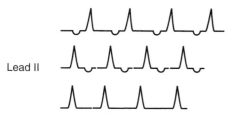

**Figure 8-13.** Accelerated junctional rhythm will appear as a continuous rhythm at a rate of 60–100 beats per minute in any of the above three patterns.

Retrograde stimulation of the atria by the AV node impulse produces a rhythm with the following characteristics:

**1.** Negative P waves in Lead II that occur immediately before the QRS, immediately after the QRS, or are hidden within the QRS complex

**2.** A short PR interval of 0.10 seconds or less

**3.** A QRS complex that is identical or very similar to the normally conducted beats

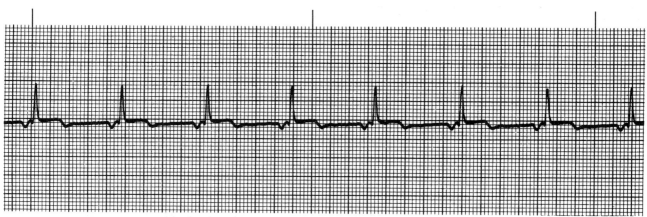

**Figure 8-14.** Accelerated Junctional Rhythm

| | |
|---|---|
| *Rhythm:* | Regular |
| *Rate:* | 65 |
| *P waves:* | Inverted before each QRS |
| *PR:* | 0.08 to 0.10 seconds |
| *QRS:* | 0.08 seconds |
| *Comment:* | ST segment elevation and T wave inversion are present. |

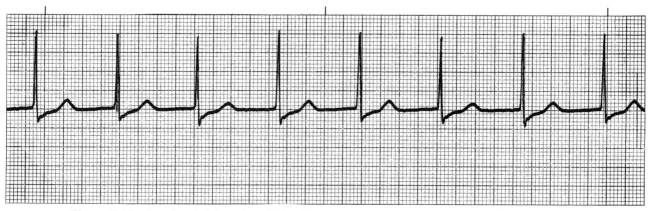

**Figure 8-15.** Accelerated Junctional Rhythm

| | |
|---|---|
| *Rhythm:* | Regular |
| *Rate:* | 68 |
| *P waves:* | Hidden in QRS complex |
| *PR:* | Not measurable |
| *QRS:* | 0.06–0.08 seconds |

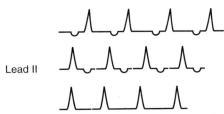

Lead II

**Figure 8-16.** Paroxysmal junctional tachycardia will appear as a continuous rhythm at a rate exceeding 100 per minute in any of the above three patterns.

Accelerated junctional rhythm is a continuous rhythm, usually transient in nature, with the same ECG characteristics as junctional rhythm and junctional tachycardia. This rhythm is differentiated from the other junctional rhythms by the heart rate (60 to 100).

Accelerated junctional rhythm is commonly a result of digitalis toxicity. Other causes include damage to the AV node secondary to acute inferior wall MI, heart failure, acute rheumatic fever, valvular heart disease, and myocarditis. It may also occur after cardiac surgery.

As a rule, the heart rate associated with accelerated junctional rhythm is not a problem because it corresponds to that of the sinus node (60 to 100). Problems are more likely to occur as a result of the loss of normal atrial depolarization (atrial kick) resulting in a decrease in cardiac output. Treatment is directed at reversing the consequences of reduced cardiac output as well as identifying and correcting the underlying cause of the rhythm. All medications should be reviewed and discontinued, if indicated.

# PAROXYSMAL JUNCTIONAL TACHYCARDIA (PJT)

Paroxysmal junctional tachycardia (Figures 8-16 and 8-17; Box 8-4) is an arrhythmia originating in the AV junction with a heart rate that exceeds 100 beats per minute. The mechanism responsible for this rhythm is believed to be enhanced automaticity of the junctional tissue or conduction of the ectopic impulse through a reentry circuit involving the AV node. Like PAT, junctional tachycardia is regular and commonly starts and ends abruptly in a paroxysmal manner.

| Box 8-4. Paroxysmal Junctional Tachycardia: Identifying ECG Features | |
| --- | --- |
| Rhythm: | Regular |
| Rate: | Over 100 per minute |
| P waves: | Inverted in Lead II and occurs immediately before the QRS, immediately after the QRS, or is hidden within the QRS complex |
| PR: | Short (0.10 seconds or less) |
| QRS: | Normal (0.10 seconds or less) |

Retrograde stimulation of the atria by the AV node impulse produces a rhythm with the following characteristics:

**1.** Negative P waves in Lead II that occur immediately before the QRS, immediately after the QRS, or are hidden within the QRS complex

**2.** A short PR interval of 0.10 seconds or less

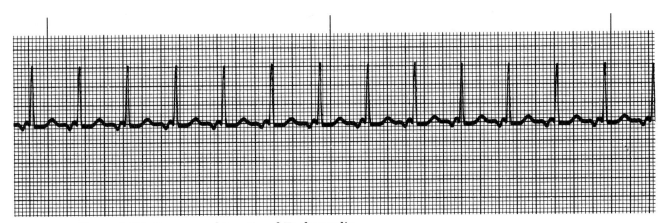

**Figure 8-17. Paroxysmal Junctional Tachycardia**

| | |
| --- | --- |
| *Rhythm:* | Regular |
| *Rate:* | 115 |
| *P waves:* | Inverted before each QRS |
| *PR:* | 0.08 seconds |
| *QRS:* | 0.06 to 0.08 seconds |

**3.** A QRS complex that is identical or very similar to the normally conducted beats

Junctional tachycardia has the same ECG characteristics as junctional rhythm and accelerated junctional rhythm. This rhythm is differentiated from the other junctional rhythms by the heart rate (greater than 100 per minute).

It may be difficult at times to distinguish PJT from PAT electrocardiographically. The P waves are often hidden in both these rhythms—in PAT, the P wave is hidden in the preceding T wave, and, in PJT, the P wave may be hidden in the QRS complex. If a differentiation cannot be made between the two, the term *paroxysmal supraventricular tachycardia* (PSVT) may be used. This term implies that the tachycardia is paroxysmal in nature (either PAT or PJT) and has a supraventricular origin (above the bifurcation of the bundle of His) with a narrow QRS complex. The term *PSVT* should not be confused with the general term *supraventricular,* which refers to any rhythm above the bifurcation of the bundle of His. In adults, true junctional tachycardia is rare. PAT is much more common than PJT. Therefore, if the tachycardia is supraventricular and paroxysmal in nature, the rhythm is most likely PAT.

Junctional tachycardia is usually a manifestation of digitalis toxicity or exogenous catecholamines or theophylline, best treated by the reduction or removal of such medications. It may also be precipitated by an increase in sympathetic tone, overexertion, ingestion of stimulants (coffee, alcohol, and tobacco), electrolyte or acid–base abnormalities, hyperventilation, or emotional stress.

Junctional tachycardia may lead to a decrease in cardiac output owing to the faster rate as well as the loss of normal atrial depolarization (atrial kick). Treatment involves identifying and correcting the underlying cause of the rhythm, and reversing the consequences of reduced cardiac output, if present. Treatment of PJT is managed in a similar manner as PAT. If the patient is hemodynamically stable, try vagal maneuvers first. If vagal maneuvers fail, administer adenosine IV per protocols. Additional treatment options include beta blockers and calcium channel blockers for patients with normal left ventricular function and amiodarone for patients with impaired LV function. Electrical cardioversion is the initial treatment of choice for patients who are hemodynamically unstable.

## AV HEART BLOCKS

The term *heart block* is used to describe arrhythmias in which there is delayed or failed conduction of supraventricular impulses through the AV node into the ventricles. This conduction disturbance may be transient or permanent. The site of pathology is at the level of the AV node or just below the AV node in the bundle of His or in the bundle branches.

AV heart blocks are classified into first-degree, second-degree (type I and type II), and third-degree. The classification system is based on the site of the block and the severity of the conduction disturbance. In first-degree AV block (the mildest form), the electrical impulses are delayed in the AV node longer than normal, but all impulse are conducted to the ventricles. In second-degree AV block, some impulses are conducted to the ventricles and some are blocked. The most extreme form of heart block is third-degree AV block, in which no impulses are conducted from the atria to the ventricles.

The ability to accurately diagnose AV blocks depends on the use of a systematic approach. The following steps are suggested:

**1.** Assess regularity of the rhythm (both atrial and ventricular).

**2.** Identify the P wave or P waves if more than one.

**3.** Assess QRS width (narrow or wide?).

**4.** Assess relationship of the P waves to the QRS complexes. (Is the PR interval consistent or does it vary?)

## FIRST-DEGREE AV BLOCK

In first-degree AV block (Figure 8-18; Box 8-5), the sinus impulse is conducted normally to the AV node, where it is delayed longer than usual before being conducted to the ventricles. This delay in the AV node results in a prolonged PR interval (greater than 0.20 seconds in duration). This rhythm is reflected on the ECG by a regular rhythm (both atrial and ventricular), one P wave preceding each QRS complex, a consistent but prolonged PR interval, and a narrow QRS. Anatomically, this conduction disorder is located at the level of the AV node (thus, the narrow QRS complex) and is not a serious form of heart block. First-degree heart block is simply a normal sinus rhythm with a prolonged PR interval.

There are numerous causes of first-degree AV block, most of which are associated with second-degree and third-degree AV block also. Causes include: drugs (digitalis, beta blockers, calcium channel blockers), increased vagal tone, hyperkalemia, rheumatic fever, myocarditis, degeneration of the conducting pathways associated with aging, and idiopathic causes. Varying degrees of heart block are

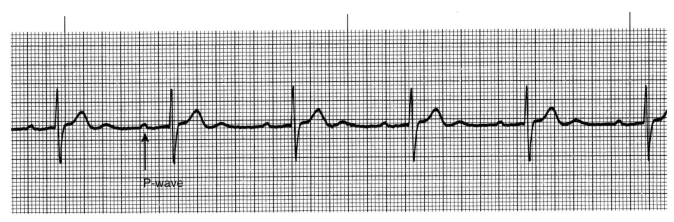

**Figure 8-18. Sinus Bradycardia with First Degree AV Block**

| | |
|---|---|
| *Rhythm:* | Regular |
| *Rate:* | 48 |
| *P waves:* | Sinus P waves present; one P wave to each QRS |
| *PR:* | 0.28 to 0.32 seconds (remains constant) |
| *QRS:* | 0.08 to 0.10 seconds. |
| *Note:* | A U wave is present. |

common with inferior wall MI because the right coronary artery, which generally supplies the inferior wall, also usually supplies the AV node.

### Box 8-5. First-Degree AV Block: Identifying ECG Features

| | |
|---|---|
| Rhythm: | Regular |
| Rate: | Heart rate is that of underlying rhythm (usually sinus); both atrial and ventricular rates will be the same |
| P waves: | Sinus; one P wave to each QRS |
| PR: | Prolonged (greater than 0.20 seconds); remains constant |
| QRS: | Normal (0.10 seconds or less) |

First-degree AV block produces no symptoms and requires no treatment. Because first-degree heart block can progress to a higher degree of AV block, the rhythm should continue to be monitored until the block resolves or stabilizes. Drugs causing AV block should be reviewed and discontinued, if indicated.

## SECOND-DEGREE AV BLOCK, TYPE I (MOBITZ I OR WENCKEBACH)

Second-degree AV block, type I (commonly known as Mobitz I or Wenckebach) (Figures 8-19 and 8-20; Box 8-6) is characterized by a failure of some of the sinus impulses to be conducted to the ventricles. In this rhythm, the sinus impulse is conducted normally to the AV node but each successive impulse has more and more

difficulty passing through the AV node, until finally an impulse does not pass through (ie, it is blocked or not conducted). This rhythm is reflected on the ECG by regularly occurring P waves and progressively lengthening PR intervals until a P wave appears that is not followed by a QRS; instead, it is followed by a pause. The dropped QRS causes the ventricular rhythm to be irregular. After each dropped beat, the cycle repeats itself. The overall appearance of the rhythm demonstrates group beating (ie, groups of beats separated by pauses) and is a distinguishing characteristic of Mobitz I. Escape beats (atrial, junctional, or ventricular) may occur during the pause in the ventricular rhythm. Escape beats can confuse the diagnosis a little because it spoils the group beating pattern. The location of the conduction disturbance is at the level of the AV node, and, therefore, the QRS complex will be narrow.

### Box 8-6. Second-Degree AV Block (Mobitz I): Identifying ECG Features

| | |
|---|---|
| Rhythm: | Atrial: Regular<br>Ventricular: Irregular |
| Rate: | Atrial: Rate is that of underlying rhythm (usually sinus)<br>Ventricular: Rate will depend on number of impulses conducted through AV node—will be less than the atrial rate |
| P waves: | Sinus |
| PR: | PR varies. PR progressively lengthens until a P wave occurs without a QRS. A pause follows the dropped QRS. |
| QRS: | Normal (0.10 seconds or less) |

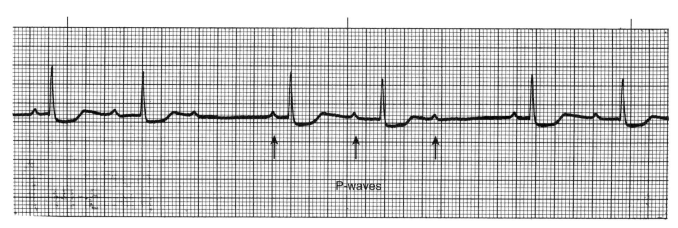

**Figure 8-19. Second-Degree AV Block, Mobitz I**

*Rhythm:*   Regular atrial rhythm; irregular ventricular rhythm

*Rate:*   Atrial: 72   Ventricular: 50

*P waves:*   Sinus P waves are present

*PR:*   Progressively lengthens from 0.20 to 0.30 seconds

*QRS:*   0.06–0.08 seconds

*Note:*   ST segment depression is present

Mobitz I can be confused with the nonconducted PAC (Figure 8-21). Both rhythms have P waves not followed by a QRS, but followed by a pause. To differentiate between the two rhythms, one must examine the configuration of the P waves and measure the P–P regularity. The nonconducted PAC will have an abnormal P wave and will occur prematurely. In Mobitz I, the P wave configuration remains the same as the sinus beats and the P wave will occur on schedule, not prematurely.

Second-degree AV block, type I is common after acute inferior wall MI, but it is usually transient and resolves spontaneously. Other causes include drugs (digitalis, beta blockers, calcium channel blockers), increased vagal tone, myocarditis, and ischemic heart disease. Mobitz I may also occur in athletes at rest because of a physiologic increase in vagal tone.

Mobitz I is seldom a serious form of heart block, although, infrequently, it can progress to a higher degree of AV block. Clinically, patients with Mobitz I

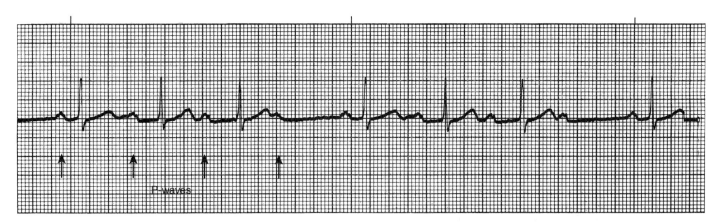

**Figure 8-20. Second-Degree AV Block, Mobitz I**

*Rhythm:*   Regular atrial rhythm; irregular ventricular rhythm

*Rate:*   Atrial: 75   Ventricular: 60

*P waves:*   Sinus P waves are present

*PR:*   Progressively lengthens from 0.24 to 0.38 seconds

*QRS:*   0.08 seconds

*Note:*   ST segment depression is present.

*Comment:*   Good example of group beating.

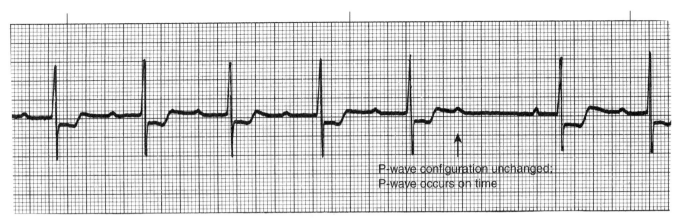

MOBITZ I      1. Pause in basic ventricular rhythm
                          2. P-P regularity unchanged (P wave occurs on time)
                          3. P wave configuration same as sinus beats
                          4. PR interval of basic rhythm varies

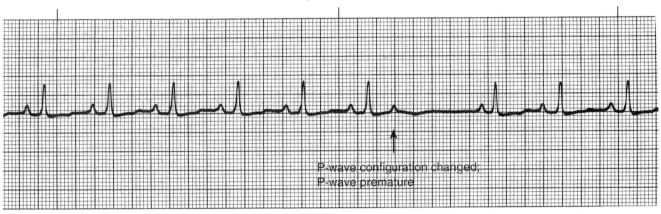

Nonconducted      1. Pause in basic ventricular rhythm
PAC                    2. P-P regularity interrupted (P wave occurs prematurely)
                          3. P wave configuration different from sinus beats
                          4. PR interval of basic rhythm remains constant

**Figure 8-21.** Differentiation of the nonconducted PAC from Mobitz I.

AV block are usually without symptoms unless the ventricular rate is very slow. If hemodynamic status is compromised because of bradycardia, atropine will often be effective in improving AV conduction. Pacemaker therapy is rarely needed. Drugs causing AV block should be reviewed and discontinued, if indicated.

## SECOND-DEGREE AV BLOCK, TYPE II (MOBITZ II)

Like Mobitz I, second-degree AV block, type II or Mobitz II (Figures 8-22 and 8-23; Box 8-7) is characterized by a failure of some of the sinus impulses to be conducted to the ventricles. There are some differences, however, in the anatomical location and severity of the conduction disturbance, as well as in the ECG features. In Mobitz II, there will be more

than one P wave before each QRS complex (usually two or three, but sometimes more), with only one of the impulses being conducted to the ventricles. The P waves will be identical and will occur regularly. The PR interval of the conducted beat may be normal or prolonged and will remain constant. The ventricular rhythm is usually regular unless the AV conduction ratio varies (alternating between 2:1, 3:1, 4:1, and so forth). The location of the conduction disturbance is below the AV node in the bundle of His or bundle branches. As a result, the QRS may be narrow (if located in the bundle of His) or wide (if located in the bundle branches). The most common location is the bundle branches.

Mobitz II is usually the result of extensive damage to the bundle branches after an acute anteroseptal MI and, unlike Mobitz I, not the result of inferior wall MI, increased vagal tone, or drug toxicity on the AV node. It can also occur with degeneration of the

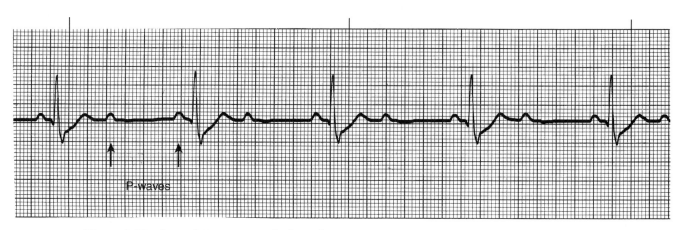

**Figure 8-22.** **Second-Degree AV Block, Mobitz II**

| | |
|---|---|
| *Rhythm:* | Regular atrial and ventricular rhythm |
| *Rate:* | Atrial: 82     Ventricular: 41 |
| *P waves:* | 2 sinus P waves to each QRS |
| *PR:* | 0.16 seconds (remains constant) |
| *QRS:* | 0.14 seconds |

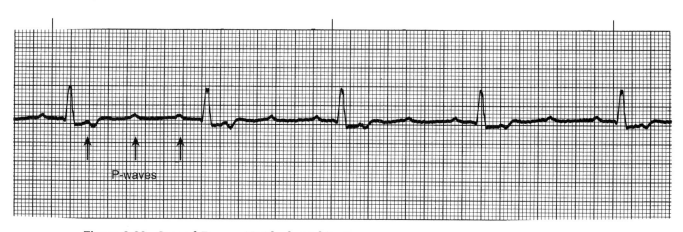

**Figure 8-23.** **Second-Degree AV Block, Mobitz II**

| | |
|---|---|
| *Rhythm:* | Regular atrial and ventricular rhythm |
| *Rate:* | Atrial: 123     Ventricular: 41 |
| *P waves:* | 3 sinus P waves to each QRS |
| *PR:* | 0.24–0.26 seconds (remains constant) |
| *QRS:* | 0.12 seconds |

electrical conduction system, which is usually age related.

Mobitz II is less common but more serious than Mobitz I. Because the anatomical location of the block is lower in the conduction system, Mobitz II has the potential to progress suddenly to third-degree AV block or ventricular standstill with little or no warning. Due to the unpredictable nature of this rhythm, a temporary transvenous pacemaker should be inserted as soon as the rhythm is recognized. If the patient is symptomatic and a transvenous pacemaker is not readily available, a transcutaneous pacemaker may be used in the interim. Atropine must be used with great cau-

tion (if at all) for treatment of second-degree AV block of the Mobitz II type (especially Mobitz II with wide QRS complexes). Administration of atropine increases sinus node discharge but usually doesn't improve conduction through the AV node. Acceleration of the atrial rate may result in paradoxical slowing of the ventricular rate. This paradoxical response is particularly likely to occur in patients with Mobitz II type second-degree AV block. If significant hypotension is present, start a dopamine infusion at 5 to 20 μg/kg/min or, if symptoms are severe, go directly to an epinephrine infusion at 2 to 10 μg/kg/min. If the rhythm doesn't resolve, permanent pacing may be necessary.

**Box 8-7. Second-Degree AV Block (Mobitz II):**
**Identifying ECG Features**

| | |
|---|---|
| Rhythm: | Atrial: Regular<br>Ventricular: Will be regular unless the AV conduction ratio varies |
| Rate: | Atrial: Rate is that of underlying rhythm (usually sinus)<br>Ventricular: Rate will depend on number of impulses conducted through AV node—will be less than the atrial rate |
| P waves: | Sinus; two or three P waves (sometimes more) before each QRS |
| PR: | May be normal or prolonged; remains constant |
| QRS: | Normal (if block located in bundle of His)<br>Wide (if block located in bundle branches) |

## THIRD-DEGREE AV BLOCK (COMPLETE HEART BLOCK)

Third-degree AV block (Figures 8-24 and 8-25; Box 8-8) represents complete absence of conduction between the atria and ventricles. This rhythm is also called *complete heart block.* With third-degree heart block, the atria and ventricles beat independently of each other and there is no relationship between atrial activity and ventricular activity (AV dissociation). The atria continue to be paced by the sinus node at its inherent rate of 60 to 100, whereas the ventricles are either paced by an escape pacemaker located in the AV node at the rate of 40 to 60 or in the ventricles at rates of 40 or below. The P waves will appear at one rate, and the QRS complexes at a slower rate, resulting in P waves that march through QRS complexes (hiding at times inside the QRS and within the T wave) and PR intervals that vary greatly. Although independent beating between the atria and the ventricles is occurring, both the atrial rhythm and the ventricular rhythm will usually be regular. Both the QRS width and the ventricular rate reflect the location of the blockage. If the block is at the level of the AV node or bundle of His, the QRS will be narrow and the heart rate will be between 40 and 60. If the blockage is in the bundle branches, the QRS will be wide and the heart rate will be much slower (usually 30 to 40).

**Box 8-8. Third-Degree AV Block (Complete**
**Heart Block): Identifying ECG Features**

| | |
|---|---|
| Rhythm: | Atrial: Regular<br>Ventricular: Regular |
| Rate: | Atrial: Rate is that of underlying rhythm (usually sinus)<br>Ventricular: Rate is between 40 and 60 if paced by AV node<br>Rate is between 30 and 40 if paced by ventricles |
| P waves: | Sinus P waves—no constant relationship between P waves and QRS. (P waves can be seen marching through QRS complexes and T waves.) |
| PR: | Varies greatly |
| QRS: | Normal (if block located at level of AV node or bundle of His)<br>Wide (if block located at level of bundle branches) |

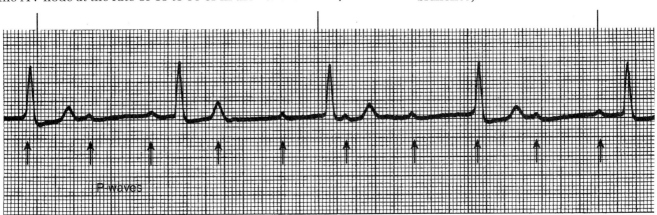

**Figure 8-24. Third-Degree AV block**

*Rhythm:* Regular atrial and ventricular rhythm

*Rate:* Atrial: 88    Ventricular: 38

*P waves:* Sinus P waves present; bear no relationship to QRS (found hidden in QRS and T waves)

*PR:* Varies greatly

*QRS:* 0.08 to 0.10 seconds

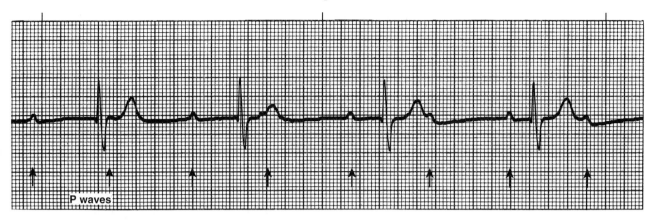

**Figure 8-25. Third-Degree AV block**

*Rhythm:* Regular atrial and ventricular rhythm

*Rate:* Atrial: 72 Ventricular: 40

*P waves:* Sinus P waves present; bear no constant relationship to QRS complexes (found hidden in QRS and T waves)

*PR:* Varies greatly

*QRS:* 0.12 seconds

Complete heart block may be transient or permanent and may occur for a number of reasons. Transient third-degree AV block is usually associated with inferior wall MI, increased vagal tone, acute myocarditis, digitalis toxicity, or after cardiac surgery. Permanent or chronic third-degree heart block is most commonly seen in older patients who have chronic degenerative changes in their electrical conduction systems. Permanent complete heart block can also occur as a complication of acute anteroseptal MI.

Regardless of its cause, complete heart block is a serious and potentially life-threatening arrhythmia. Like Mobitz II, complete heart block can progress to ventricular standstill suddenly, with little or no warning. If third-degree AV block occurs gradually, as seen in age-related degeneration of the electrical conduction system, the patient may have no significant symptoms and may only require cardiac monitoring with a transcutaneous pacemaker on standby until a permanent pacemaker is implanted. However, if complete heart block occurs suddenly (usually as a complication of acute MI), the patient may develop symptoms of hemodynamic compromise (dyspnea, heart failure, hypotension, chest pain, fainting) related to reduced cardiac output secondary to the slow ventricular rate and loss of the "atrial kick." The fainting spells associated with complete heart block are called *Stokes-Adams attacks* or *Stokes-Adams syncope.* Once the rhythm is recognized, a transcutaneous pacemaker should be applied while preparations are made for insertion of a temporary transvenous pacemaker. Atropine may be

effective in accelerating the sinus rate and AV node conduction in narrow complex third-degree heart block (AV node level), but it has little or no effect on wide complex third-degree heart block (bundle branch level). For significant hypotension, start a dopamine infusion at 5 to 20 µg/kg/min, or, if symptoms are severe, go directly to an epinephrine infusion at 2 to 10 µg/kg/min. Unresolved third-degree AV block will require a permanent pacemaker.

Table 8-1 compares the ECG characteristics of each type of AV block and will assist in interpretation of the different heart block rhythms.

**Table 8-1. AV Block Comparisons**

| PR Constant *(First-degree)* | PR Varies *(Second-degree, Mobitz I)* |
|---|---|
| PR constant | PR varies |
| PR prolonged One P wave to each QRS | PR progressively gets longer until a QRS is dropped |
| Regular atrial rhythm; regular ventricular rhythm | Regular atrial rhythm; irregular ventricular rhythm |
| *(Second-degree, Mobitz II)* | *(Third-degree)* |
| PR constant | PR varies |
| PR normal or prolonged Two, three, four P waves (or more) to each QRS | P waves have no constant relationship to QRS (found hidden in QRS complexes and T waves) |
| Regular atrial rhythm; regular ventricular rhythm (unless conduction ratios vary) | Regular atrial rhythm; regular ventricular rhythm |

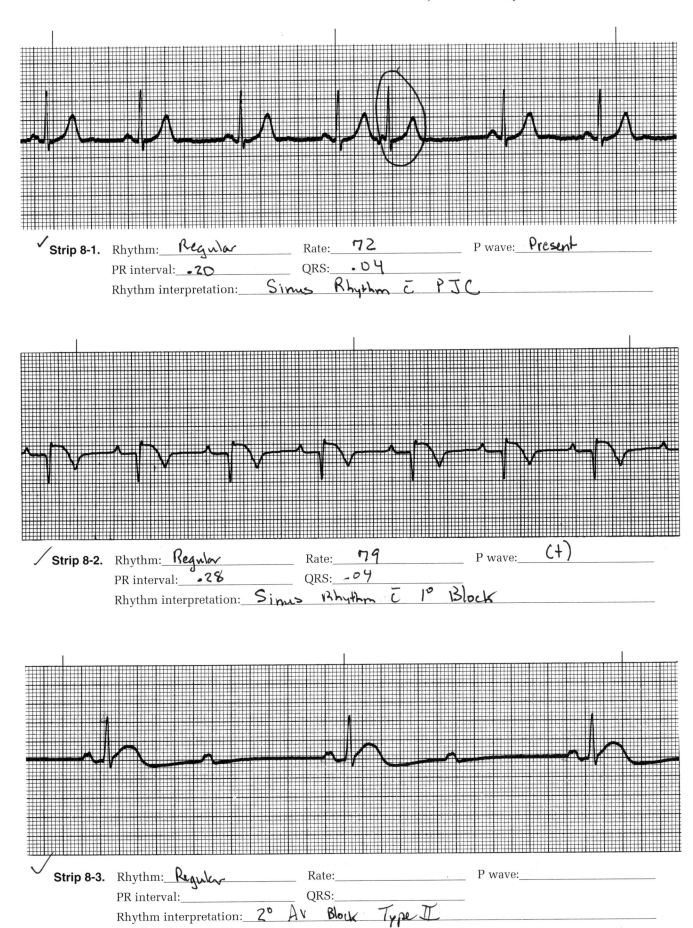

✓ **Strip 8-1.** Rhythm: _Regular_    Rate: _72_    P wave: _Present_
PR interval: _.20_    QRS: _.04_
Rhythm interpretation: _Sinus Rhythm c̄ PJC_

✓ **Strip 8-2.** Rhythm: _Regular_    Rate: _79_    P wave: _(+)_
PR interval: _.28_    QRS: _.04_
Rhythm interpretation: _Sinus Rhythm c̄ 1° Block_

✓ **Strip 8-3.** Rhythm: _Regular_    Rate: ___    P wave: ___
PR interval: ___    QRS: ___
Rhythm interpretation: _2° AV Block Type II_

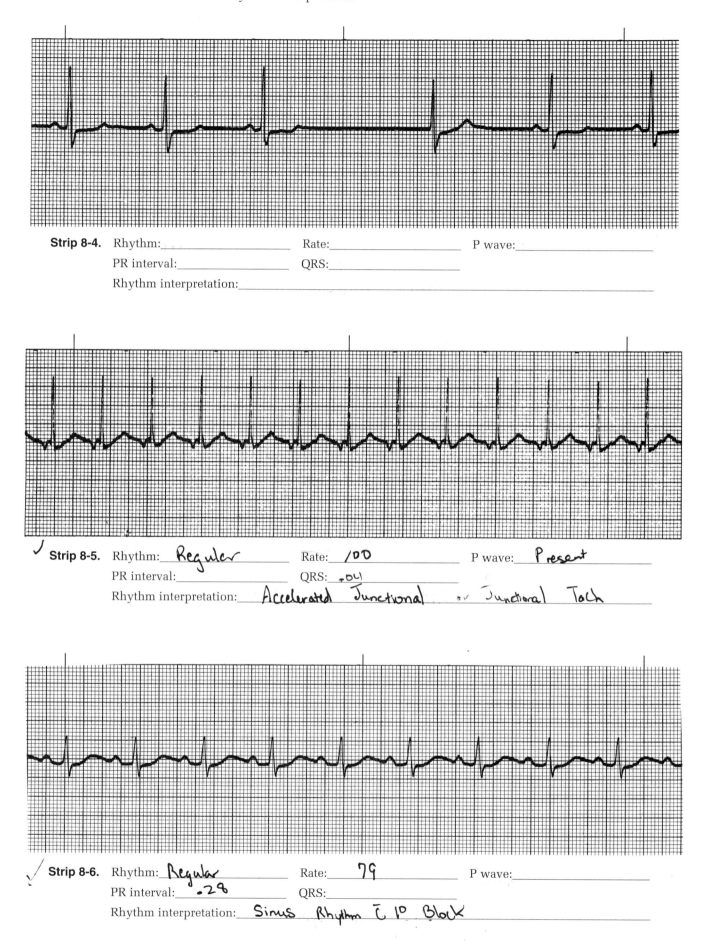

**Strip 8-4.** Rhythm: _____ Rate: _____ P wave: _____

PR interval: _____ QRS: _____

Rhythm interpretation: _____

**Strip 8-5.** Rhythm: _Regular_ Rate: _100_ P wave: _Present_

PR interval: _____ QRS: _.04_

Rhythm interpretation: _Accelerated Junctional  or Junctional Tach_

**Strip 8-6.** Rhythm: _Regular_ Rate: _79_ P wave: _____

PR interval: _.28_ QRS: _____

Rhythm interpretation: _Sinus Rhythm c̄ 1° Block_

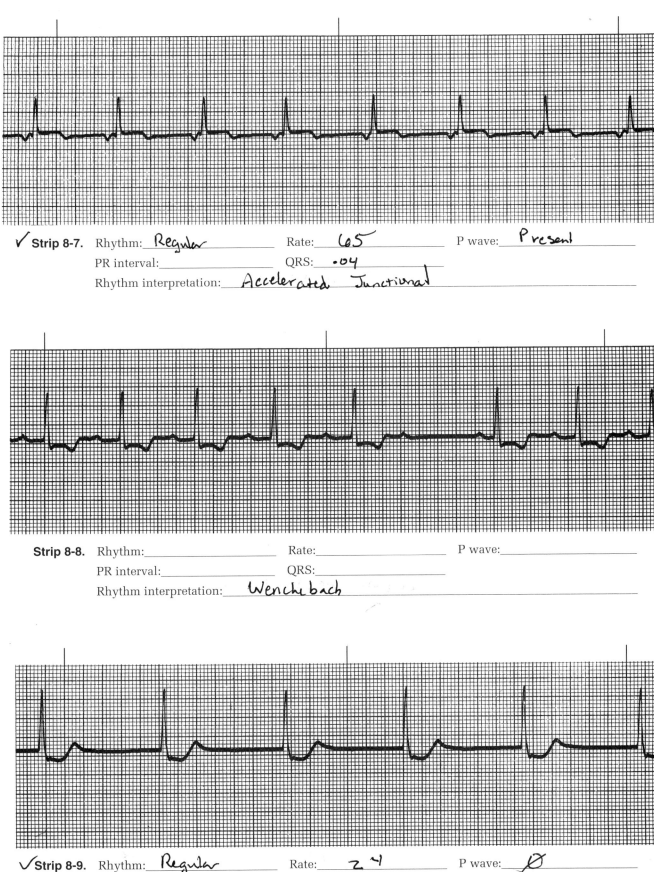

✓ **Strip 8-7.**  Rhythm: _Regular_  Rate: _65_  P wave: _Present_
PR interval: _____  QRS: _.04_
Rhythm interpretation: _Accelerated Junctional_

**Strip 8-8.**  Rhythm: _____  Rate: _____  P wave: _____
PR interval: _____  QRS: _____
Rhythm interpretation: _Wenchebach_

✓ **Strip 8-9.**  Rhythm: _Regular_  Rate: _2 4_  P wave: _Ø_
PR interval: _____  QRS: _____
Rhythm interpretation: _Junctional Rhythm_

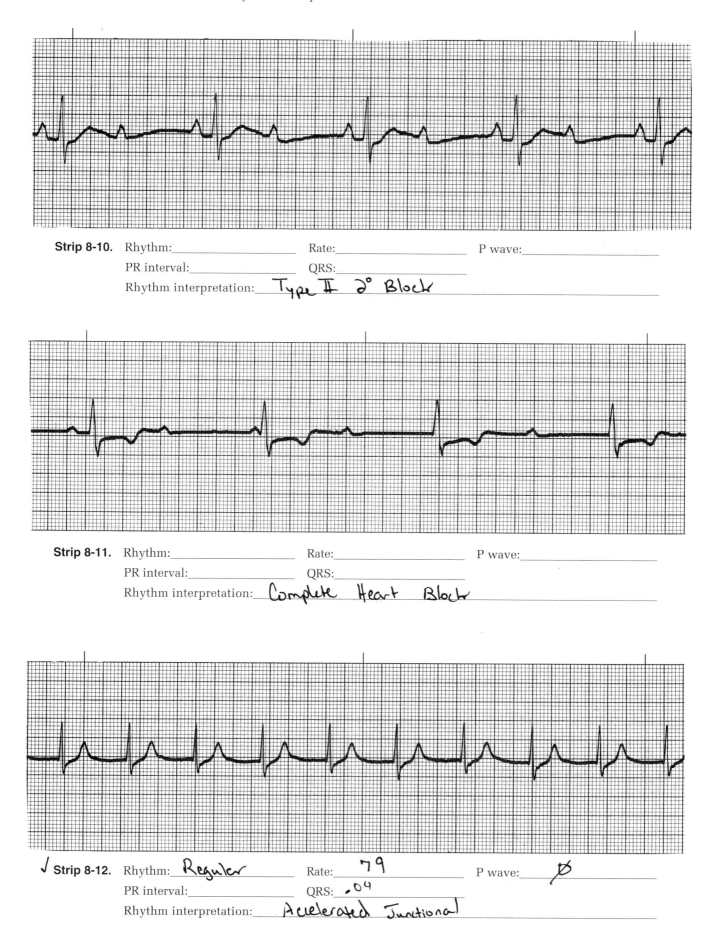

**Strip 8-10.** Rhythm:_____ Rate:_____ P wave:_____

PR interval:_____ QRS:_____

Rhythm interpretation:___Type II 2° Block_____

**Strip 8-11.** Rhythm:_____ Rate:_____ P wave:_____

PR interval:_____ QRS:_____

Rhythm interpretation:___Complete Heart Block_____

✓ **Strip 8-12.** Rhythm:___Regular___ Rate:___79___ P wave:___∅___

PR interval:_____ QRS:___.04___

Rhythm interpretation:___Accelerated Junctional_____

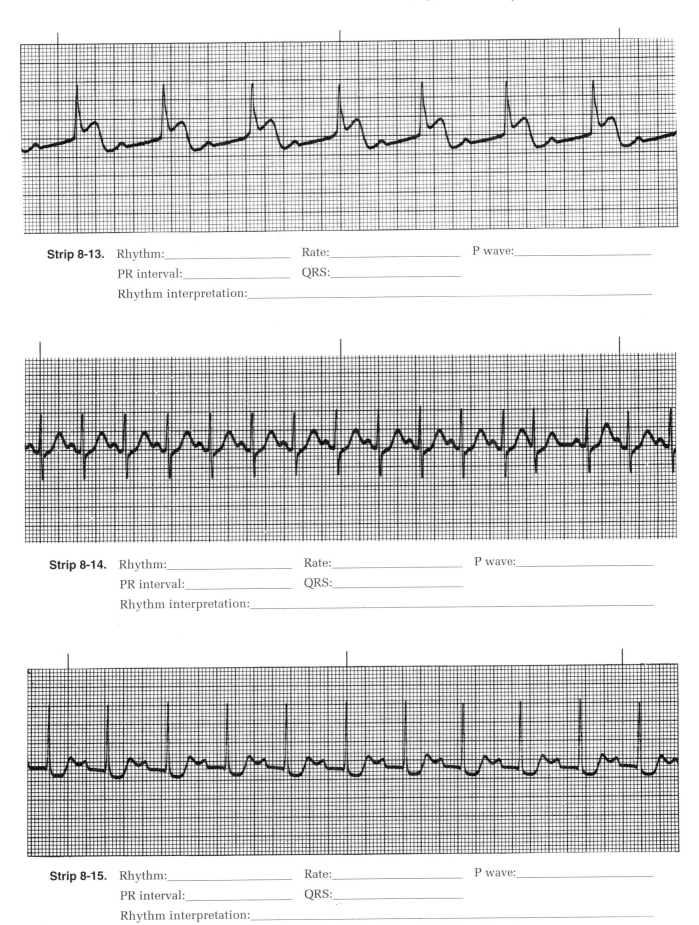

**Strip 8-13.** Rhythm:_____ Rate:_____ P wave:_____

PR interval:_____ QRS:_____

Rhythm interpretation:_____

**Strip 8-14.** Rhythm:_____ Rate:_____ P wave:_____

PR interval:_____ QRS:_____

Rhythm interpretation:_____

**Strip 8-15.** Rhythm:_____ Rate:_____ P wave:_____

PR interval:_____ QRS:_____

Rhythm interpretation:_____

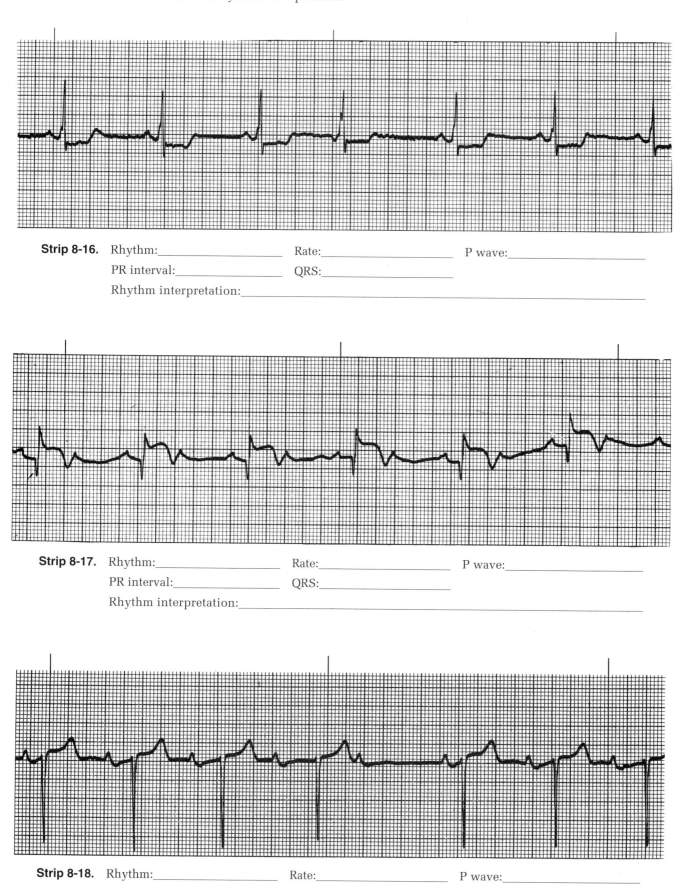

**Strip 8-16.** Rhythm:_____ Rate:_____ P wave:_____

PR interval:_____ QRS:_____

Rhythm interpretation:_____

**Strip 8-17.** Rhythm:_____ Rate:_____ P wave:_____

PR interval:_____ QRS:_____

Rhythm interpretation:_____

**Strip 8-18.** Rhythm:_____ Rate:_____ P wave:_____

PR interval:_____ QRS:_____

Rhythm interpretation:_____

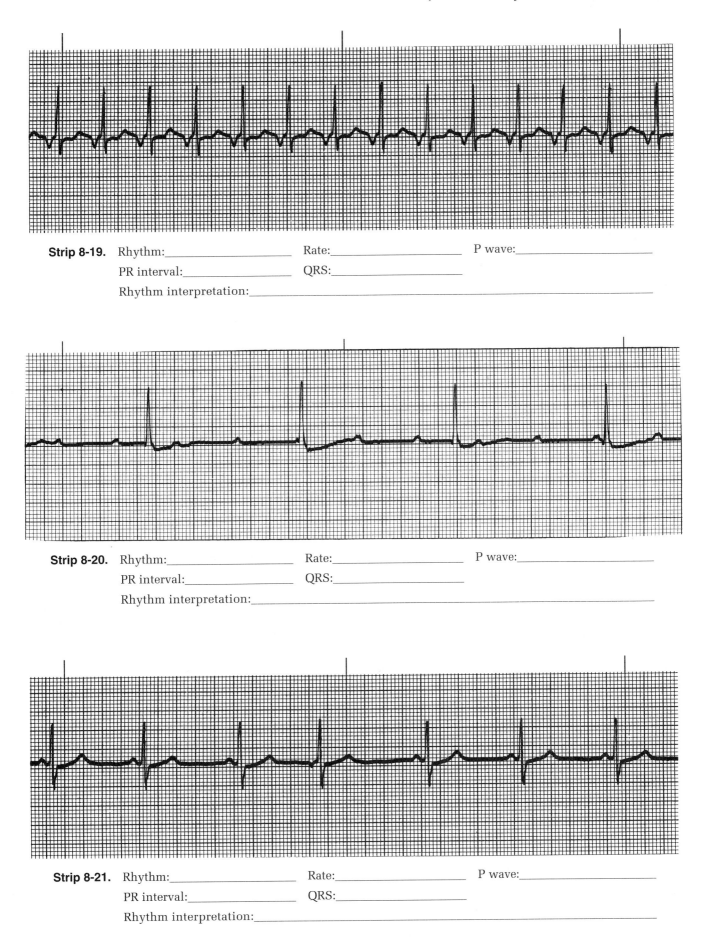

**Strip 8-19.** Rhythm:_____ Rate:_____ P wave:_____

PR interval:_____ QRS:_____

Rhythm interpretation:_____

**Strip 8-20.** Rhythm:_____ Rate:_____ P wave:_____

PR interval:_____ QRS:_____

Rhythm interpretation:_____

**Strip 8-21.** Rhythm:_____ Rate:_____ P wave:_____

PR interval:_____ QRS:_____

Rhythm interpretation:_____

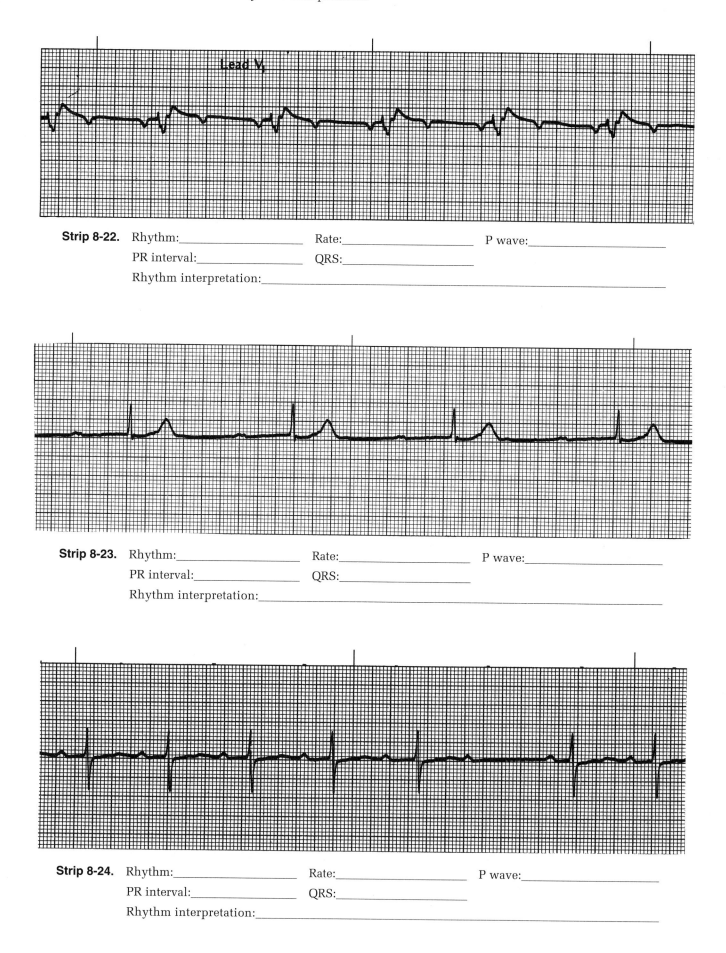

Lead V₁

**Strip 8-22.** Rhythm:_____ Rate:_____ P wave:_____

PR interval:_____ QRS:_____

Rhythm interpretation:_____

**Strip 8-23.** Rhythm:_____ Rate:_____ P wave:_____

PR interval:_____ QRS:_____

Rhythm interpretation:_____

**Strip 8-24.** Rhythm:_____ Rate:_____ P wave:_____

PR interval:_____ QRS:_____

Rhythm interpretation:_____

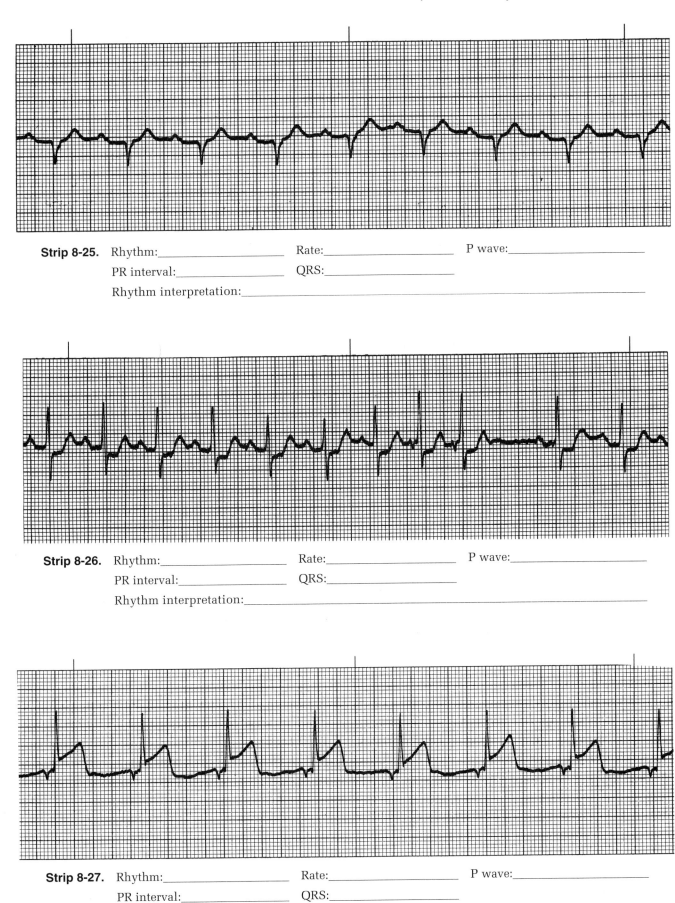

**Strip 8-25.** Rhythm:_____ Rate:_____ P wave:_____

PR interval:_____ QRS:_____

Rhythm interpretation:_____

**Strip 8-26.** Rhythm:_____ Rate:_____ P wave:_____

PR interval:_____ QRS:_____

Rhythm interpretation:_____

**Strip 8-27.** Rhythm:_____ Rate:_____ P wave:_____

PR interval:_____ QRS:_____

Rhythm interpretation:_____

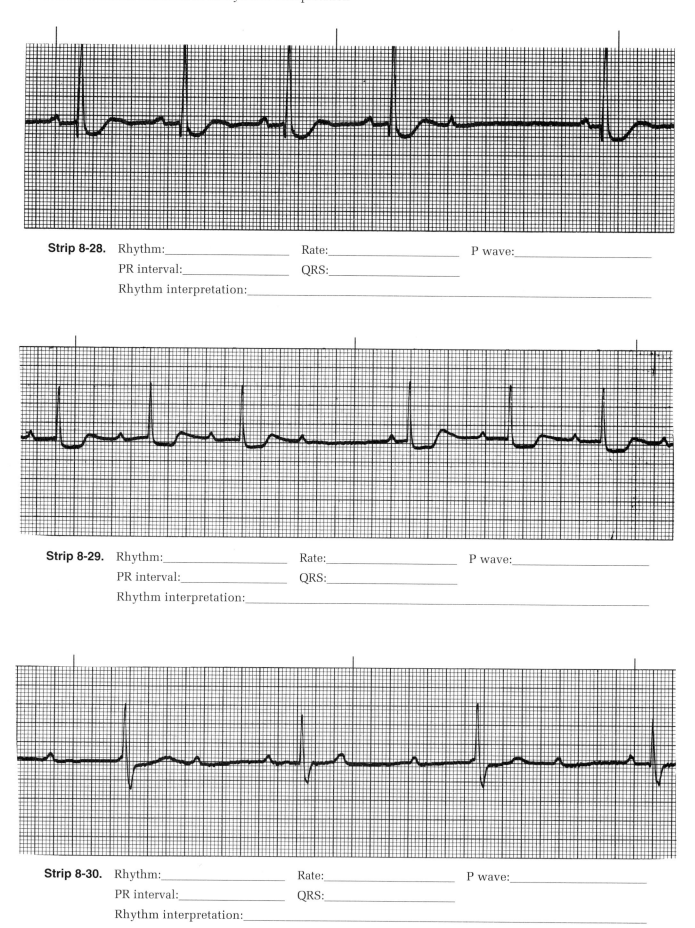

**Strip 8-28.** Rhythm:_____ Rate:_____ P wave:_____

PR interval:_____ QRS:_____

Rhythm interpretation:_____

**Strip 8-29.** Rhythm:_____ Rate:_____ P wave:_____

PR interval:_____ QRS:_____

Rhythm interpretation:_____

**Strip 8-30.** Rhythm:_____ Rate:_____ P wave:_____

PR interval:_____ QRS:_____

Rhythm interpretartion:_____

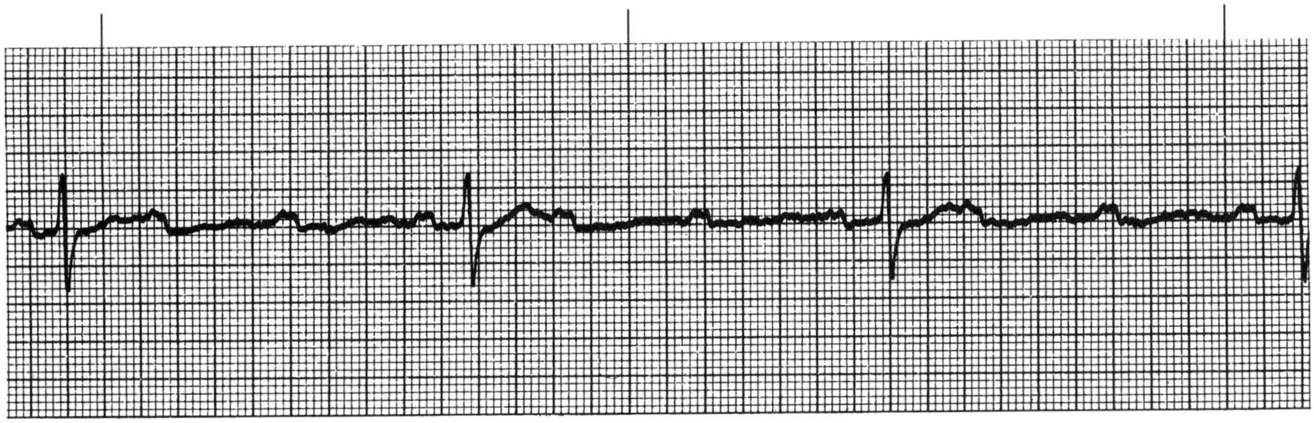

**Strip 8-31.** Rhythm:_____ Rate:_____ P wave:_____

PR interval:_____ QRS:_____

Rhythm interpretation:_____

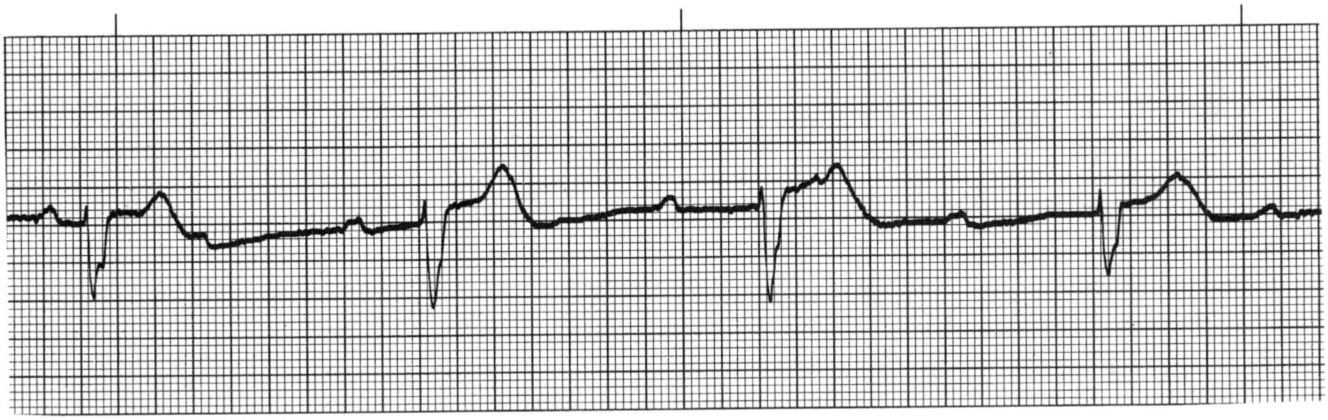

**Strip 8-32.** Rhythm:_____ Rate:_____ P wave:_____

PR interval:_____ QRS:_____

Rhythm interpretation:_____

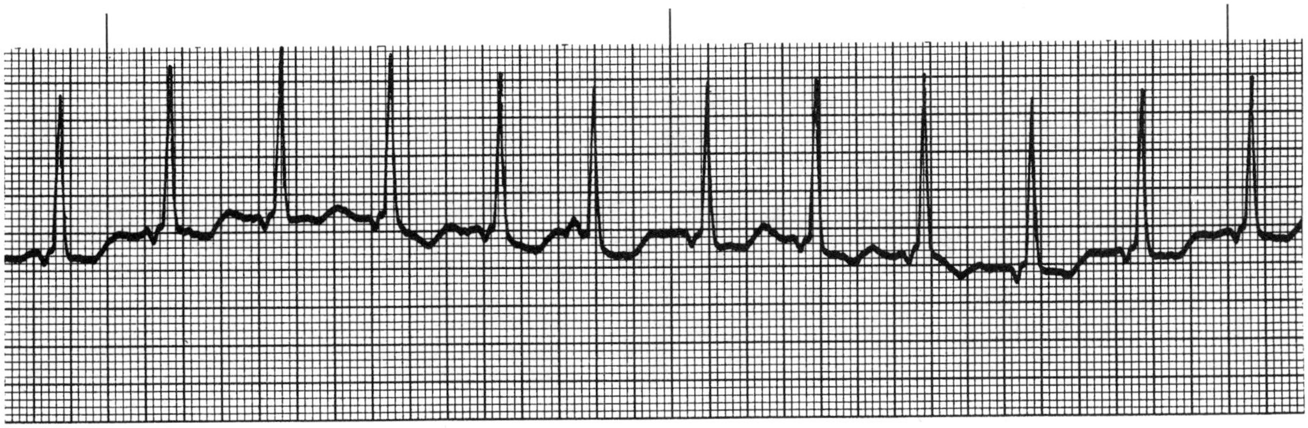

**Strip 8-33.** Rhythm:_____ Rate:_____ P wave:_____

PR interval:_____ QRS:_____

Rhythm interpretation:_____

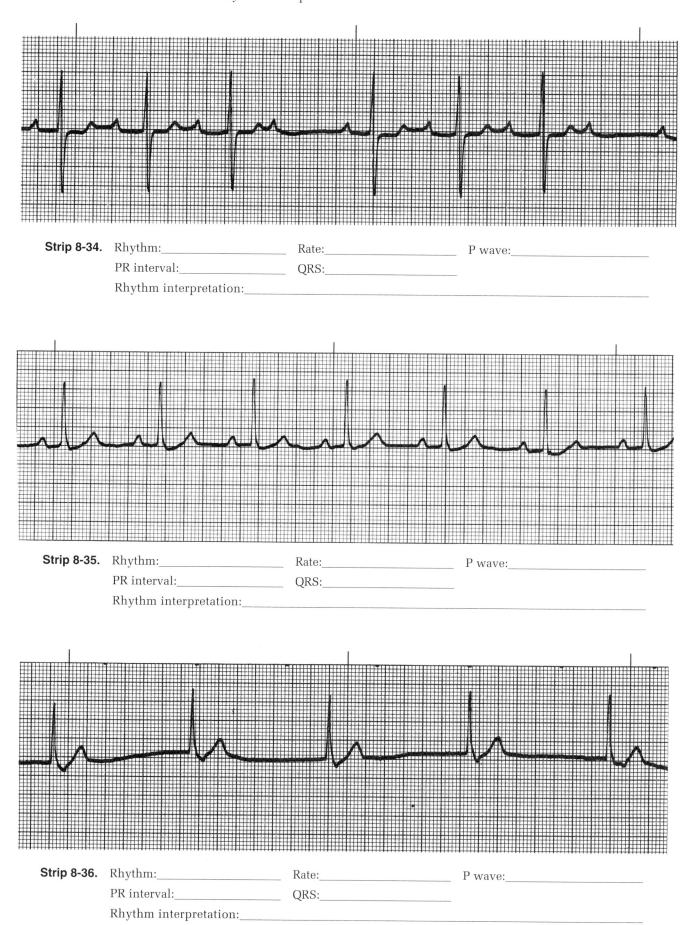

**Strip 8-34.** Rhythm:_____ Rate:_____ P wave:_____

PR interval:_____ QRS:_____

Rhythm interpretation:_____

**Strip 8-35.** Rhythm:_____ Rate:_____ P wave:_____

PR interval:_____ QRS:_____

Rhythm interpretation:_____

**Strip 8-36.** Rhythm:_____ Rate:_____ P wave:_____

PR interval:_____ QRS:_____

Rhythm interpretation:_____

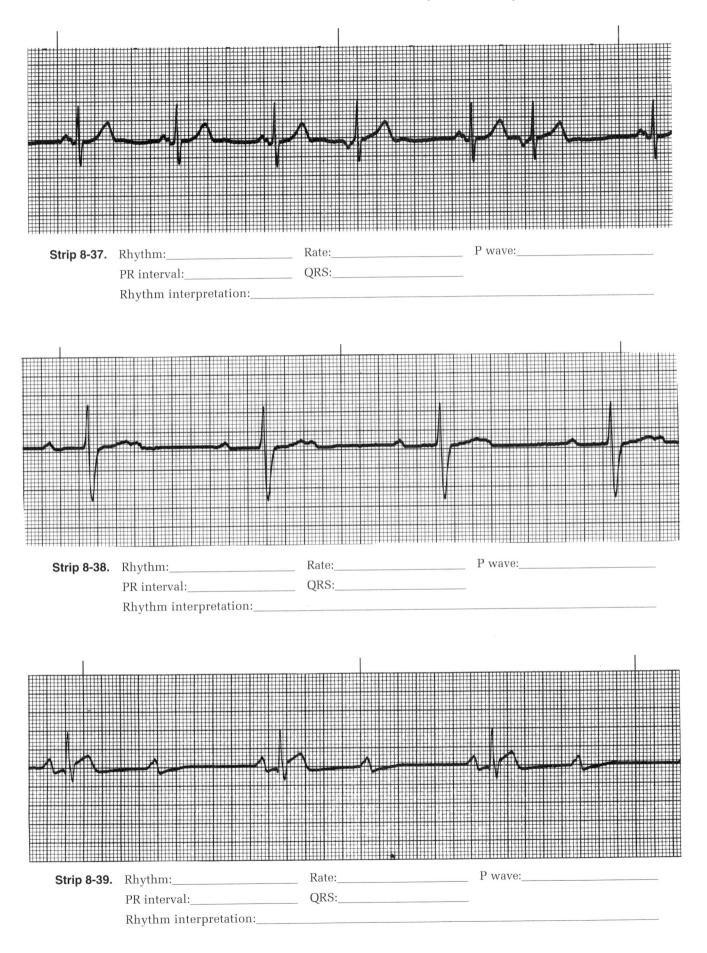

**Strip 8-37.** Rhythm:_____ Rate:_____ P wave:_____

PR interval:_____ QRS:_____

Rhythm interpretation:_____

**Strip 8-38.** Rhythm:_____ Rate:_____ P wave:_____

PR interval:_____ QRS:_____

Rhythm interpretation:_____

**Strip 8-39.** Rhythm:_____ Rate:_____ P wave:_____

PR interval:_____ QRS:_____

Rhythm interpretation:_____

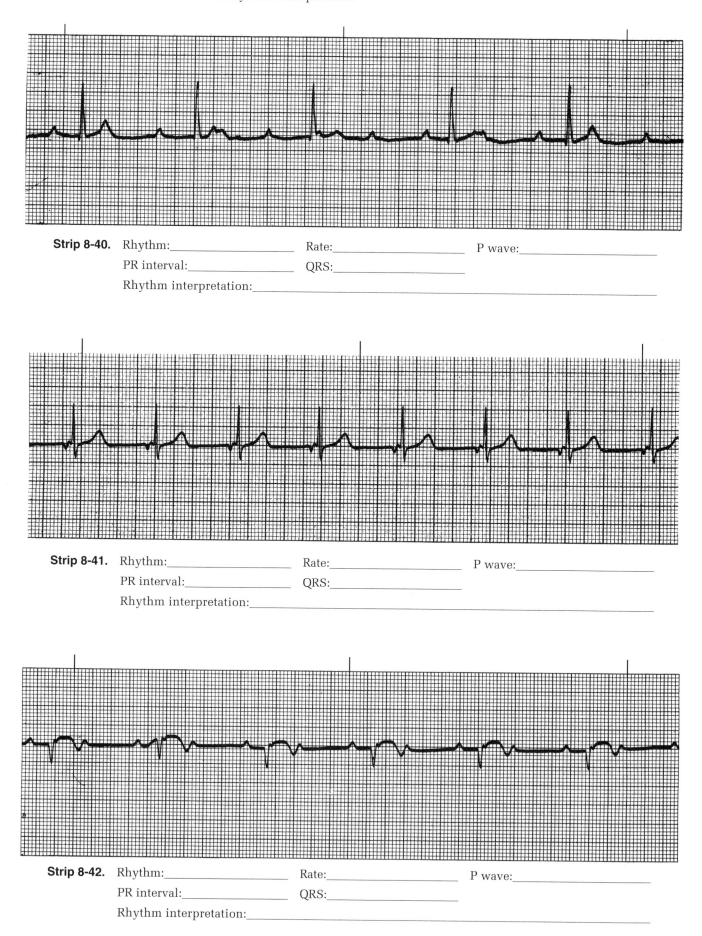

**Strip 8-40.** Rhythm:_____ Rate:_____ P wave:_____

PR interval:_____ QRS:_____

Rhythm interpretation:_____

**Strip 8-41.** Rhythm:_____ Rate:_____ P wave:_____

PR interval:_____ QRS:_____

Rhythm interpretation:_____

**Strip 8-42.** Rhythm:_____ Rate:_____ P wave:_____

PR interval:_____ QRS:_____

Rhythm interpretation:_____

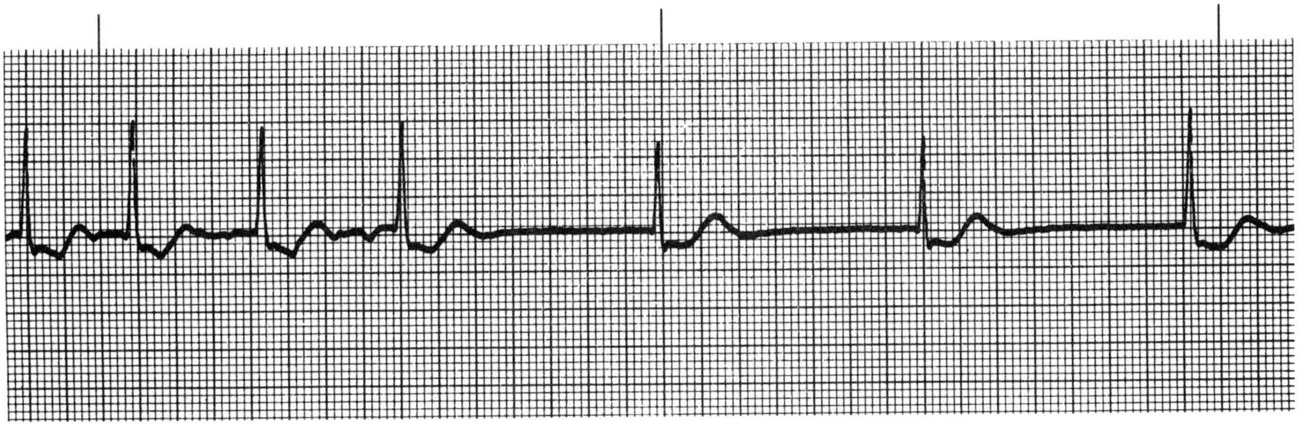

**Strip 8-43.** Rhythm:_____ Rate:_____ P wave:_____

PR interval:_____ QRS:_____

Rhythm interpretation:_____

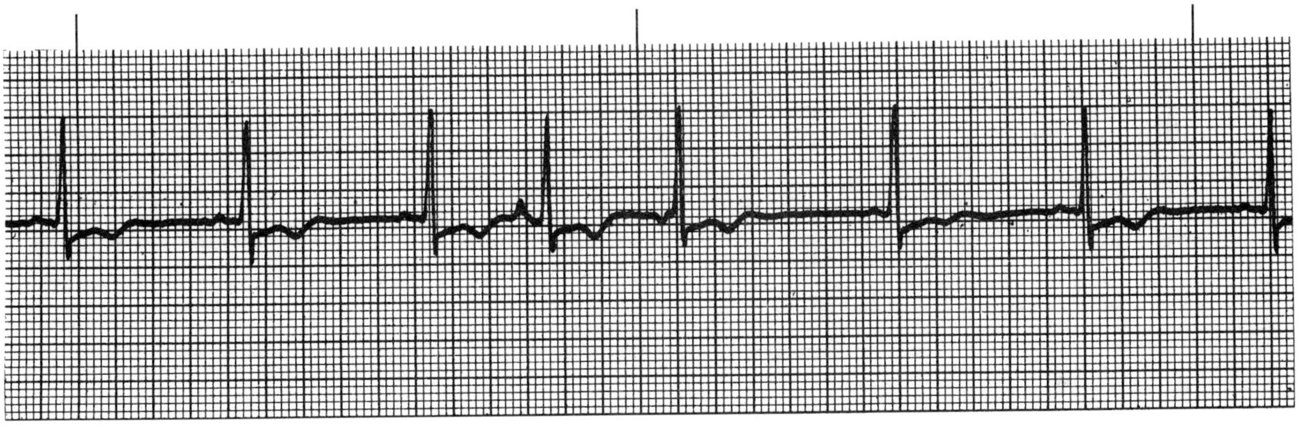

**Strip 8-44.** Rhythm:_____ Rate:_____ P wave:_____

PR interval:_____ QRS:_____

Rhythm interpretation:_____

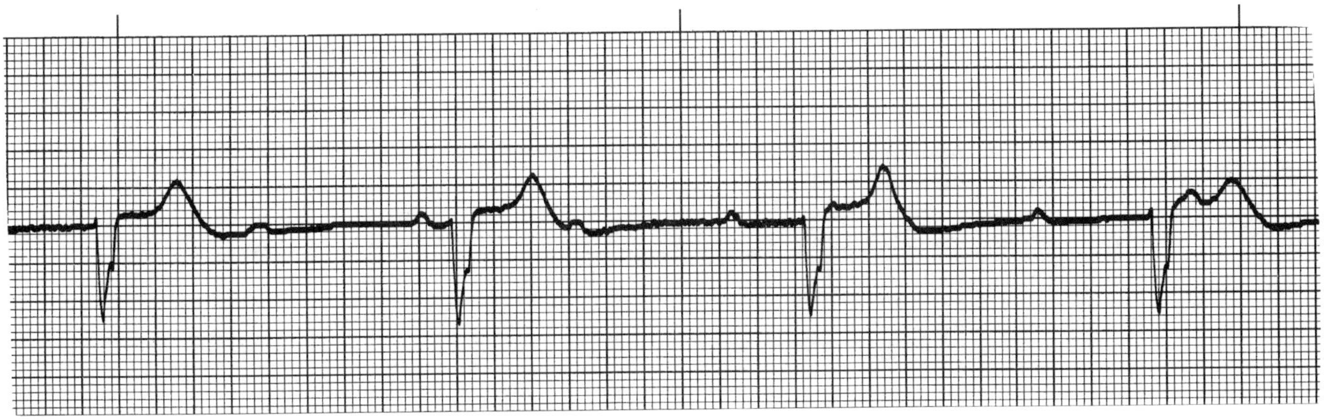

**Strip 8-45.** Rhythm:_____ Rate:_____ P wave:_____

PR interval:_____ QRS:_____

Rhythm interpretation:_____

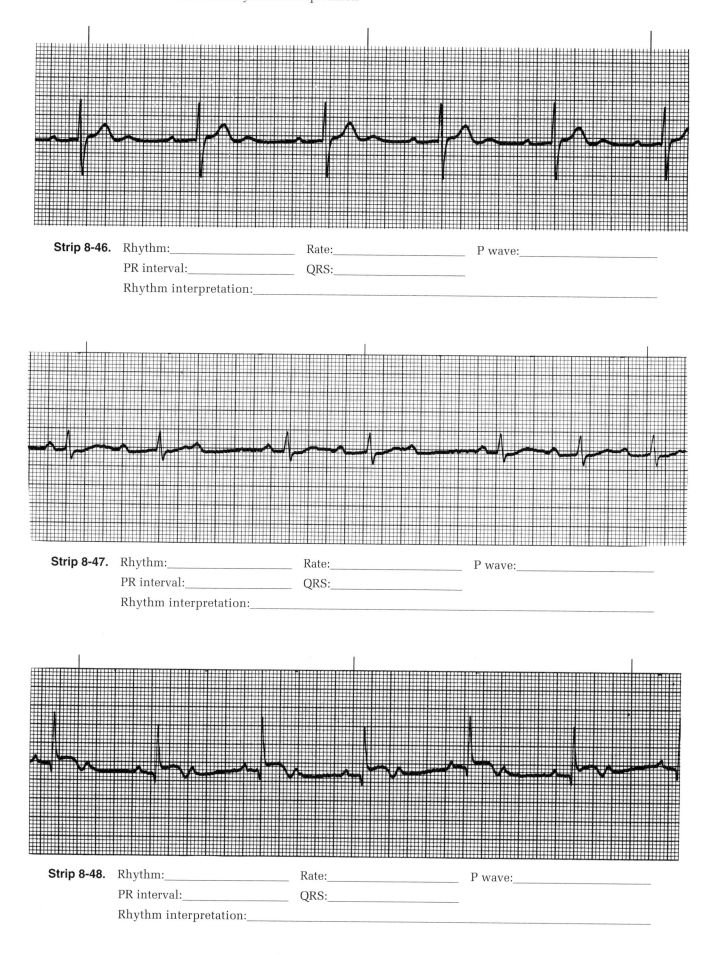

**Strip 8-46.** Rhythm:_____ Rate:_____ P wave:_____

PR interval:_____ QRS:_____

Rhythm interpretation:_____

**Strip 8-47.** Rhythm:_____ Rate:_____ P wave:_____

PR interval:_____ QRS:_____

Rhythm interpretation:_____

**Strip 8-48.** Rhythm:_____ Rate:_____ P wave:_____

PR interval:_____ QRS:_____

Rhythm interpretation:_____

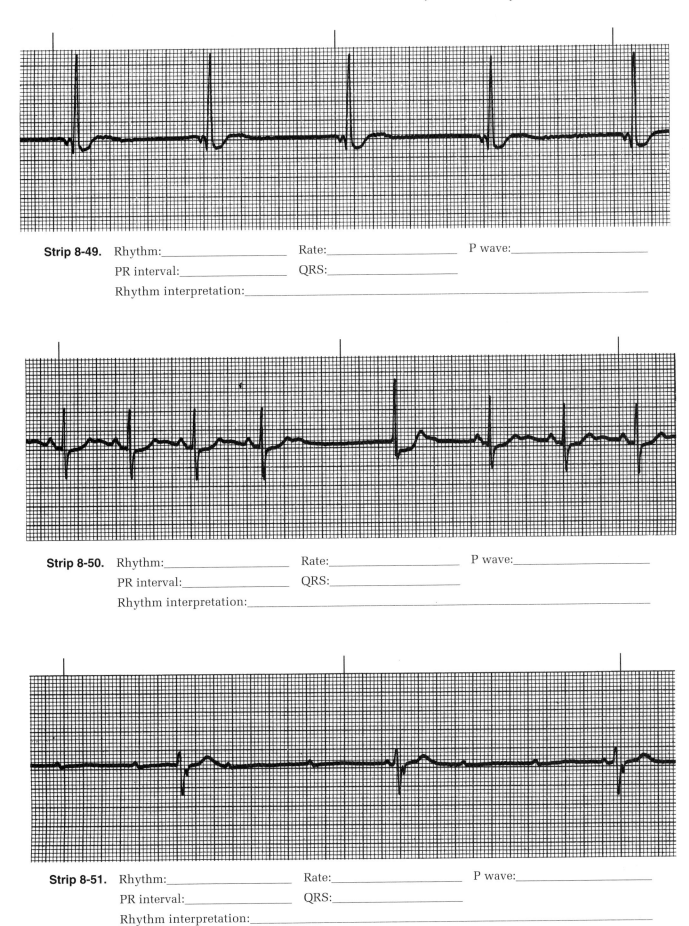

**Strip 8-49.** Rhythm:_____ Rate:_____ P wave:_____

PR interval:_____ QRS:_____

Rhythm interpretation:_____

**Strip 8-50.** Rhythm:_____ Rate:_____ P wave:_____

PR interval:_____ QRS:_____

Rhythm interpretation:_____

**Strip 8-51.** Rhythm:_____ Rate:_____ P wave:_____

PR interval:_____ QRS:_____

Rhythm interpretation:_____

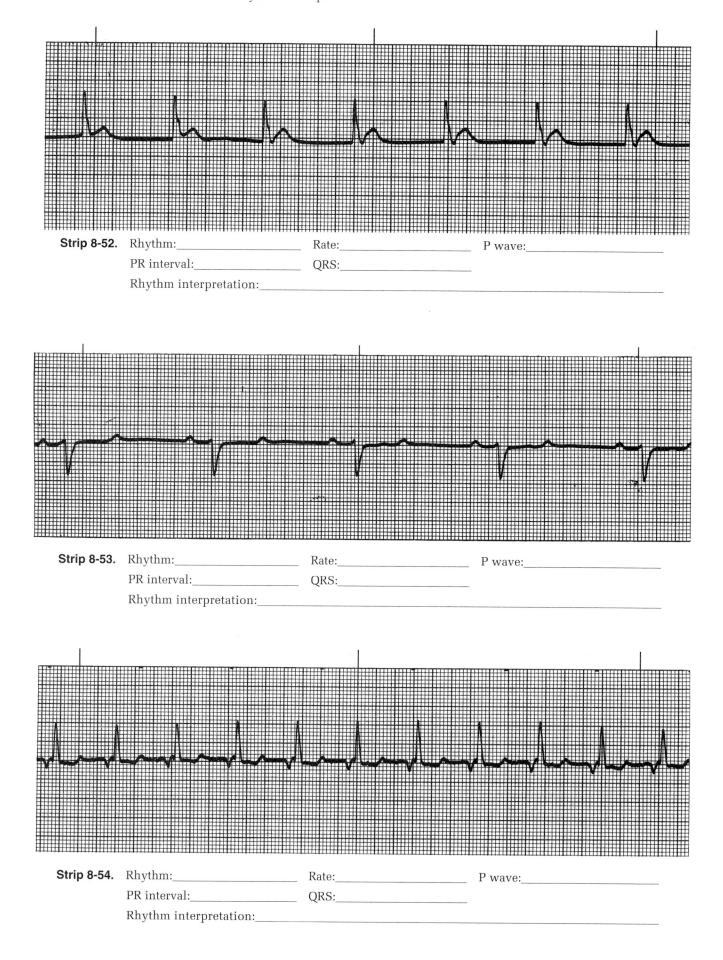

**Strip 8-52.** Rhythm:_____ Rate:_____ P wave:_____

PR interval:_____ QRS:_____

Rhythm interpretation:_____

**Strip 8-53.** Rhythm:_____ Rate:_____ P wave:_____

PR interval:_____ QRS:_____

Rhythm interpretation:_____

**Strip 8-54.** Rhythm:_____ Rate:_____ P wave:_____

PR interval:_____ QRS:_____

Rhythm interpretation:_____

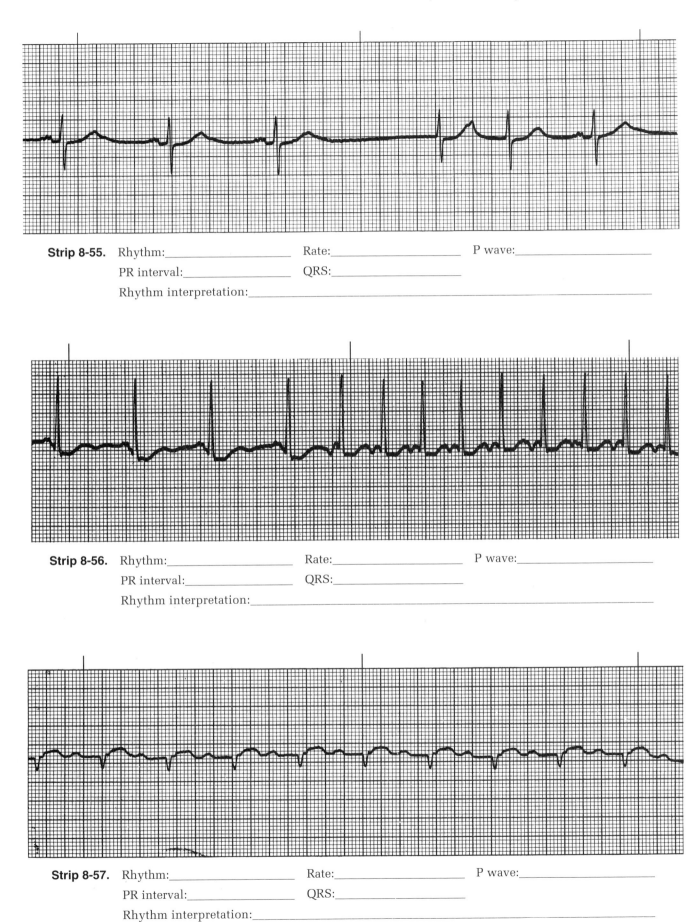

**Strip 8-55.** Rhythm:_____ Rate:_____ P wave:_____

PR interval:_____ QRS:_____

Rhythm interpretation:_____

**Strip 8-56.** Rhythm:_____ Rate:_____ P wave:_____

PR interval:_____ QRS:_____

Rhythm interpretation:_____

**Strip 8-57.** Rhythm:_____ Rate:_____ P wave:_____

PR interval:_____ QRS:_____

Rhythm interpretation:_____

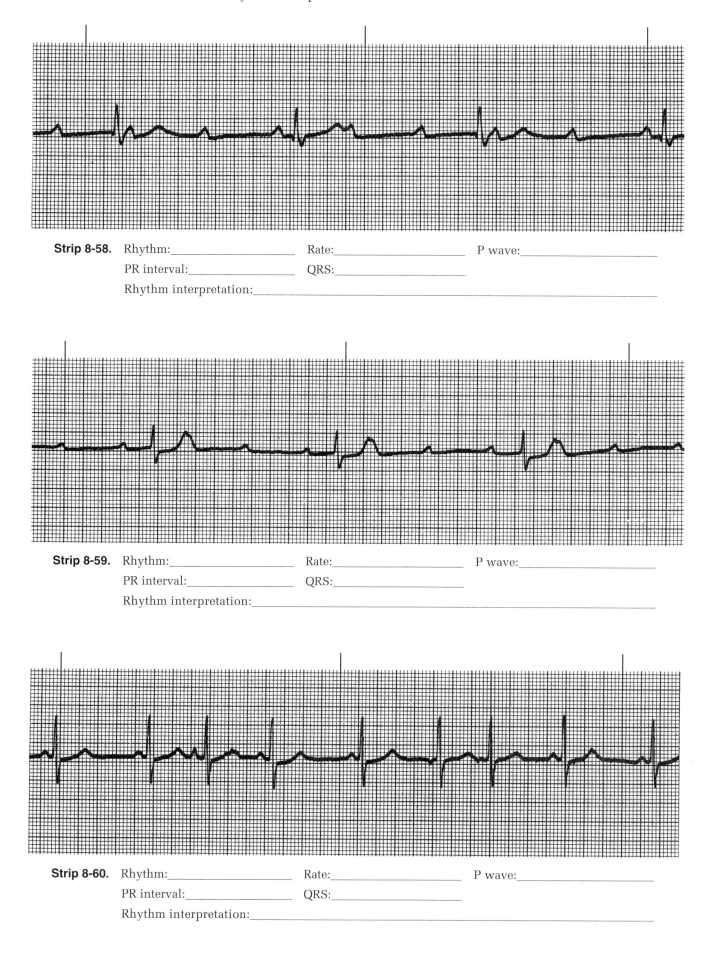

**Strip 8-58.** Rhythm:_____ Rate:_____ P wave:_____

PR interval:_____ QRS:_____

Rhythm interpretation:_____

**Strip 8-59.** Rhythm:_____ Rate:_____ P wave:_____

PR interval:_____ QRS:_____

Rhythm interpretation:_____

**Strip 8-60.** Rhythm:_____ Rate:_____ P wave:_____

PR interval:_____ QRS:_____

Rhythm interpretation:_____

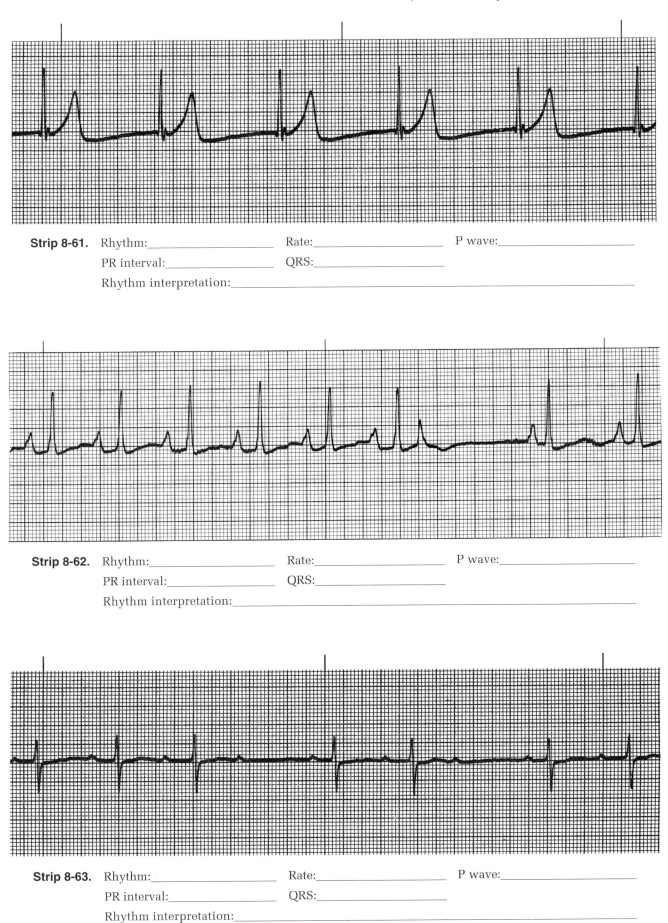

**Strip 8-61.** Rhythm:_____ Rate:_____ P wave:_____

PR interval:_____ QRS:_____

Rhythm interpretation:_____

**Strip 8-62.** Rhythm:_____ Rate:_____ P wave:_____

PR interval:_____ QRS:_____

Rhythm interpretation:_____

**Strip 8-63.** Rhythm:_____ Rate:_____ P wave:_____

PR interval:_____ QRS:_____

Rhythm interpretation:_____

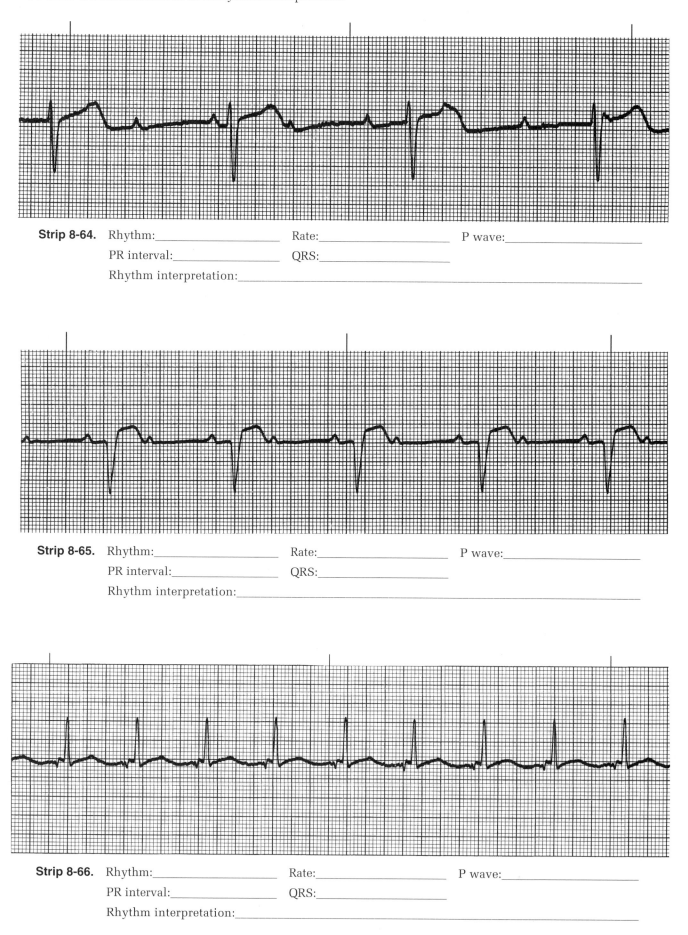

**Strip 8-64.** Rhythm:_____ Rate:_____ P wave:_____

PR interval:_____ QRS:_____

Rhythm interpretation:_____

**Strip 8-65.** Rhythm:_____ Rate:_____ P wave:_____

PR interval:_____ QRS:_____

Rhythm interpretation:_____

**Strip 8-66.** Rhythm:_____ Rate:_____ P wave:_____

PR interval:_____ QRS:_____

Rhythm interpretation:_____

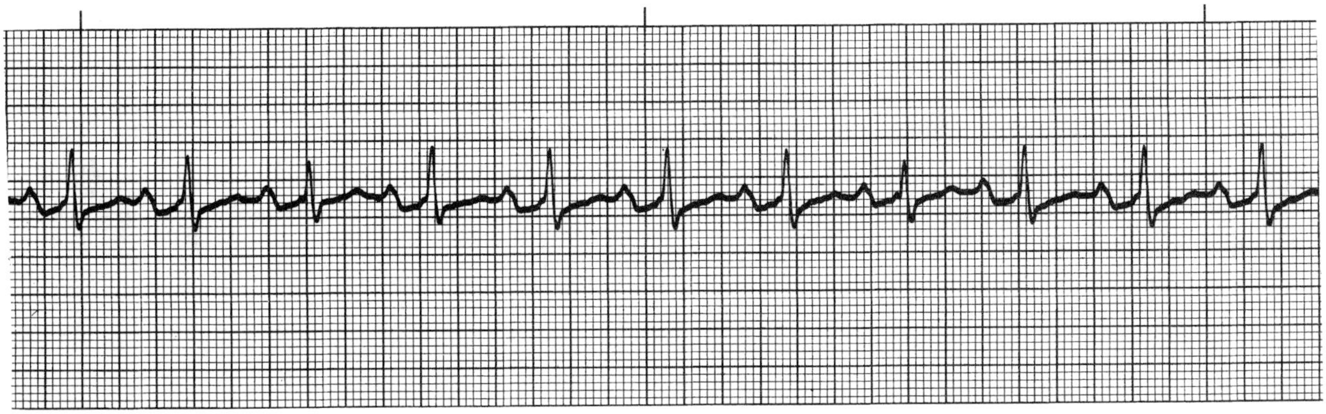

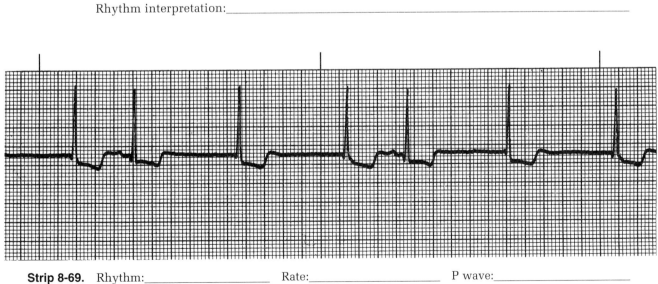

**Strip 8-67.** Rhythm:_____ Rate:_____ P wave:_____

PR interval:_____ QRS:_____

Rhythm interpretation:_____

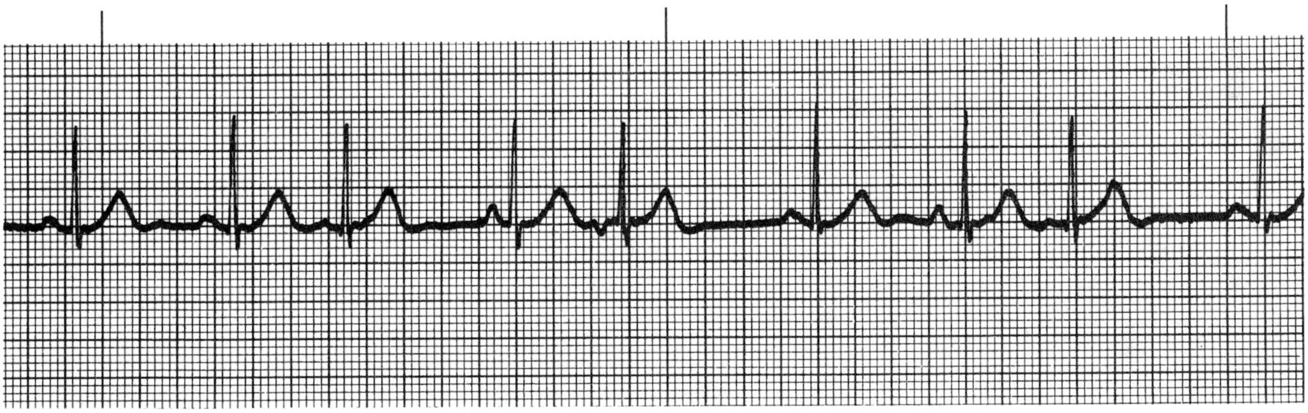

**Strip 8-68.** Rhythm:_____ Rate:_____ P wave:_____

PR interval:_____ QRS:_____

Rhythm interpretation:_____

**Strip 8-69.** Rhythm:_____ Rate:_____ P wave:_____

PR interval:_____ QRS:_____

Rhythm interpretation:_____

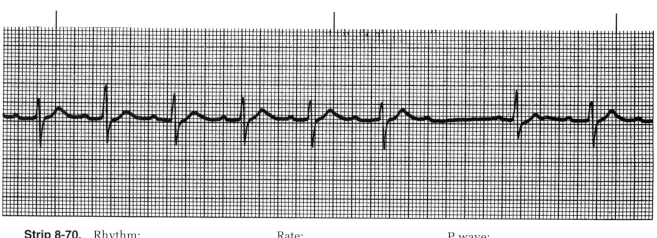

**Strip 8-70.** Rhythm:_____ Rate:_____ P wave:_____

PR interval:_____ QRS:_____

Rhythm interpretation:_____

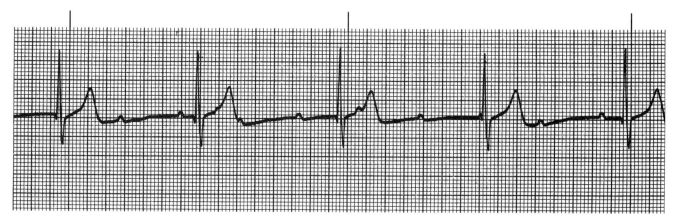

**Strip 8-71.** Rhythm:_____ Rate:_____ P wave:_____

PR interval:_____ QRS:_____

Rhythm interpretation:_____

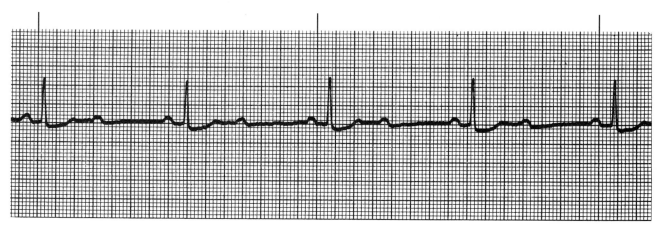

**Strip 8-72.** Rhythm:_____ Rate:_____ P wave:_____

PR interval:_____ QRS:_____

Rhythm interpretation:_____

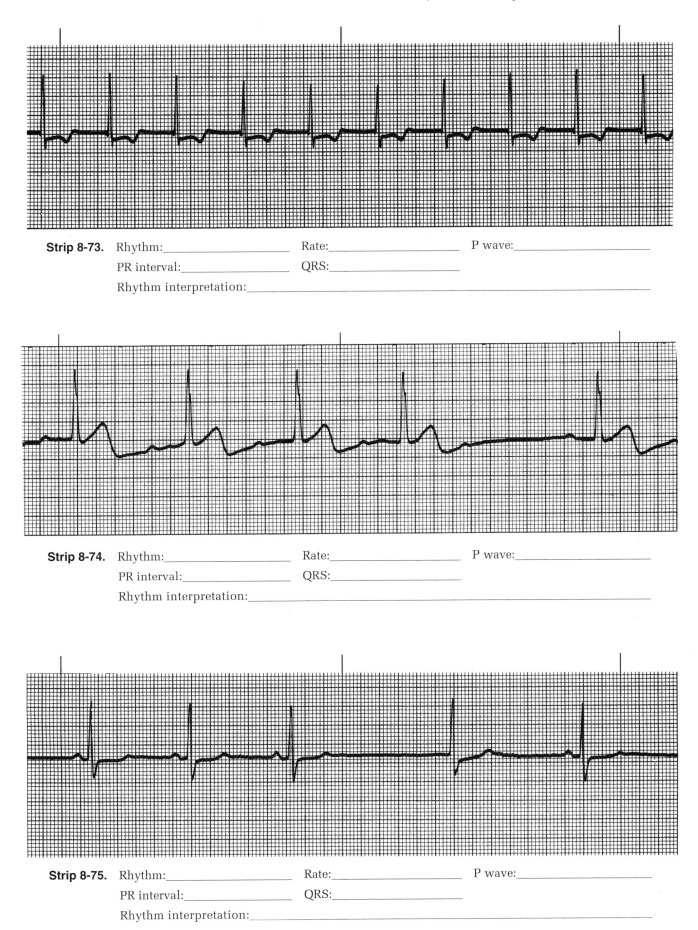

**Strip 8-73.** Rhythm:_____ Rate:_____ P wave:_____

PR interval:_____ QRS:_____

Rhythm interpretation:_____

**Strip 8-74.** Rhythm:_____ Rate:_____ P wave:_____

PR interval:_____ QRS:_____

Rhythm interpretation:_____

**Strip 8-75.** Rhythm:_____ Rate:_____ P wave:_____

PR interval:_____ QRS:_____

Rhythm interpretation:_____

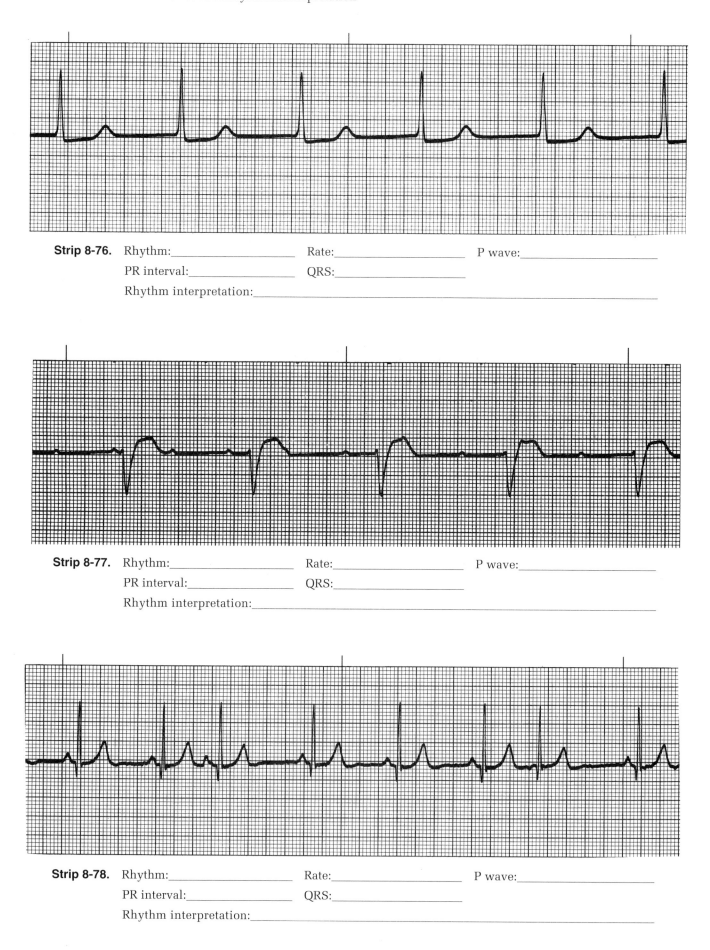

**Strip 8-76.** Rhythm:_____ Rate:_____ P wave:_____

PR interval:_____ QRS:_____

Rhythm interpretation:_____

**Strip 8-77.** Rhythm:_____ Rate:_____ P wave:_____

PR interval:_____ QRS:_____

Rhythm interpretation:_____

**Strip 8-78.** Rhythm:_____ Rate:_____ P wave:_____

PR interval:_____ QRS:_____

Rhythm interpration:_____

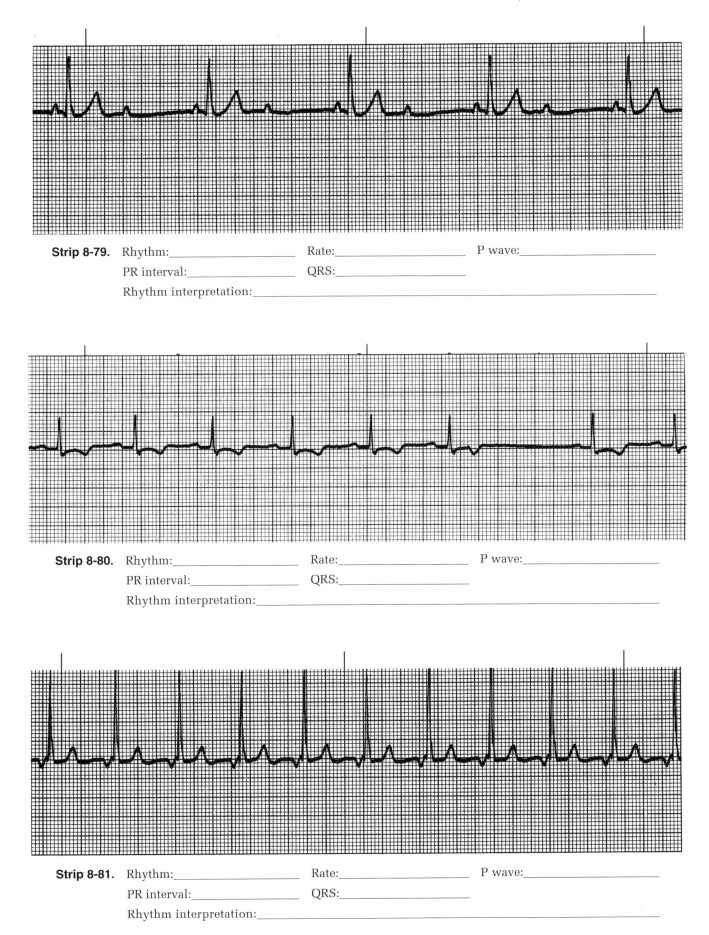

**Strip 8-79.** Rhythm:_____ Rate:_____ P wave:_____

PR interval:_____ QRS:_____

Rhythm interpretation:_____

**Strip 8-80.** Rhythm:_____ Rate:_____ P wave:_____

PR interval:_____ QRS:_____

Rhythm interpretation:_____

**Strip 8-81.** Rhythm:_____ Rate:_____ P wave:_____

PR interval:_____ QRS:_____

Rhythm interpretation:_____

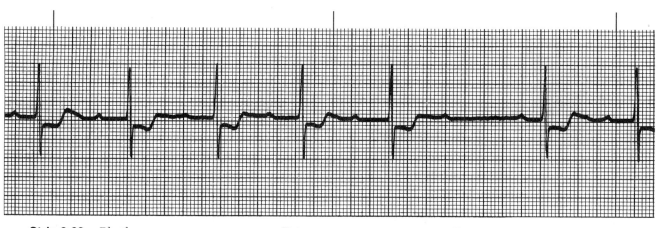

**Strip 8-82.** Rhythm:_____ Rate:_____ P wave:_____

PR interval:_____ QRS:_____

Rhythm interpretation:_____

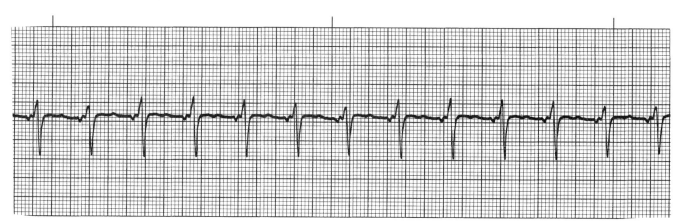

**Strip 8-83.** Rhythm:_____ Rate:_____ P wave:_____

PR interval:_____ QRS:_____

Rhythm interpretation:_____

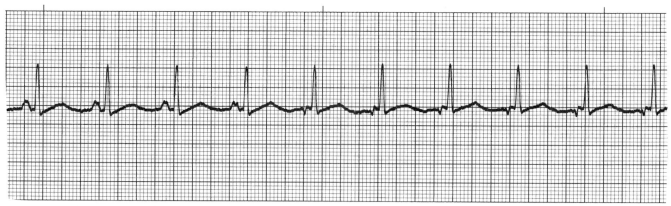

**Strip 8-84.** Rhythm:_____ Rate:_____ P wave:_____

PR interval:_____ QRS:_____

Rhythm interpretation:_____

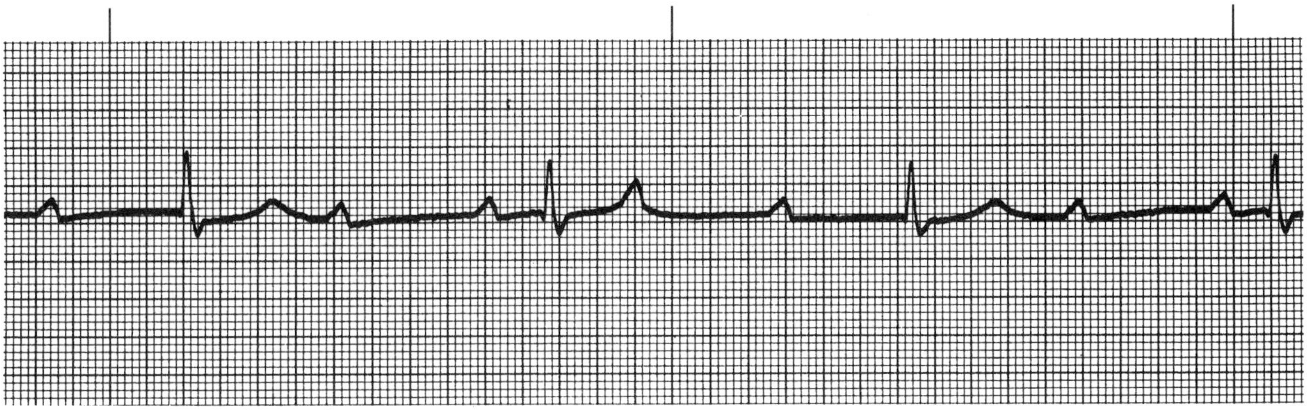

**Strip 8-85.** Rhythm:_____ Rate:_____ P wave:_____

PR interval:_____ QRS:_____

Rhythm interpretation:_____

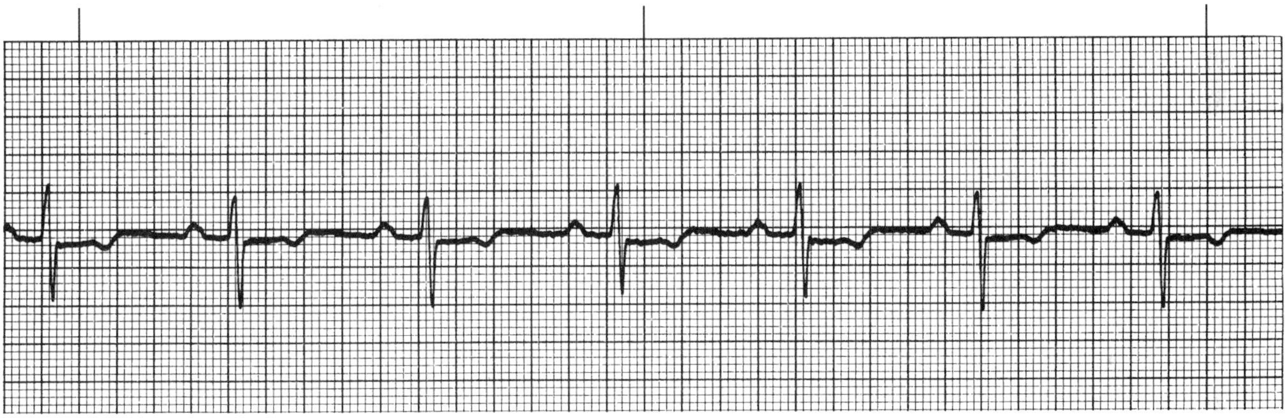

**Strip 8-86.** Rhythm:_____ Rate:_____ P wave:_____

PR interval:_____ QRS:_____

Rhythm interpretation:_____

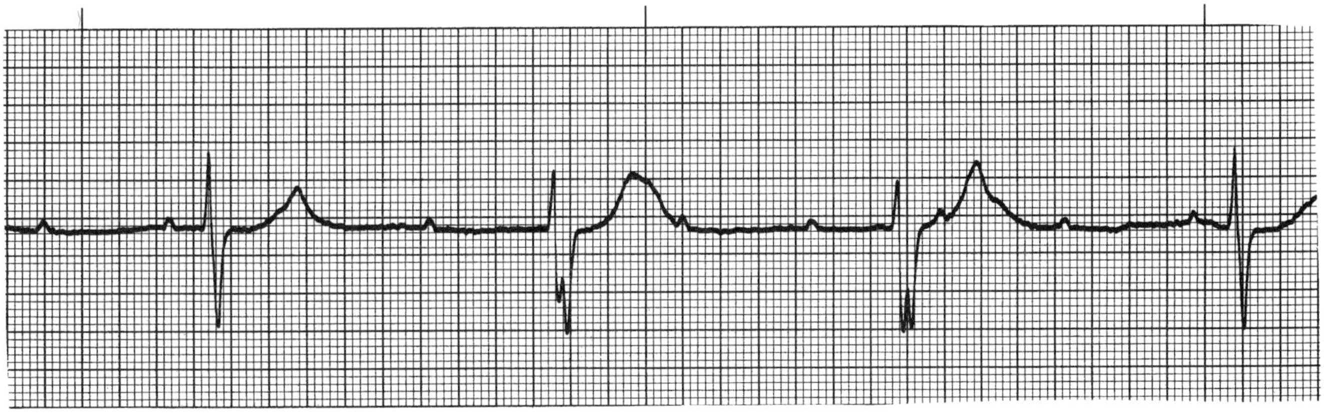

**Strip 8-87.** Rhythm:_____ Rate:_____ P wave:_____

PR interval:_____ QRS:_____

Rhythm interpretation:_____

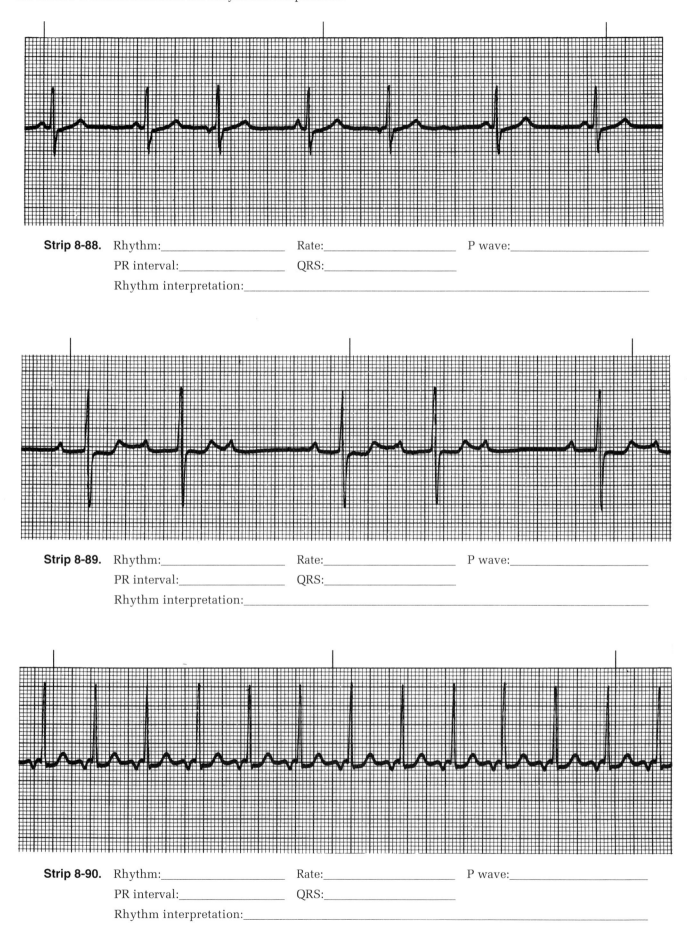

**Strip 8-88.** Rhythm:_____ Rate:_____ P wave:_____

PR interval:_____ QRS:_____

Rhythm interpretation:_____

**Strip 8-89.** Rhythm:_____ Rate:_____ P wave:_____

PR interval:_____ QRS:_____

Rhythm interpretation:_____

**Strip 8-90.** Rhythm:_____ Rate:_____ P wave:_____

PR interval:_____ QRS:_____

Rhythm interpretation:_____

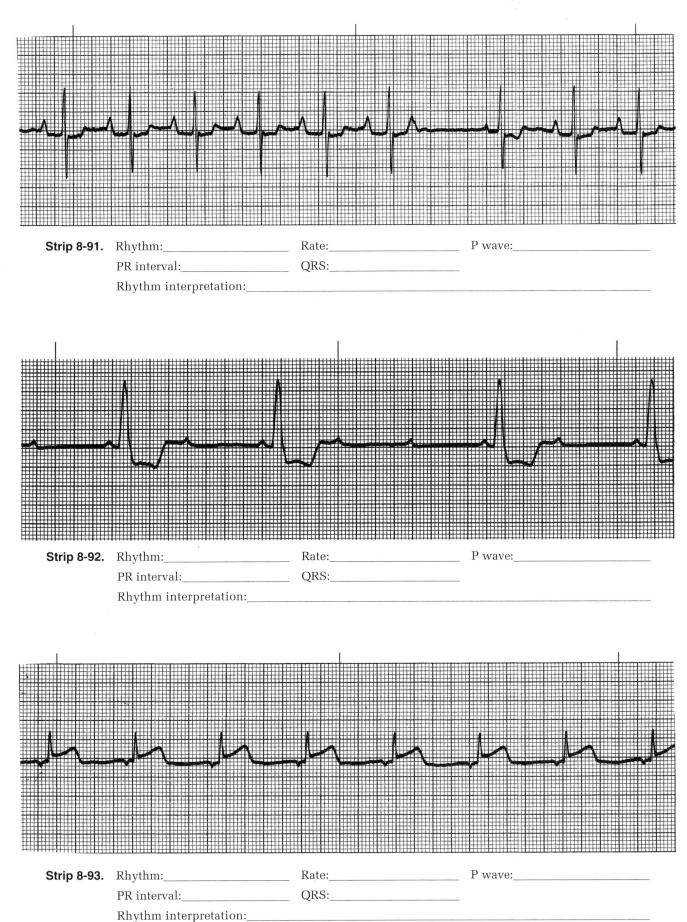

**Strip 8-91.** Rhythm:_____ Rate:_____ P wave:_____

PR interval:_____ QRS:_____

Rhythm interpretation:_____

**Strip 8-92.** Rhythm:_____ Rate:_____ P wave:_____

PR interval:_____ QRS:_____

Rhythm interpretation:_____

**Strip 8-93.** Rhythm:_____ Rate:_____ P wave:_____

PR interval:_____ QRS:_____

Rhythm interpretation:_____

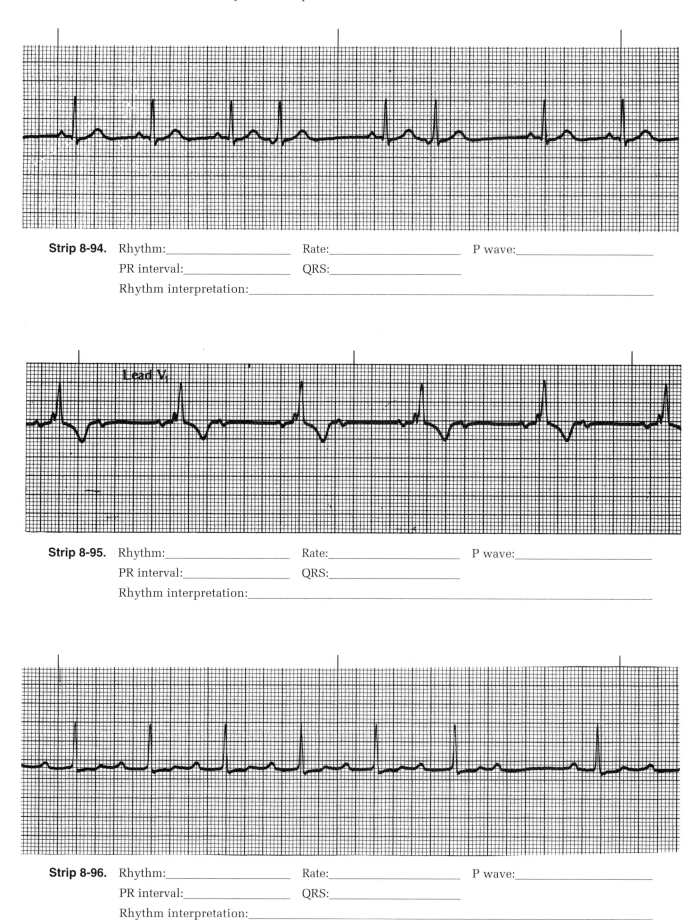

**Strip 8-94.** Rhythm:_____ Rate:_____ P wave:_____

PR interval:_____ QRS:_____

Rhythm interpretation:_____

Lead V₁

**Strip 8-95.** Rhythm:_____ Rate:_____ P wave:_____

PR interval:_____ QRS:_____

Rhythm interpretation:_____

**Strip 8-96.** Rhythm:_____ Rate:_____ P wave:_____

PR interval:_____ QRS:_____

Rhythm interpretation:_____

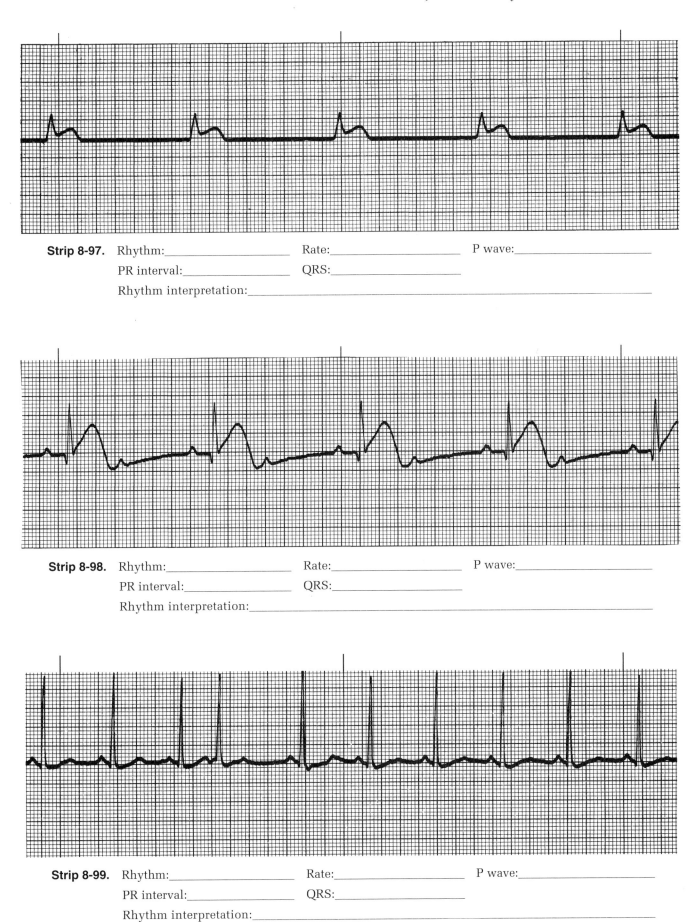

**Strip 8-97.** Rhythm:_____ Rate:_____ P wave:_____

PR interval:_____ QRS:_____

Rhythm interpretation:_____

**Strip 8-98.** Rhythm:_____ Rate:_____ P wave:_____

PR interval:_____ QRS:_____

Rhythm interpretation:_____

**Strip 8-99.** Rhythm:_____ Rate:_____ P wave:_____

PR interval:_____ QRS:_____

Rhythm interpretation:_____

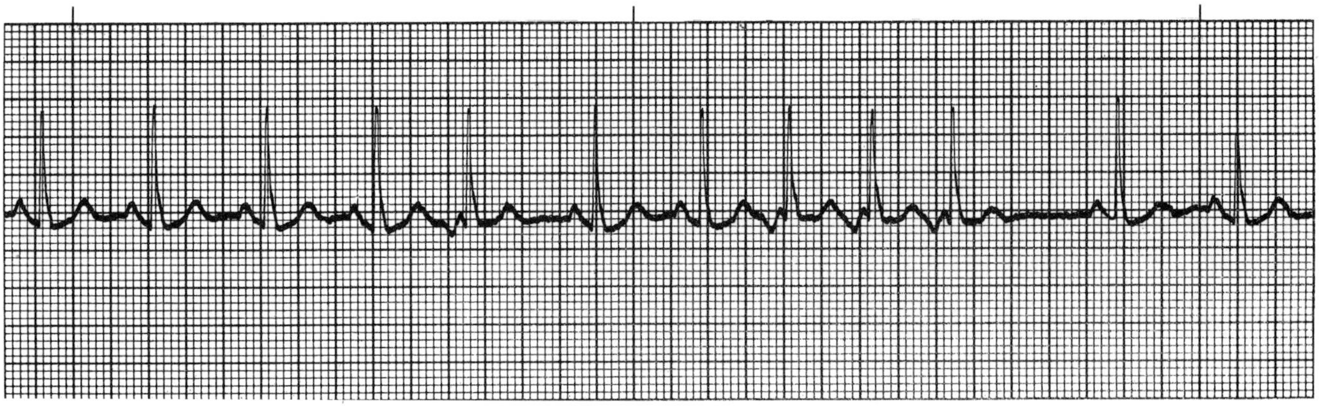

**Strip 8-100.** Rhythm:_____ Rate:_____ P wave:_____

PR interval:_____ QRS:_____

Rhythm interpretation:_____

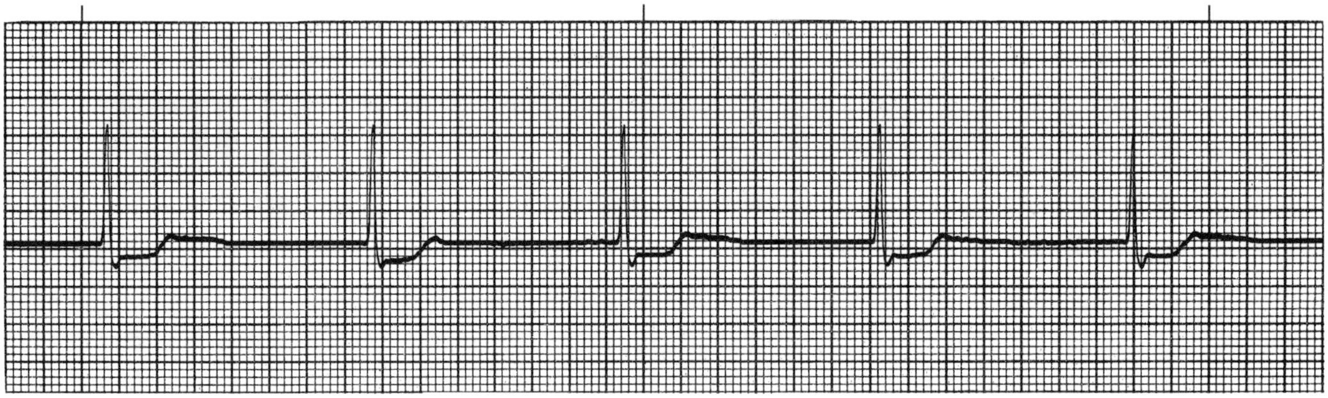

**Strip 8-101.** Rhythm:_____ Rate:_____ P wave:_____

PR interval:_____ QRS:_____

Rhythm interpretation:_____

# 9

# VENTRICULAR ARRHYTHMIAS AND BUNDLE BRANCH BLOCK

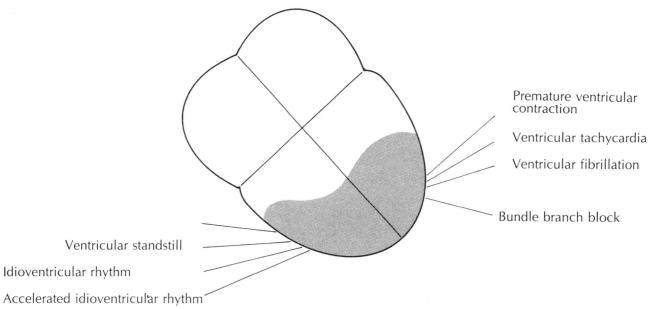

**Figure 9-1.** Ventricular arrhythmias and bundle branch block.

The three preceding chapters have focused on supraventricular arrhythmias—rhythm disturbances arising above the bundle of His in the sinus node, the atria, or the AV node. With these rhythms, the electrical impulse spreads normally through the bundle branches into the ventricles, resulting in a normal QRS complex. Ventricular arrhythmias (Figure 9-1) originate below the bundle of His in the right or left ventricle. The electrical stimulus arises from ventricular tissue and spreads through the ventricles in an abnormal manner, resulting in an abnormal QRS complex. Ventricular arrhythmias include premature ventricular contractions (PVCs), ventricular tachycardia, ventricular fibrillation, idioventricular rhythm, accelerated idioventricular rhythm, and ventricular standstill. All of these rhythms are associated with a wide QRS complex (except ventricular fibrillation and ventricular standstill). The impulse focus in bundle branch block does not originate in ventricular tissue, but it is included in this rhythm group because of the location of the block within the intraventricular system and the resulting wide QRS complex. Most of these rhythms are, or have the potential to be, life-threatening and demand prompt recognition and treatment.

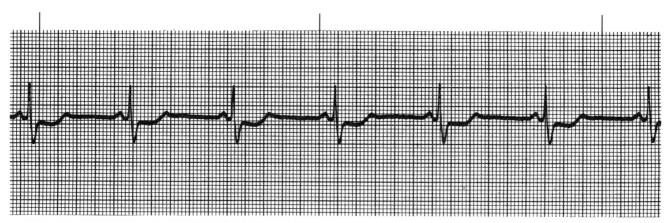

**Figure 9-2.** **Sinus Bradycardia with Bundle Branch Block**

*Rhythm:* Regular

*Rate:* 54

*P waves:* Sinus P waves are present

*PR:* 0.14 to 0.16 seconds

*QRS:* 0.12 seconds

*Comment:* ST segment depression is present.

## BUNDLE BRANCH BLOCK

A bundle branch block (Figures 9-2 through 9-4; Box 9-1) refers to an obstruction in the transmission of the electrical impulse through one of the branches (either right or left) of the bundle of His. Normally, the electrical impulses travel through the right bundle branch and the left bundle branch and their fascicles simultaneously, causing synchronous depolarization of the right and left ventricles. Normal ventricular depolarization is completed within 0.10 seconds or less. A block in one bundle branch causes the ventricle on that side to be depolarized later than the ventricle on the intact side. This delay results in an abnormal QRS complex—one that is wide (0.12 seconds or more in duration) and bizarre in size and shape. The presence of a bundle branch block can be recognized by a single monitoring lead by the appearance of the wide, bizarre QRS complex. However, differentiating between right and left bundle branch block requires a 12-lead ECG.

Right bundle branch block (RBBB) may be present in people with organic heart disease, or it may occur in normal people without any underlying heart disease. RBBB may be permanent or transient.

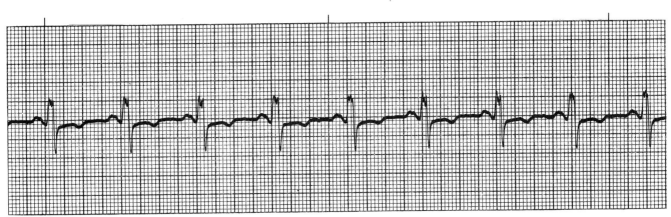

**Figure 9-3.** **Normal Sinus Rhythm with Bundle Branch Block**

| | |
|---|---|
| *Rhythm:* | Regular |
| *Rate:* | 75 |
| *P waves:* | Sinus P waves are notched which could indicate left atrial enlargement |
| *PR:* | 0.14 to 0.16 seconds |
| *QRS:* | 0.12 seconds |
| *Comment:* | A notched QRS complex is a common pattern with RBBB. |

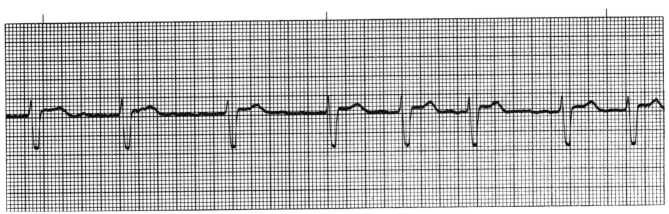

**Figure 9-4.** **Atrial Fibrillation with Bundle Branch Block**

| | |
|---|---|
| *Rhythm:* | Irregular |
| *Rate:* | 60 |
| *P waves:* | Wavy fibrillation waves |
| *PR:* | Not measurable |
| *QRS:* | 0.12–0.14 seconds |

Sometimes, it appears only when the heart rate exceeds a certain critical value (rate-related bundle branch block). Common causes of RBBB are: anteroseptal myocardial infarction, pulmonary embolism, congestive heart failure, pericarditis, myocarditis, hypertensive heart disease, cardiac tumors, cardiomyopathy, congenital right bundle branch block, and chronic degenerative disease of the electrical conduction system. It may also occur after cardiac surgery and in syphilitic, rheumatic, and congenital heart disease.

---

**Box 9-1. Bundle Branch Block: Identifying ECG Features**

| | |
|---|---|
| Rhythm: | Regular |
| Rate: | Rate is that of underlying rhythm (usually sinus) |
| P waves: | Sinus |
| PR: | Normal (0.12–0.20 seconds) |
| QRS: | Wide (0.12 seconds or greater) |

---

Unlike RBBB, left bundle branch block (LBBB) is almost always a sign of organic heart disease. LBBB may also be permanent or transient and may be rate-related. Common causes of LBBB are anteroseptal myocardial infarction, congestive heart failure, pericarditis, myocarditis, hypertensive heart disease (the most common cause), cardiac tumors, cardiomyopathy, chronic degenerative disease of the electrical conduction system, aortic stenosis, and syphilitic, rheumatic and congenital heart disease.

A bundle branch block by itself is not significant and usually requires no treatment. However, a temporary transvenous pacemaker is indicated for the treatment of a right or left bundle branch block under the following conditions:

**1.** If a new right or left bundle branch block develops as a result of an acute myocardial infarction (MI)

**2.** If a bundle branch block is complicated by second-degree AV block or third-degree AV block, especially in the setting of an anterior MI

**3.** If a new RBBB is complicated by a block in one of the fascicles of the left bundle branch (left anterior or left posterior fascicular block)

**4.** In left bundle branch block with first-degree AV block

## PREMATURE VENTRICULAR CONTRACTIONS (PVCs)

A premature ventricular contraction (PVC; Figures 9-5 through 9-14; Box 9-2) is a premature, ectopic impulse that originates somewhere in one of the ventricles and is usually caused by enhanced automaticity. The stimulus will depolarize the ventricles abnormally, resulting in an abnormal QRS complex with the following characteristics:

**1.** The QRS is premature.

**2.** A P wave is not associated with the PVC. However, P waves associated with the underlying sinus rhythm can occasionally be seen before the PVC, or after the PVC in the ST segment or T wave (see Figure 9-8).

**3.** The QRS is wide (0.12 seconds or greater), distorted and bizarre, often notched, and appears different from the QRS complexes of the underlying rhythm.

**4.** The ST segment and T wave are usually opposite the main QRS deflection. Because depolarization is abnormal, repolarization is also abnormal.

**5.** The pause associated with the PVC is usually compensatory—that is, the measurement between the R wave preceding the PVC and the R wave after the PVC is equal to two R-R intervals of the underlying regular rhythm (see Figure 9-5). The compensatory pause occurs because the SA node is not depolarized by the ectopic ventricular beat, the discharge timing of the sinus node remains unchanged, and the basic underlying rhythm will resume on time after the PVC. Rarely, the sinus node will be depolarized by the PVC, resetting the discharge timing of the SA node and resulting in a non-compensatory pause (the measurement between the R wave preceding the PVC and the R wave after the PVC will be less than two R-R intervals of the underlying regular rhythm).

---

**Box 9-2. Premature Ventricular Contraction (PVC): Identifying ECG Features**

| | |
|---|---|
| Rhythm: | Underlying rhythm usually regular; irregular with PVC |
| Rate: | Rate is that of underlying rhythm |
| P waves: | None associated with PVC; however, P waves associated with the underlying rhythm can occasionally be seen before the PVC or after the PVC in the ST segment or T wave |
| PR: | Not measurable |
| QRS: | Premature, wide (0.12 seconds or greater), and abnormal (differ from the QRS complexes of the underlying rhythm) |

---

PVCs occur in addition to the patient's underlying rhythm and appear in various combinations. They may appear as a single beat, every other beat (bigeminal pattern, see Figure 9-6), every third beat

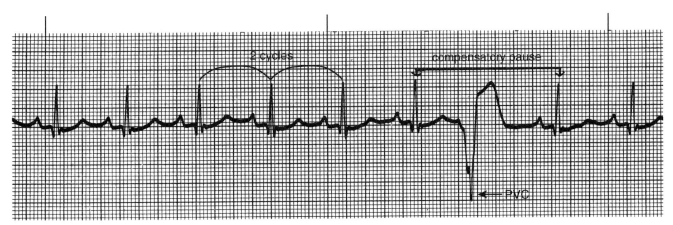

**Figure 9-5.  Normal Sinus Rhythm with One PVC**

*Rhythm:*  Basic rhythm regular; irregular with PVC

*Rate:*  Basic rhythm rate 79

*P waves:*  Sinus P waves with basic rhythm

*PR:*  0.16 to 0.20 seconds (basic rhythm)

*QRS:*  0.08 to 0.10 seconds (basic rhythm) 0.14 to 0.16 seconds (PVC)

*Comment:*  The interval between the beat preceding the PVC and the beat following the PVC is equal to the time of two normal beats and represents a full compensatory pause.

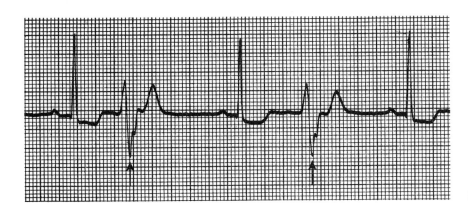

**Figure 9-6.**  Bigeminal PVCs.

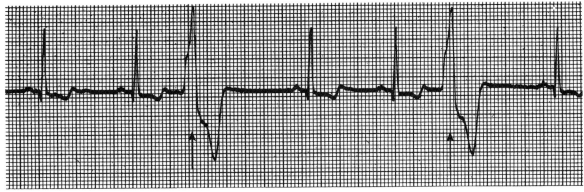

**Figure 9-7.**  Trigeminal PVCs.

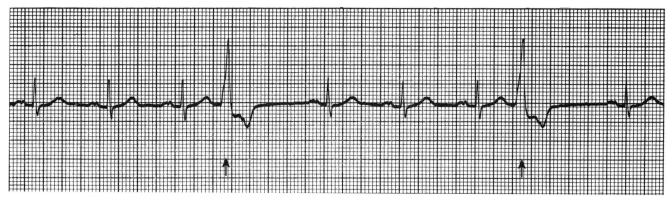

**Figure 9-8.** Quadrigeminal PVCs; the notched P wave associated with the underlying sinus rhythm can be seen after the PVCs in the ST segment.

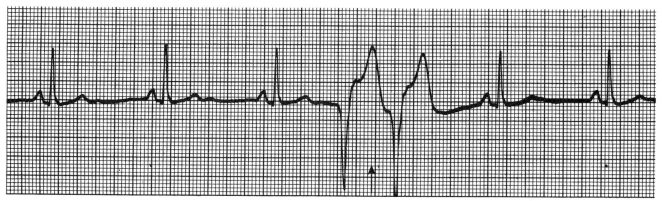

**Figure 9-9.** Paired PVCs.

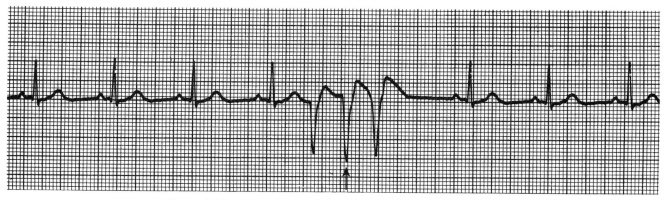

**Figure 9-10.** Run of PVCs (a burst of ventricular tachycardia).

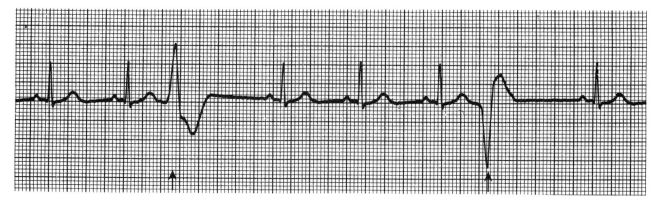

**Figure 9-11.** Multifocal PVCs.

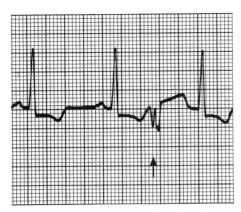

**Figure 9-12.** Interpolated PVC.

(trigeminal pattern, see Figure 9-7), every fourth beat (quadrigeminal pattern, see Figure 9-8), in pairs (also called *couplets,* see Figure 9-9), or in runs (see Figure 9-10). A run of three or more consecutive PVCs is termed *ventricular tachycardia.* PVCs that are identical in size, shape, and direction arise from the same focus in the ventricles and are called *uniform* or *unifocal PVCs.* PVCs from different ectopic sites will differ in size, shape, and direction and are called *multiform* or *multifocal PVCs* (see Figure 9-11). A PVC sandwiched between two normally conducted sinus beats, without greatly disturbing the regularity of the underlying rhythm, is called an *interpolated*

*PVC* (see Figure 9-12). The compensatory pause, usually associated with the PVC, is absent.

The *R-on-T phenomenon* (see Figure 9-13) is a term used to indicate a PVC that has occurred during the vulnerable period of ventricular repolarization (on or near the peak of the T wave). During this period, the myocardial fibers have repolarized enough to respond to a strong stimulus. Stimulation of the ventricle at this time may precipitate repetitive ventricular contractions, resulting in ventricular tachycardia or fibrillation.

Like premature atrial contractions, PVCs are very common, becoming more frequent with age. They may occur in healthy hearts as well as in people with underlying heart disease. Some of the causes of PVCs include anxiety; ingestion of caffeine, tobacco, or alcohol; certain drugs (digitalis, epinephrine, isoproterenol, aminophylline); hypoxia; acidosis; electrolyte imbalance (hypokalemia, hypomagnesemia); congestive heart failure; myocardial infarction; valvular, hypertensive, or ischemic heart disease; cardiomyopathy; reperfusion after thrombolytic therapy or angioplasty; after heart surgery or contact of the endocardium with catheters (pacing leads, pulmonary artery catheters).

Treatment of PVCs should be guided by the clinical setting. Because occasional PVCs are a normal finding in healthy people, no treatment may be indi-

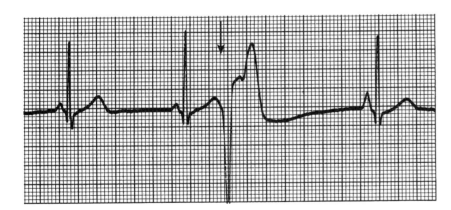

**Figure 9-13.** R-on-T PVC.

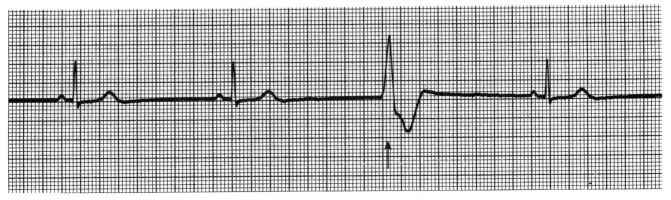

**Figure 9-14.** Ventricular escape beat.

cated. Initially, a search should be made for possible reversible causes. Elimination of certain drugs; omission of stimulants; oxygen therapy for hypoxia; treatment of congestive heart failure, hypokalemia, and hypomagnesemia may be effective in some patients. Most physicians elect not to treat PVCs unless they result in hemodynamic instability or symptomatic ventricular tachycardia. However, some may treat significant PVCs (couplets, "R-on-T" PVCs, or nonsustained runs of PVCs) in the first 24 to 48 hours after an acute MI or after cardiac surgery. Intravenous amiodarone, procainamide, or lidocaine can be used to treat significant PVCs. Oral antiarrhythmics have also been shown to be effective for PVC suppression. All antiarrhythmic agents have some degree of proarrhythmic effects and may actually worsen the rhythm problem (may induce torsades de pointes type ventricular tachycardia due to QT prolongation) making some physicians wary of using antiarrhythmics for the sole purpose of PVC suppression.

On some occasions, a ventricular beat may occur late instead of early. These beats are called *ventricular escape beats* (see Figure 9-14). Escape beats are more likely to occur as the result of an increased vagal effect on the SA node rather than to enhanced automaticity as is associated with the premature ventricular beat. Escape beats occur commonly after a pause in the underlying rhythm. The morphologic characteristics of the late beat will be the same as for the PVC. No treatment is required.

# VENTRICULAR TACHYCARDIA (VT)

Ventricular tachycardia (Figures 9-15 through 9-19; Box 9-3) is an arrhythmia originating in an ectopic focus in the ventricles, discharging impulses at a rate of 140 to 250 per minute. The rhythm is usually associated with enhanced automaticity or reentry. On the ECG, the rhythm appears as a series of wide QRS complexes at a rapid rate. Impulses originating from ventricular tissue do not produce P waves. However, the sinus node continues to beat independently, and sinus P waves may occasionally be seen between the wide QRS complexes—usually the sinus P waves are hidden in the QRS complexes. The QRS complexes are distorted and bizarre, often notched, with a duration of 0.12 seconds or greater. As a rule, the QRS complexes are identical (monomorphic). When the QRS complexes differ, the ventricular tachycardia is considered to be polymorphic. The QRS complexes are followed by large T waves, opposite in direction to the main QRS deflection. The rhythm is usually regular but may be slightly irregular. Ventricular tachycardia may occa-

sionally occur at rates greater than 250 beats per minute. At such extreme rates, the QRS complexes appear sawtooth in morphology and the rhythm is often referred to as *ventricular flutter* (see Figure 9-16). The patient becomes hemodynamically compromised very quickly because there is virtually no cardiac output. Ventricular tachycardia of this type is commonly an immediate forerunner to ventricular fibrillation.

---

**Box 9-3. Ventricular Tachycardia: Identifying ECG Features**

| | |
|---|---|
| Rhythm: | Regular |
| Rate: | 140–250 |
| P waves: | No P waves are associated with ventricular tachycardia. However, the SA node continues to beat independently and sinus P waves may occasionally be seen between the QRS complexes. Usually the P waves are hidden in the QRS. |
| PR: | Not measurable |
| QRS: | Wide (0.12 seconds or greater) |

---

Ventricular tachycardia usually occurs in patients with underlying heart disease. Common causes include myocardial ischemia, cardiomyopathy, mitral valve prolapse, congestive heart failure, or digitalis toxicity. Other causes include electrolyte disturbances (especially hypokalemia and hypomagnesemia), mechanical stimulation of the endocardium by a pacing catheter or pulmonary artery catheter, and reperfusion after thrombolytic therapy or angioplasty. The most common cause of sustained monomorphic ventricular tachycardia is coronary artery disease, usually with prior myocardial infarction. Certain medications (quinidine, procainamide, disopyramide, phenothiazines, tricyclic antidepressants, amiodarone, flecainide , ibutilide, propafenone, and sotalol) may prolong the QT interval, causing the ventricles to be particularly vulnerable to polymorphic ventricular tachycardia (torsades de pointes; see Figure 9-18).

Ventricular tachycardia is most often preceded by frequent and repetitive ventricular ectopy. Ventricular tachycardia may appear as a sustained rhythm (lasting longer than 30 seconds) or as a nonsustained rhythm (lasting less than 30 seconds) occurring in short bursts or paroxysms (see Figures 9-10 and 9-17). Three PVCs in a row are technically considered a burst of nonsustained ventricular tachycardia. Nonsustained ventricular tachycardia, unless frequent, usually does not cause hemodynamic compromise, but can progress into sustained VT. Sustained VT is a life-threatening arrhythmia for two major reasons. First, the rapid ventricular rate and loss of atrial kick reduce cardiac output, leading

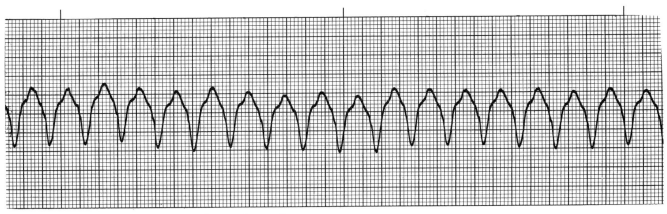

**Figure 9-15. Ventricular Tachycardia**

| | |
|---|---|
| *Rhythm:* | Regular |
| *Rate:* | 150 |
| *P waves:* | None identified |
| *PR:* | Not measurable |
| *QRS:* | 0.14–0.16 seconds |

to hypotension and decreased perfusion to vital organs. Second, the condition may degenerate into ventricular fibrillation.

Treatment of VT depends on how well the rhythm is tolerated by the patient. Patient tolerance is related to the ventricular rate and the underlying left ventricular function. As part of the initial assessment, you should check for a pulse. If there is no pulse (pulseless VT), the rhythm must be treated as ventricular fibrillation. If there is a pulse, protocols for VT with a pulse are followed and fall under stable and unstable categories.

### Stable Monomorphic VT With a Pulse

If there is a pulse and the patient is stable (eg, adequate level of consciousness, warm skin, acceptable blood pressure [usually 90 mmHg systolic or greater], no chest pain or dyspnea), the following guidelines are suggested:

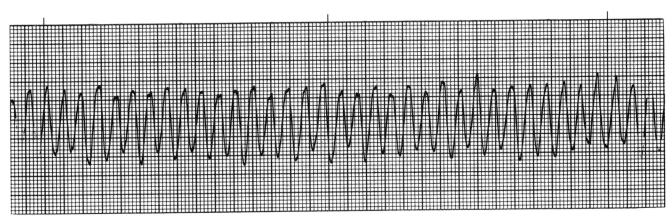

**Figure 9-16. Ventricular Flutter**

| | |
|---|---|
| *Rhythm:* | Regular |
| *Rate:* | 375 |
| *P waves:* | Not seen |
| *PR:* | Not measurable |
| *QRS:* | 0.12–0.14 seconds |
| *Comment:* | Ventricular flutter is a form of ventricular tachycardia. The ventricular rate is so fast the QRS complexes have a sawtooth appearance. |

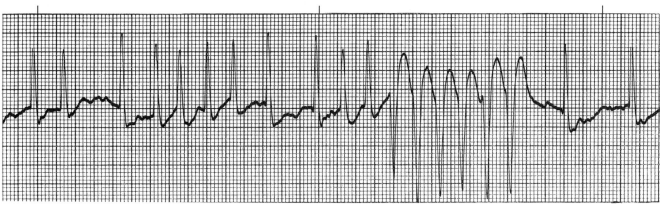

**Figure 9-17. Atrial Fibrillation with a Burst of Ventricular Tachycardia**

| | |
|---|---|
| *Rhythm:* | Basic rhythm irregular; ventricular tachycardia regular |
| *Rate:* | 160 (basic rhythm) 250 (VT rate) |
| *P waves:* | Fibrillation waves in basic rhythm; none with VT |
| *PR:* | Not measurable |
| *QRS:* | 0.08–0.10 seconds (basic rhythm); 0.12 seconds (VT) |

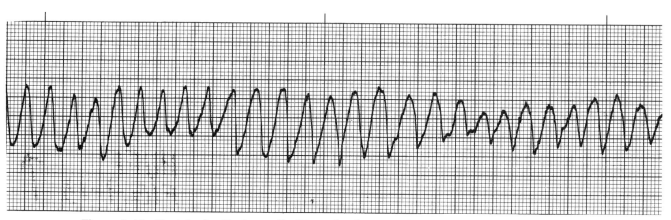

**Figure 9-18. Ventricular Tachycardia (Torsades de pointes)**

| | |
|---|---|
| *Rhythm:* | Regular |
| *Rate:* | 250 |
| *P waves:* | None identified |
| *PR:* | Not measurable |
| *QRS:* | 0.12–0.22 seconds (some much wider than others) |
| *Comment:* | This type of ventricular tachycardia is called torsades de pointes (twists of points). The QRS changes from negative to positive polarity and appears to twist around the isoelectric line. It is associated with a prolonged QT interval and is refractory to antiarrhythmics. Intravenous magnesium or overdrive pacing has been successful in the treatment of this rhythm. |

1. Use any ONE of the following medications:
   a. Amiodarone is given as a 150-mg IV bolus over 10 minutes followed by a 1-mg/min infusion over 6 hours, and then a 0.5-mg/min infusion for 18 hours. Additional 150-mg IV bolus doses can be repeated for recurrent or resistant arrhythmias to a maximum dose of 2.2 g in 24 hours (maximum includes bolus and infusion doses). The major side effects from amiodarone are bradycardia and hypotension. Amiodarone can also induce torsades de pointes VT, although the drug has a lower incidence of proarrhythmic effects than other

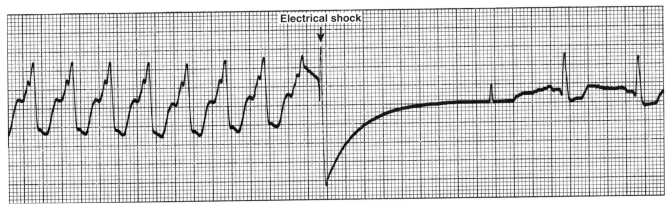

**Figure 9-19.** Electrical cardioversion of ventricular tachycardia to sinus rhythm.

antiarrhythmic drugs under similar circumstances.

**b.** Lidocaine is given as a 1- to 1.5-mg/kg IV bolus followed by one half the initial dose (0.5 to 0.75-mg/kg IV bolus) every 5 to 10 minutes to a maximum dose of 3 mg/kg. The maintenance infusion rate is 1 to 4 mg/min. Reappearance of the arrhythmia during a continuous infusion of lidocaine should be treated with a small IV bolus dose (0.5 mg/kg) and an increase in the infusion rate. The half-life of lidocaine increases after 24 to 48 hours. Therefore, after 24 hours, the dosage should be reduced or blood levels should be monitored. Signs of toxicity include slurred speech, altered consciousness, muscle twitching, seizures, and bradycardia.

**c.** Procainamide can be given in an infusion of 20 to 30 mg/min until the arrhythmia is suppressed, significant hypotension occurs, the QRS complex doubles its pretreatment width, or a total dose of 17 mg/kg is given. The maintenance infusion rate is 1 to 4 mg per minute. Rapid administration of procainamide exacerbates hypotension. Procainamide also prolongs the QT interval.

**d.** Sotalol is approved only in oral form in the United States for ventricular arrhythmias. The initial dose is 80 mg orally twice a day for 3 days, then 160 mg twice a day for 3 days, and may be increased to 240 to 320 mg twice a day, if necessary. Sotalol can cause bradycardia or hypotension, and can prolong the QT interval.

**2.** If the rhythm is unresponsive to drug therapy, sedate the patient and perform electrical cardioversion beginning at 100 joules (or equivalent biphasic energy level), increasing joules (200, 300, 360) with subsequent attempts.

If the patient has an ejection fraction of less than 40% or has congestive heart failure, the recommended guidelines are:

**1.** Use ONE of the following medications:
**a.** Amiodarone—same dose as above
**b.** Lidocaine is given in a reduced dose of 0.5 to 0.75 mg/kg IV bolus, and this dose can be repeated every 5 to 10 minutes to a maximum dose of 3 mg/kg.

**2.** If the rhythm is unresponsive to drug therapy, sedate the patient and perform electrical cardioversion.

All antiarrhythmic medications have some degree of proarrhythmic effects. Sequential use of more than one antiarrhythmic agent compounds the adverse effects, particularly for bradycardia, hypotension, and torsades de pointes. Never use more than one agent unless absolutely necessary. When an appropriate dose of a single antiarrhythmic medication fails to terminate an arrhythmia, turn to electrical cardioversion rather than a second antiarrhythmic medication. Figure 9-19 shows electrical cardioversion of ventricular tachycardia to a sinus rhythm.

### Unstable Monomorphic VT With a Pulse

If there is a pulse and the patient is unstable (eg, decreased level of consciousness; cool, clammy skin; blood pressure less than 90 mmHg systolic; dyspneic, complaining of chest pain; or, in extreme situations, unconscious, cyanotic, having seizures), the following guidelines are suggested:

**1.** Sedate the patient (if conscious).

**2.** Cardiovert the rhythm at 100 joules initially (or equivalent biphasic energy level), increasing the joules (200, 300, 360) with subsequent attempts. Once electrical cardioversion has terminated the rhythm, antiarrhythmic medication is usually started to prevent reoccurrence of the arrhythmia.

Treatment of chronic, recurrent ventricular tachycardia includes therapy with oral antiarrhythmic drugs. Further evaluation may include specialized electrophysiologic testing and endocardial mapping, with long-term options including use of the implantable cardioverter defibrillator (ICD) or reentry circuit ablation. The ICD is a special, surgically implanted device developed to deliver an electric shock directly to the heart during a life-threatening tachycardia. Destruction (ablation) of the reentry circuit involves delivering short pulses of radiofrequency current through an intracardiac catheter. It produces a small burn that effectively blocks the part of the circuit supporting the reentrant-type wave.

A special type of polymorphic ventricular tachycardia is called *torsades de pointes* (see Figure 9-18), a French term meaning "twisting of the points." In this arrhythmia, the direction of the QRS complexes seems to rotate, pointing downward for a series of beats and then twisting and pointing upward in the same lead. The ventricular rate is extremely rapid (much faster than monomorphic VT), and the patient usually becomes hemodynamically compromised very quickly. Ventricular tachycardia of this type is commonly an immediate forerunner to ventricular fibrillation.

Torsades de pointes classically occurs in the setting of delayed ventricular repolarization, evidenced by prolongation of the QT interval or the presence of prominent U waves. It can be caused by certain antiarrhythmic drugs (eg, procainamide, quinidine, disopyramide, amiodarone, propafenone, and sotalol) used in the treatment of "ordinary" or monomorphic VT. Hypocalcemia, hypokalemia, hypomagnesemia, and bradycardias can also initiate torsades de pointes as well as psychotropic drugs (eg, phenothiazines, tricyclic antidepressants), liquid protein diets, and congenital disorders that cause a prolonged QT interval.

Recognition of torsades de pointes is critical because the treatment plan differs greatly from the treatment of monomorphic VT. Drugs conventionally used in treating monomorphic VT can cause torsades de pointes and, if given, are usually ineffective and may make the rhythm worse. Treatment of torsades de pointes includes:

**1.** Removing or correcting causative factors (eg, drug effects, electrolyte imbalances, underlying bradycardia)—the rhythm has a tendency to recur unless the precipitating factors are eliminated.

**2.** Magnesium may be administered as a loading dose of 1 to 2 g in 50 cc D5W over 5 minutes followed by a maintenance infusion of 0.5 to 1.0 g per hour. Rapid administration of magnesium may cause significant hypotension or asystole and should be avoided.

**3.** If the rhythm is believed to be precipitated by bradycardia, a temporary pacemaker may be inserted to accomplish "overdrive" suppression of the arrhythmia by increasing the underlying heart rate and thereby increasing ventricular repolarization time.

**4.** Drug therapy with isoproterenol, phenytoin, or lidocaine may be used in select cases.

## VENTRICULAR FIBRILLATION

In ventricular fibrillation (Figures 9-20 and 9-21; Box 9-4), a disorganized, chaotic, electrical focus in the ventricles takes over control of the heart. The ventricles do not beat in any coordinated fashion but, instead, quiver asynchronously and ineffectively just

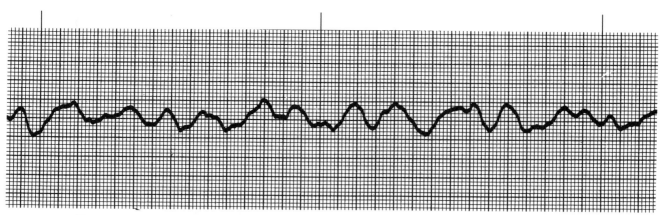

**Figure 9-20. Ventricular Fibrillation ("coarse" wave forms)**

| | |
|---|---|
| *Rhythm:* | Chaotic |
| *Rate:* | 0 (no QRS complexes are present) |
| *P waves:* | None; wave deflections are chaotic and vary in size, shape, and height |
| *PR:* | Not measurable |
| *QRS:* | Absent |

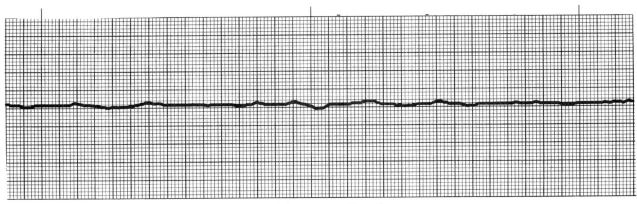

**Figure 9-21. Ventricular Fibrillation ("fine" wave forms)**

*Rhythm:* Chaotic

*Rate:* 0 (no QRS complexes are present)

*P waves:* Absent; wave deflections are chaotic and vary in size, shape, and height

*PR:* Not measurable

*QRS:* Absent

as the atria respond in atrial fibrillation. The ECG tracing shows an undulating, wavy baseline composed of irregular waveforms that vary in amplitude and morphology. Ventricular fibrillation waves represent chaotic, incomplete, and haphazard depolarization of small groups of muscle fibers in the ventricles. Because organized depolarization of the atria and ventricles is absent, P waves and QRS complexes are also absent. If the fibrillatory waves are large, the arrhythmia is considered to be "coarse" ventricular fibrillation (see Figure 9-20). If the fibrillatory waves are small, the arrhythmia is considered to be "fine" ventricular fibrillation (see Figure 9-21). The distinction between the two may be significant because coarse ventricular fibrillation usually indicates a more recent onset and is more likely to be reversed by defibrillation alone. Fine ventricular fibrillation usually indicates that the arrhythmia has been present longer and may require drug therapy first, then defibrillation, before the arrhythmia can be reversed. Fine ventricular fibrillation will progress to ventricular asystole unless defibrillation restores the cardiac rhythm.

**Box 9-4. Ventricular Fibrillation: Identifying ECG Features**

Rhythm: Chaotic; irregular deflections

Rate: 0 (P waves and QRS complexes are absent)

P waves: Absent; deflections seen are chaotic, irregular undulations that vary in size, shape, and height; deflections may be small (described as "fine") or large (described as "coarse")

PR: Not measurable

QRS: Absent

Ventricular fibrillation can occur in patients with heart disease of any type. It may be preceded by significant PVCs (occurring in pairs, runs, multifocal, R-on-T type) or ventricular tachycardia, but can also occur spontaneously. It is the most common cause of sudden cardiac death in patients with an acute myocardial infarction. Other causes of ventricular fibrillation include myocardial ischemia, cardiomyopathy, mitral valve prolapse, cardiac trauma, hypoxia, cocaine toxicity, electrolyte imbalances, acidosis, and drug toxicity (especially digitalis and proarrhythmic agents). Ventricular fibrillation may also occur during anesthesia, cardiac catheterization procedures, pacemaker implantation, placement of a Swan-Ganz pulmonary artery catheter, or after accidental electrocution.

Once ventricular fibrillation occurs, there is no cardiac output, peripheral pulses and blood pressure are absent, and the patient becomes unconscious immediately. Cyanosis and seizure activity may also be present. Death is imminent unless the arrhythmia is treated immediately. Treatment protocols include:

1. Check the pulse and rapidly assess the patient—if there is a pulse and/or the patient is conscious, ventricular fibrillation is not the problem. ECG artifacts produced by loose or dry electrodes, patient movement, or muscle tremors, may resemble ventricular fibrillation.

2. If there is no pulse and the patient is unconscious, defibrillate up to three times (200 joules, 300 joules, 360 joules or equivalent biphasic).

3. If unsuccessful, start CPR; establish an IV line; intubate patient.

4. Administer epinephrine 1 mg IV push and re-

peat every 3 to 5 minutes OR vasopressin 40 units IV push, single dose, one time only (in 10–20 minutes, if single dose vasopressin is ineffective, may continue with epinephrine 1 mg IV push every 3 to 5 minutes).

**5.** Continue CPR for 1 minute to circulate drug; defibrillate at 360 joules × 1.

**6.** Consider ONE of the following antiarrhythmics:

    **a.** Amiodarone 300 mg IV push (cardiac arrest dose); if ventricular fibrillation is refractory or recurs, consider additional administration of 150 mg IV push; if drug therapy is successful, a maintenance infusion of amiodarone can be started at 1 mg/min for 6 hours followed by 0.5 mg/min for 18 hours (maximum cumulative dose: 2.2 g in 24 hours).

    **b.** Lidocaine 1 to 1.5 mg/kg IV push followed by one half the initial dose (0.5 to 0.75 mg/kg IV push) every 5 to 10 minutes to a maximum dose of 3 mg/kg. If drug therapy is successful, a maintenance infusion of lidocaine can be started at 1 to 4 mg/min.

    **c.** Procainamide infusion of 20 to 30 mg/min to maximum dose of 17 mg/kg; procainamide is acceptable but not recommended because prolonged administration time is unsuitable for cardiac arrest.

**7.** Continue drug therapy, CPR, and defibrillation attempts (drug–CPR–shock pattern) until rhythm resolves or a decision is made to stop resuscitative efforts.

## IDIOVENTRICULAR RHYTHM (VENTRICULAR ESCAPE RHYTHM)

Idioventricular rhythm (IVR; Figure 9-22; Box 9-5) is an arrhythmia originating in a subsidiary pacemaker site in the ventricles, with a heart rate between 30 and 40 per minute (sometimes less). Because the impulse focus is in the ventricles, the ECG tracing is characterized by an absence of P waves and the presence of wide QRS complexes occurring at a regular rate.

| Box 9-5. Idioventricular Rhythm: Identifying ECG Features | |
| --- | --- |
| Rhythm: | Usually regular |
| Rate: | 30–40 (sometimes slower) |
| P waves: | Absent |
| PR: | Not measurable |
| QRS: | Wide (0.12 seconds or greater) |

Idioventricular rhythm is considered an escape rhythm. It occurs (1) when the rate of impulse formation of the dominant pacemaker (usually the sinus node) and the backup pacemaker in the AV node becomes less than the pacemaker in the ventricles or (2) when the electrical impulse from the SA node, atria, or AV node fails to reach the ventricles because of sinus arrest, sinus block, or third-degree AV block. When an electrical impulse fails to arrive in the ventricles, latent (or subsidiary) pacemaker cells in the ventricles take over pacemaker function at their inherent firing rate of 40 or below. The result may be an escape beat (see Figure 9-14) or a ventricular escape rhythm.

Ventricular escape rhythm may be transient or continuous. Transient idioventricular rhythm is seen as three or more ventricular beats lasting only a few seconds or minutes, is usually related to increased vagal effect on the higher pacing centers, and is not significant. Continuous idioventricular rhythm associated with third-degree heart block can generally be treated with pacemaker therapy and has a better prognosis than idioventricular rhythm not associated with AV block. Continuous idioventricular rhythm not associated with AV block is seen in advanced heart disease and is often the cardiac arrhythmia present just before the final arrhythmia, ventricular standstill (asystole). Continuous idioventricular rhythm is generally symptomatic because of the marked reduction in cardiac output due to the slow rate and loss of the atrial kick.

The goal of treatment is not to eradicate the rhythm with suppressive agents, but to stimulate a rhythm from a higher pacemaker site, if possible. Treatment may include:

**1.** Administer atropine 0.5 to 1.0 mg IV push; may repeat every 3 to 5 minutes until the heart rate increases or a total dose of 0.04 mg/kg is given; atropine may be ineffective for idioventricular rhythm associated with third-degree heart block.

**2.** Initiate transcutaneous pacing.

**3.** If the patient is hypotensive, start a dopamine infusion at 5 to 20 μg/kg/min; if symptoms are severe, go directly to a epinephrine infusion at 2 to 10 μg/kg/min.

**4.** Consider insertion of a temporary transvenous pacemaker; chronic idioventricular rhythm associated with third-degree AV block will require insertion of a permanent pacemaker.

## ACCELERATED IDIOVENTRICULAR RHYTHM

Accelerated idioventricular rhythm (AIVR; Figures 9-23 and 9-24; Box 9-6) is an arrhythmia originating in

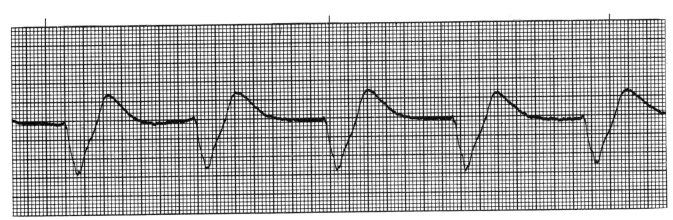

**Figure 9-22. Idioventricular Rhythm**

*Rhythm:*   Regular

*Rate:*   44

*P waves:*   Absent

*PR:*   Not measurable

*QRS:*   0.32 seconds

an ectopic pacemaker site in the ventricles with a rate between 50 and 100 per minute. The term *accelerated* denotes a rhythm that exceeds the inherent idioventricular escape rate of 30 to 40 but is not fast enough to be ventricular tachycardia. This rhythm is usually related to enhanced automaticity of the ventricular tissue. AIVR has the same ECG characteristics as idioventricular rhythm and is differentiated by the heart rate.

AIVR is common after an inferior MI and is frequently a reperfusion rhythm as a result of thrombolytic agents, angioplasty, or spontaneous reperfusion. AIVR may also result from digitalis toxicity or

cardiomyopathy. Brief episodes of AIVR frequently alternate with periods of normal sinus rhythm (see Figure 9-24).

**Box 9-6. Accelerated Idioventricular Rhythm: Identifying ECG Features**

| | |
|---|---|
| Rhythm: | Usually regular |
| Rate: | 50–100 |
| P waves: | Absent |
| PR: | Not measurable |
| QRS: | Wide (0.12 seconds or greater) |

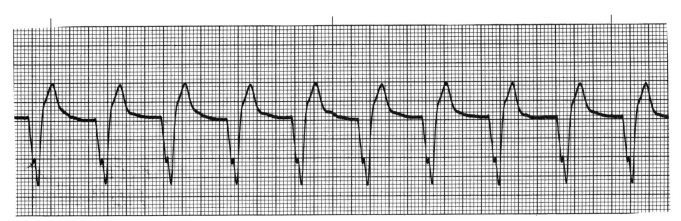

**Figure 9-23. Accelerated Idioventricular Rhythm**

*Rhythm:*   Regular

*Rate:*   84

*P waves:*   None identified

*PR:*   Not measurable

*QRS:*   0.16 seconds

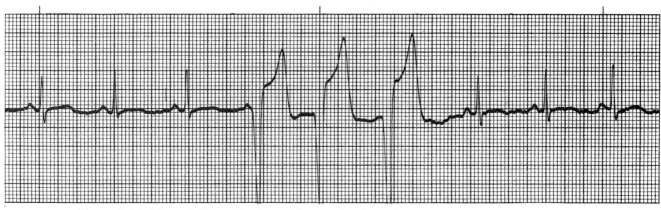

**Figure 9-24.** **Normal Sinus Rhythm with Episode of Accelerated Idioventricular Rhythm**

*Rhythm:*       Basic rhythm regular; AIVR basically regular; (off by 2 squares)

*Rate:*           79 basic rhythm; AIVR rate (around 80)

*P waves:*      Sinus P waves with basic rhythm; none with AIVR

*PR interval:* 0.12–0.16 seconds

*QRS:*           0.06–0.08 seconds (basic rhythm); 0.12 seconds AIVR

AIVR is a transient arrhythmia that is usually well tolerated and produces no hemodynamic effects. The ventricular rate is within normal limits and usually adequate to maintain cardiac output. Suppressive therapy is not recommended because abolishing the ventricular rhythm may leave an even less desirable heart rate. Treatment is usually not required.

## VENTRICULAR STANDSTILL (VENTRICULAR ASYSTOLE)

Ventricular standstill or asystole (Figures 9-25 and 9-26; Box 9-7) is the absence of all electrical ac-

tivity within the ventricles. The ECG tracing will show either P waves without QRS complexes or a straight line. If P waves are present, the arrhythmia was most likely preceded by some type of advanced AV block (Mobitz II or third-degree). Ventricular standstill with a straight line is usually the terminal arrhythmia after ventricular tachycardia, ventricular fibrillation, or idioventricular rhythm. Ventricular standstill may also occur in metabolic acidosis, hypoxia, hyperkalemia, hypokalemia, hypothermia, or drug overdose. Prognosis is extremely poor despite resuscitative efforts (usually as low as 1 to 2 people out of 100 cardiac arrests). The only hope for resuscitation of a person in asystole is to identify and treat a reversible cause.

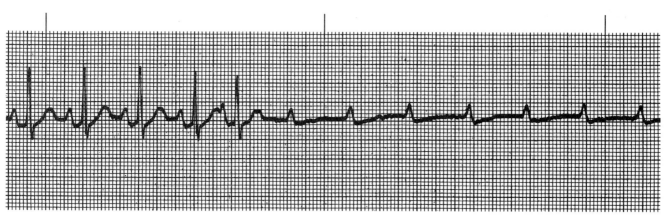

**Figure 9-25.** **Normal Sinus Rhythm with One PAC Changing to Ventricular Standstill**

*Rhythm:*    Basic rhythm regular

*Rate:*        Basic rhythm 100

*P waves:*   Sinus P waves are present

*PR:*          0.16 to 0.18 seconds (basic rhythm)

*QRS:*        0.06 seconds (basic rhythm)

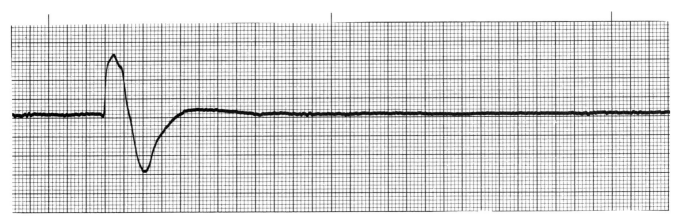

**Figure 9-26. One Wide Ventricular Complex Changing to Ventricular Standstill**

*Rhythm:*    0

*Rate:*    0

*P waves:*    None identified

*PR:*    Not measurable

*QRS:*    0.28 seconds or wider

**Box 9-7. Ventricular Standstill: Identifying ECG Features**

Rhythm:    0 (no QRS complexes are present)

Rate:    0 (no QRS complexes are present)

P waves:    ECG tracing will show either P waves without QRS complexes or a straight line.

PR:    Not measurable

QRS:    Absent

Once ventricular standstill occurs, there is no cardiac output, peripheral pulses and blood pressure are absent, and the patient becomes unconscious immediately. Cyanosis and seizure activity may also be present. Death is imminent unless the arrhythmia is treated immediately. Without ECG monitoring, ventricular standstill cannot be distinguished from ventricular fibrillation at the bedside. Treatment protocols include:

**1.** Check pulse and rapidly assess the patient. If there is a pulse and/or the patient is conscious, ventricular standstill is not the problem.

**2.** Check monitor lead system. A loose electrode pad or leadwire will show a straight line. Check monitor rhythm in two leads, if possible. Fine waveform ventricular fibrillation may mimic ventricular standstill.

**3.** Start CPR; establish IV line; intubate the patient.

**4.** Apply transcutaneous pacemaker. To be effective, this must be performed early combined with drug therapy.

**5.** Give epinephrine 1 mg IV, and continue CPR to circulate drug; drug may be repeated every 3 to 5 minutes.

**6.** Give atropine 1 mg IV, and continue CPR to circulate drug; drug may be repeated every 3 to 5 minutes until total dose of 0.04 mg/kg is given.

**7.** Continue administration of epinephrine, atropine, and CPR until rhythm is resolved or a decision is made to discontinue resuscitative efforts.

With asystole refractory to treatment, the patient is making the transition from life to death. Medical personnel should try to make that transition as sensitive and dignified as possible.

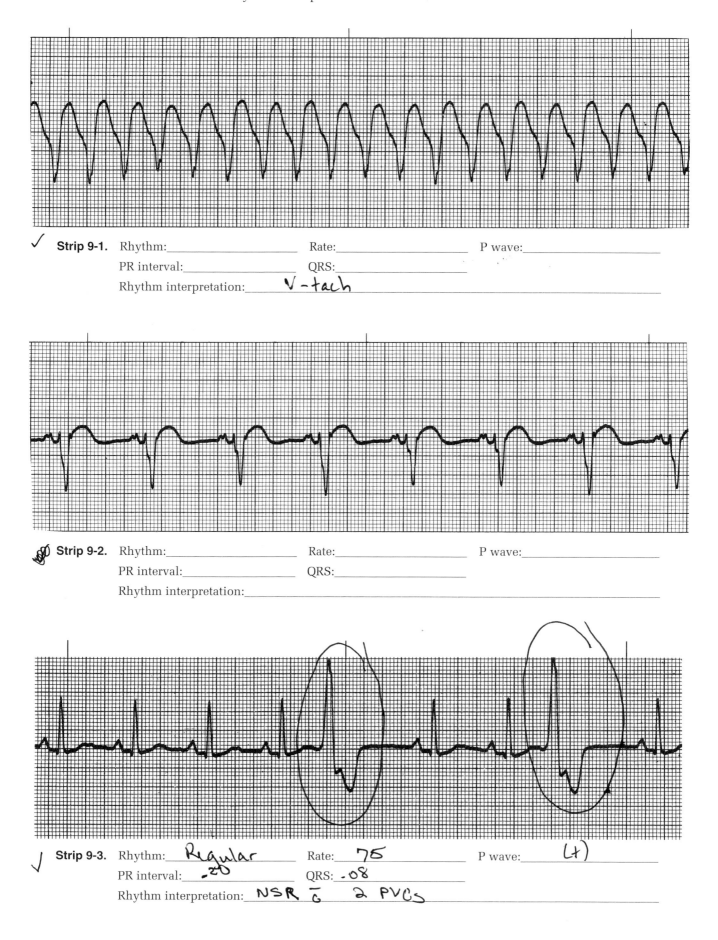

✓ **Strip 9-1.** Rhythm:_____ Rate:_____ P wave:_____

PR interval:_____ QRS:_____

Rhythm interpretation:_____V-tach_____

**Strip 9-2.** Rhythm:_____ Rate:_____ P wave:_____

PR interval:_____ QRS:_____

Rhythm interpretation:_____

✓ **Strip 9-3.** Rhythm:___Regular___ Rate:___75___ P wave:___(+)___

PR interval:___.20___ QRS:_.08_

Rhythm interpretation:___NSR c̄   2 PVCs___

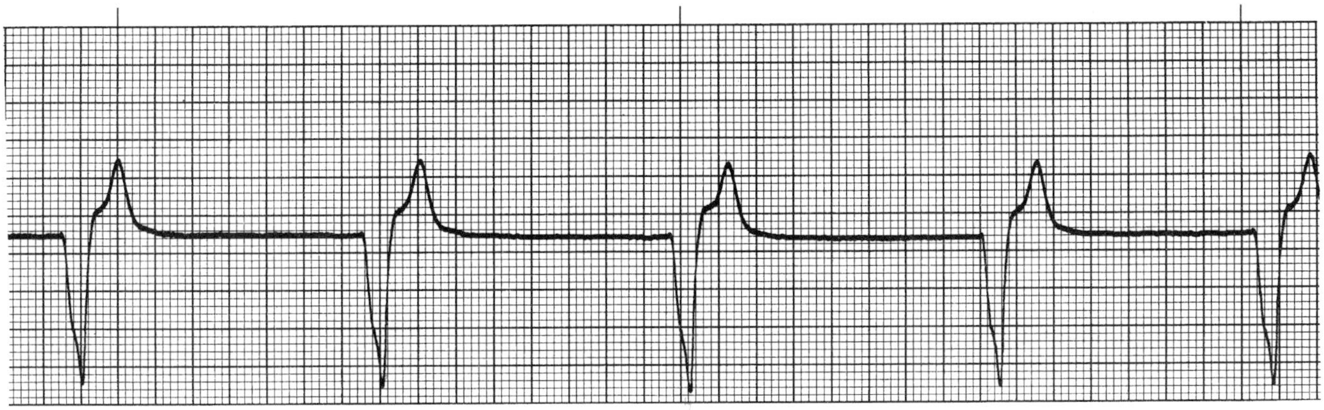

**Strip 9-4.** Rhythm: _Regular_  Rate: _37_  P wave: _____

PR interval: _Ø_  QRS: _.12_

Rhythm interpretation: _Idioventricular_

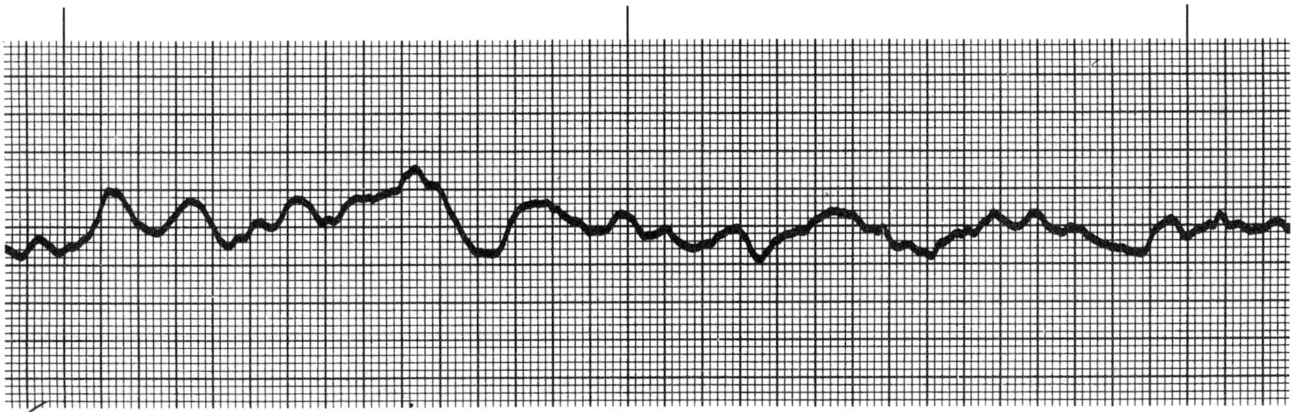

**Strip 9-5.** Rhythm: _____  Rate: _____  P wave: _____

PR interval: _____  QRS: _____

Rhythm interpretation: _Coarse V-fib_

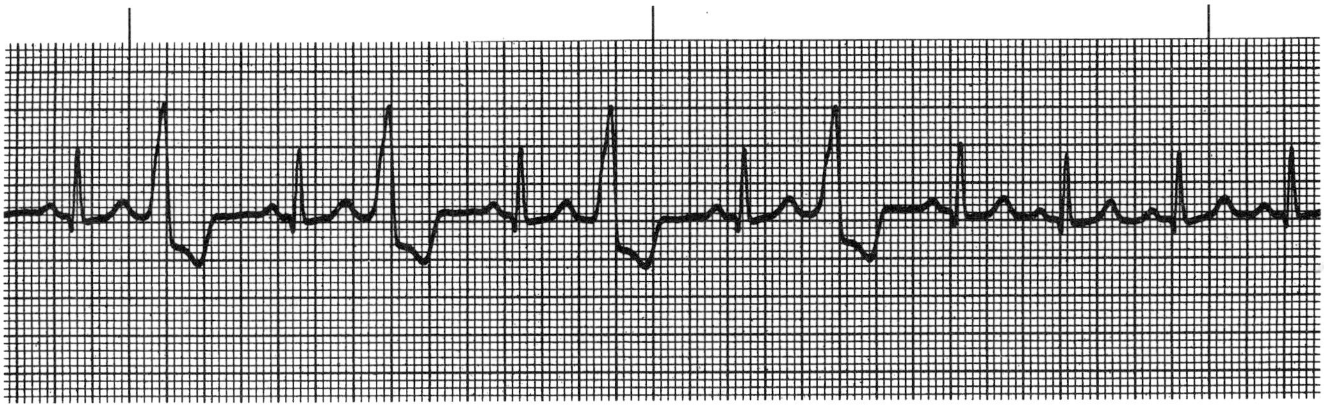

**Strip 9-6.** Rhythm: _____  Rate: _____  P wave: _____

PR interval: _____  QRS: _____

Rhythm interpretation: _____

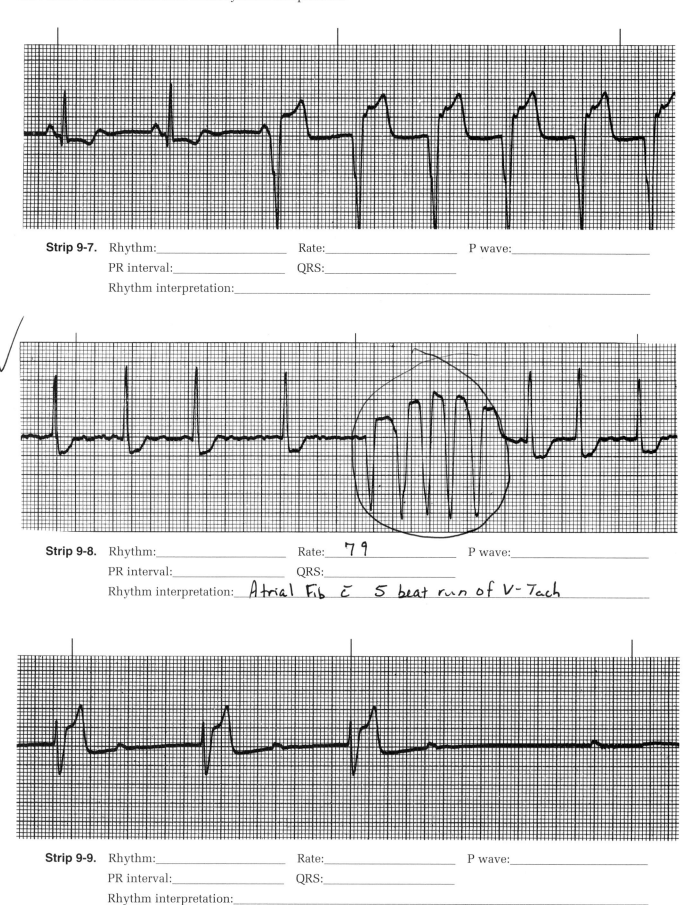

**Strip 9-7.** Rhythm:_____ Rate:_____ P wave:_____

PR interval:_____ QRS:_____

Rhythm interpretation:_____

**Strip 9-8.** Rhythm:_____ Rate: _79_____ P wave:_____

PR interval:_____ QRS:_____

Rhythm interpretation: _Atrial Fib c̄ 5 beat run of V-Tach_____

**Strip 9-9.** Rhythm:_____ Rate:_____ P wave:_____

PR interval:_____ QRS:_____

Rhythm interpretation:_____

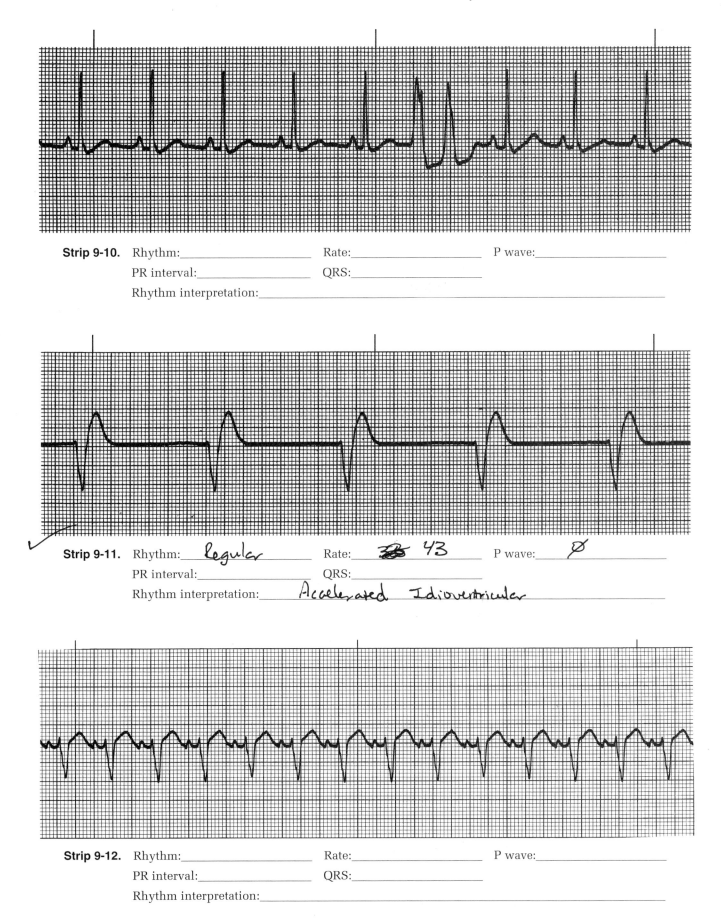

**Strip 9-10.** Rhythm:_____ Rate:_____ P wave:_____

PR interval:_____ QRS:_____

Rhythm interpretation:_____

**Strip 9-11.** Rhythm:_Regular_ Rate:_~~335~~ 43_ P wave:_Ø_

PR interval:_____ QRS:_____

Rhythm interpretation:_Accelerated Idioventricular_

**Strip 9-12.** Rhythm:_____ Rate:_____ P wave:_____

PR interval:_____ QRS:_____

Rhythm interpretation:_____

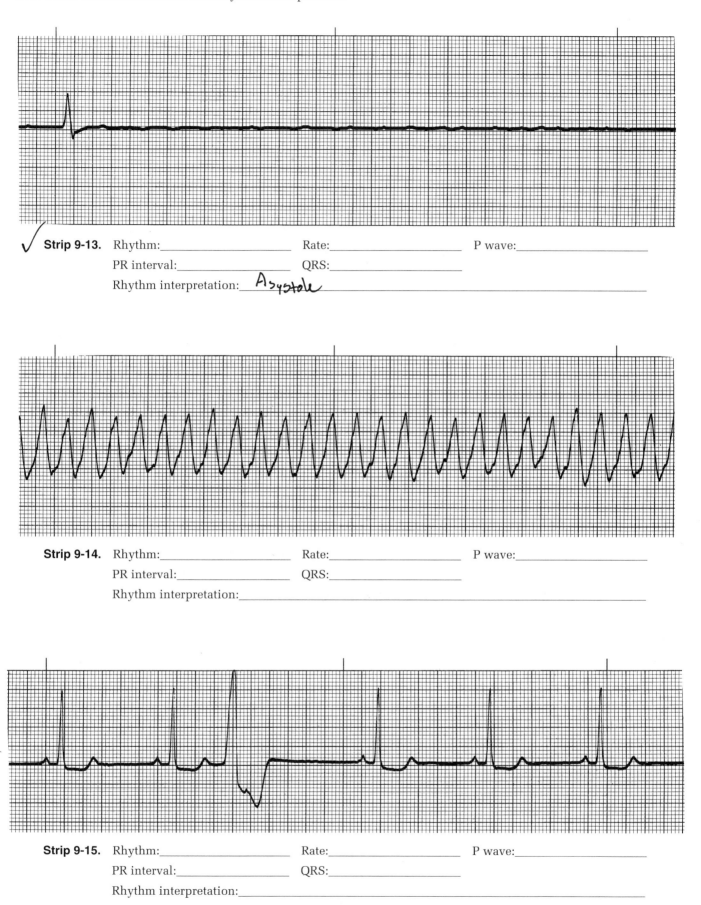

**Strip 9-13.** Rhythm:_____ Rate:_____ P wave:_____

PR interval:_____ QRS:_____

Rhythm interpretation:___Asystole_____

**Strip 9-14.** Rhythm:_____ Rate:_____ P wave:_____

PR interval:_____ QRS:_____

Rhythm interpretation:_____

**Strip 9-15.** Rhythm:_____ Rate:_____ P wave:_____

PR interval:_____ QRS:_____

Rhythm interpretation:_____

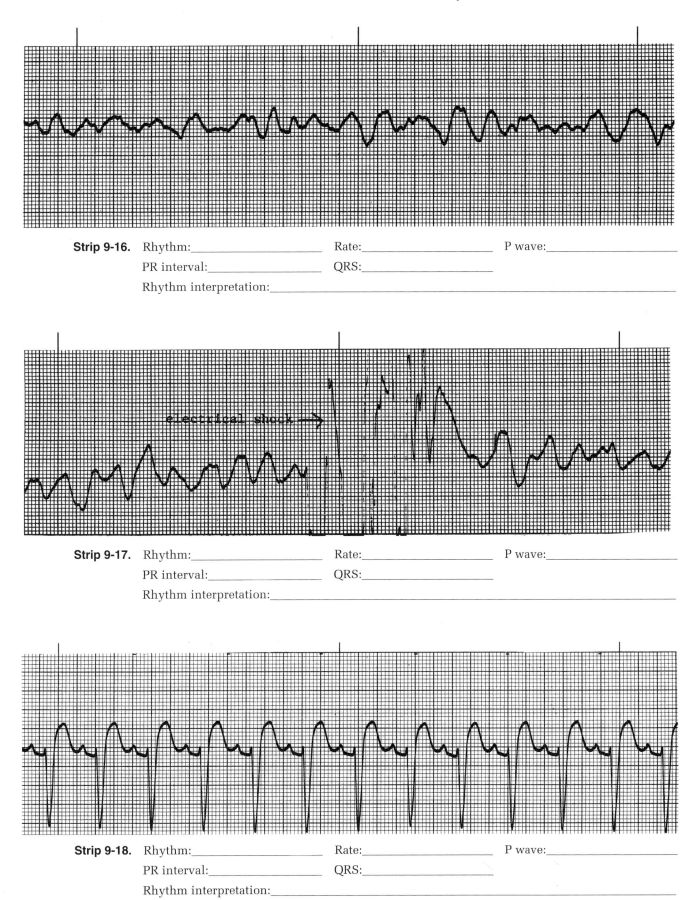

**Strip 9-16.** Rhythm:_____ Rate:_____ P wave:_____

PR interval:_____ QRS:_____

Rhythm interpretation:_____

**Strip 9-17.** Rhythm:_____ Rate:_____ P wave:_____

PR interval:_____ QRS:_____

Rhythm interpretation:_____

**Strip 9-18.** Rhythm:_____ Rate:_____ P wave:_____

PR interval:_____ QRS:_____

Rhythm interpretation:_____

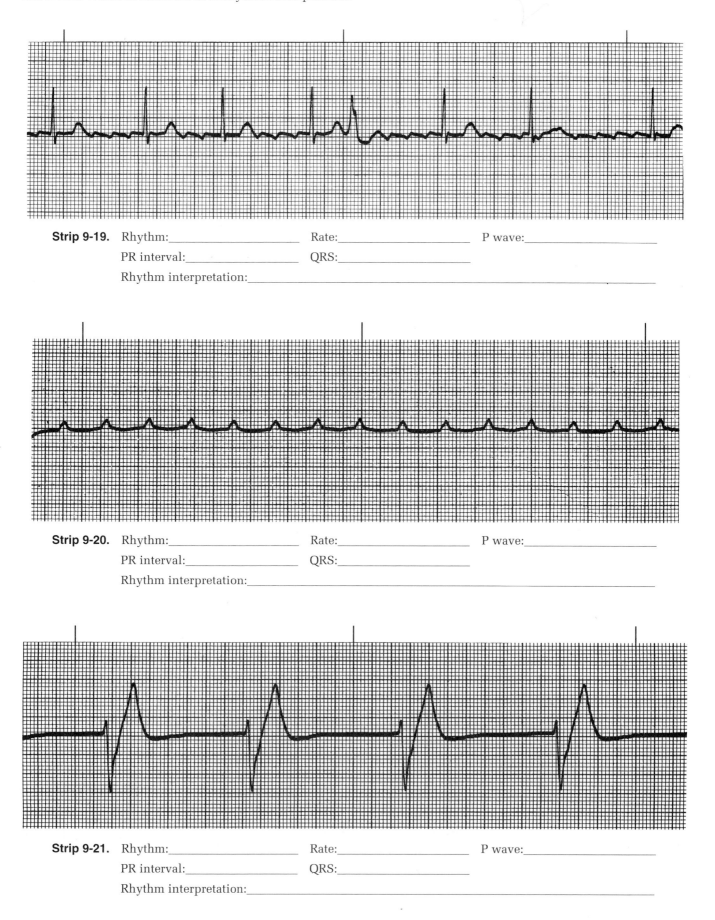

**Strip 9-19.** Rhythm:_____ Rate:_____ P wave:_____

PR interval:_____ QRS:_____

Rhythm interpretation:_____

**Strip 9-20.** Rhythm:_____ Rate:_____ P wave:_____

PR interval:_____ QRS:_____

Rhythm interpretation:_____

**Strip 9-21.** Rhythm:_____ Rate:_____ P wave:_____

PR interval:_____ QRS:_____

Rhythm interpretation:_____

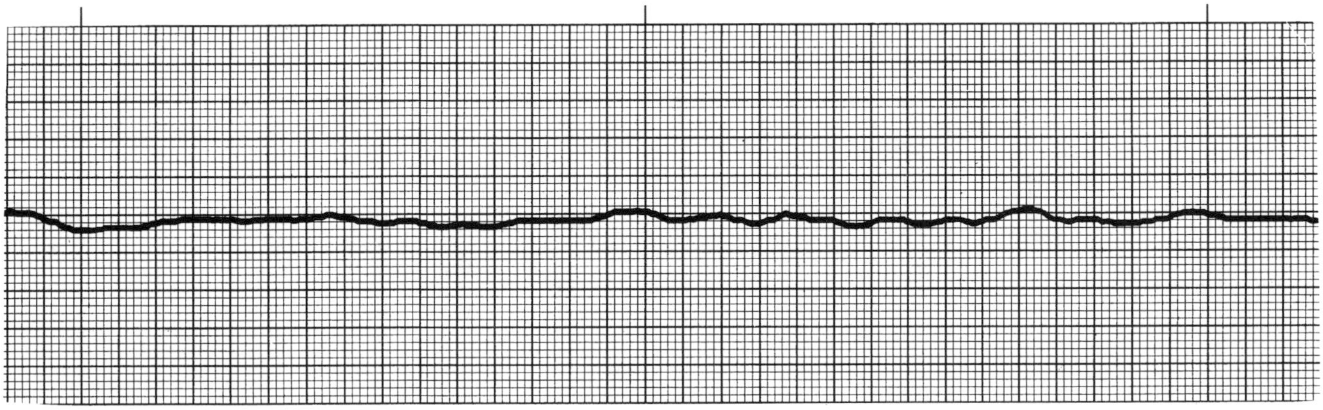

**Strip 9-22.** Rhythm:_____ Rate:_____ P wave:_____

PR interval:_____ QRS:_____

Rhythm interpretation:_____

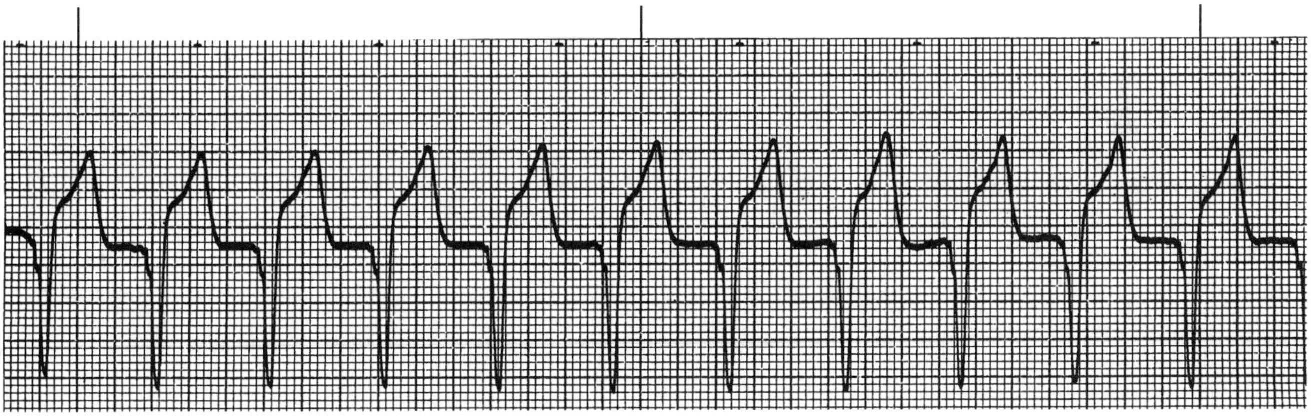

**Strip 9-23.** Rhythm:_____ Rate:_____ P wave:_____

PR interval:_____ QRS:_____

Rhythm interpretation:_____

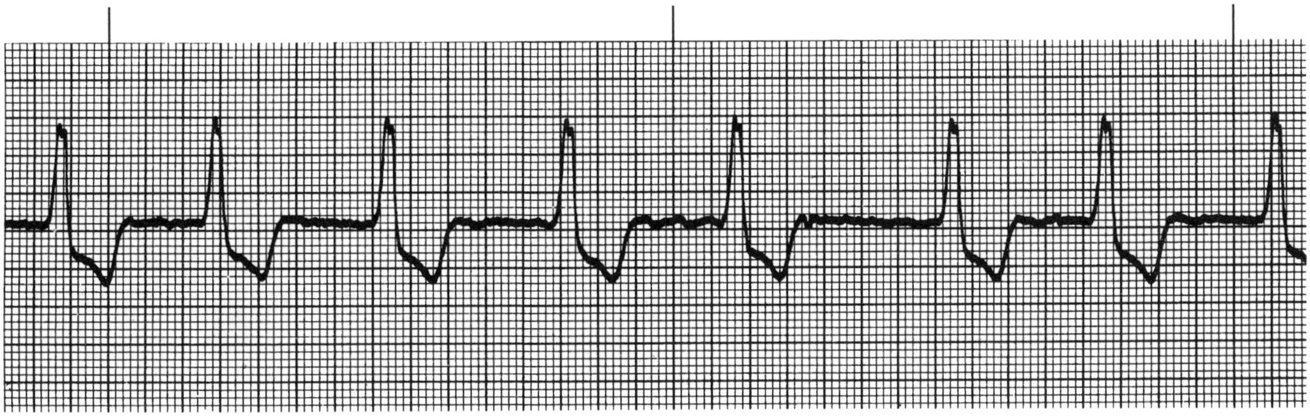

**Strip 9-24.** Rhythm:_____ Rate:_____ P wave:_____

PR interval:_____ QRS:_____

Rhythm interpretation:_____

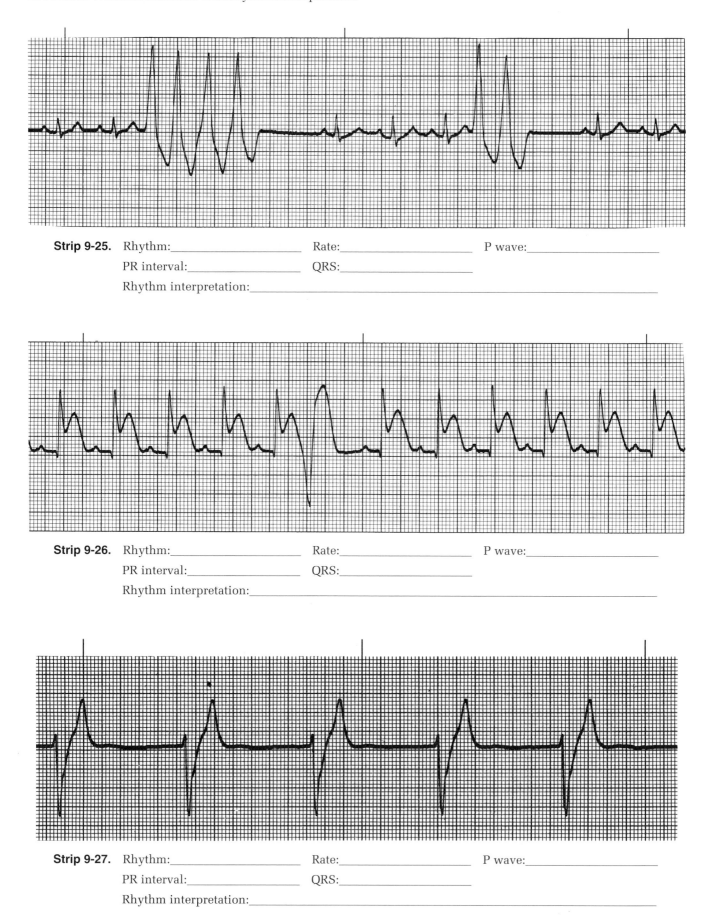

**Strip 9-25.** Rhythm:_____ Rate:_____ P wave:_____

PR interval:_____ QRS:_____

Rhythm interpretation:_____

**Strip 9-26.** Rhythm:_____ Rate:_____ P wave:_____

PR interval:_____ QRS:_____

Rhythm interpretation:_____

**Strip 9-27.** Rhythm:_____ Rate:_____ P wave:_____

PR interval:_____ QRS:_____

Rhythm interpretation:_____

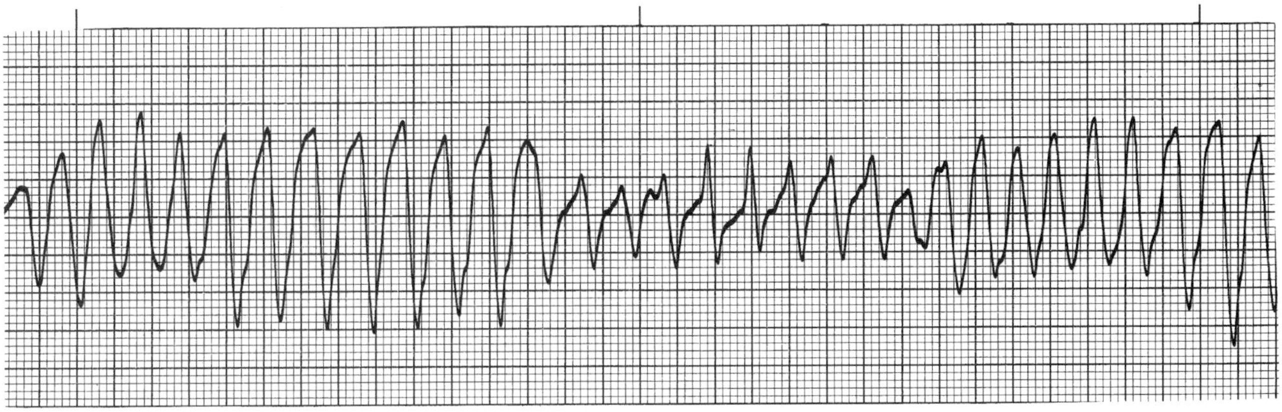

**Strip 9-28.** Rhythm:_____ Rate:_____ P wave:_____

PR interval:_____ QRS:_____

Rhythm interpretation:_____

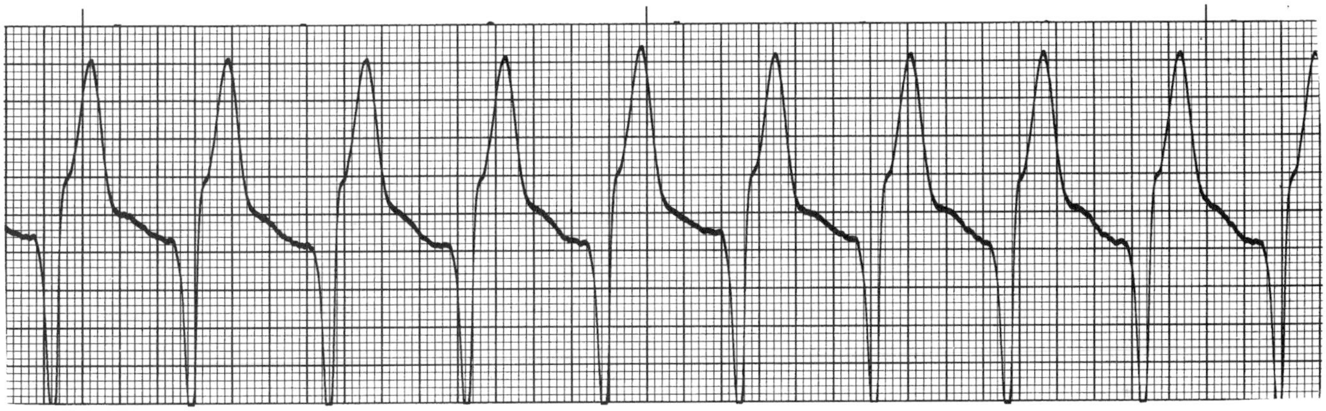

**Strip 9-29.** Rhythm:_____ Rate:_____ P wave:_____

PR interval:_____ QRS:_____

Rhythm interpretation:_____

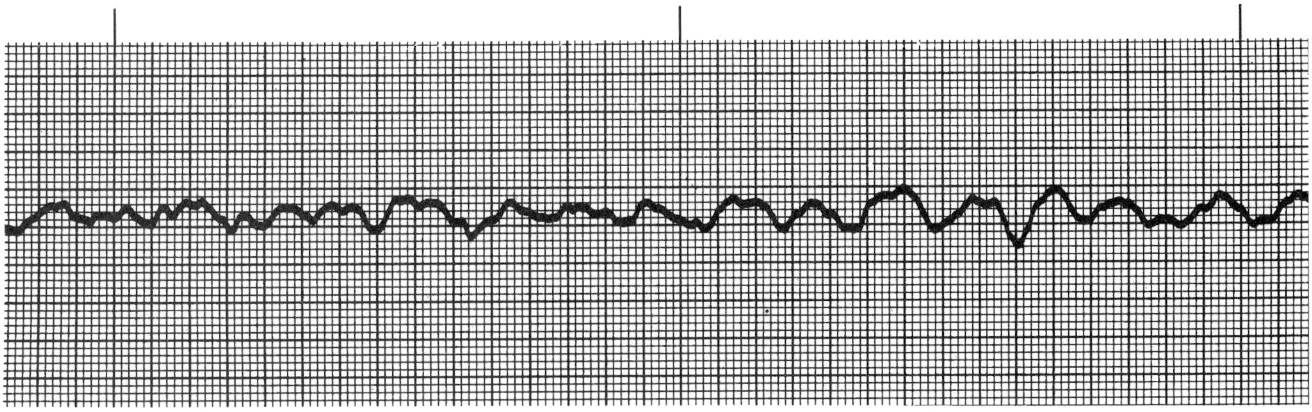

**Strip 9-30.** Rhythm:_____ Rate:_____ P wave:_____

PR interval:_____ QRS:_____

Rhythm interpretation:_____

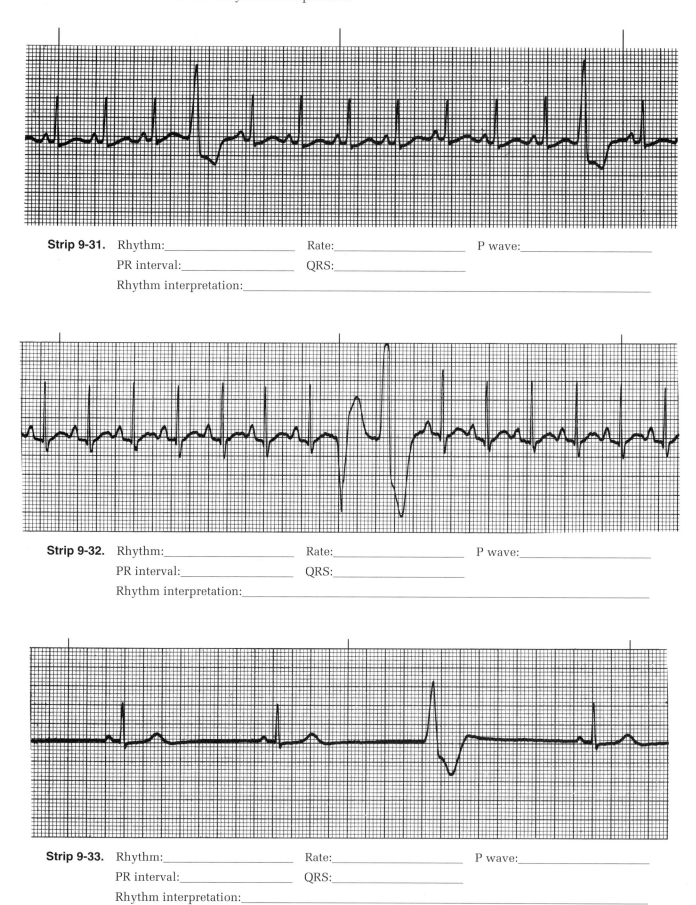

**Strip 9-31.** Rhythm:_____  Rate:_____  P wave:_____

PR interval:_____  QRS:_____

Rhythm interpretation:_____

**Strip 9-32.** Rhythm:_____  Rate:_____  P wave:_____

PR interval:_____  QRS:_____

Rhythm interpretation:_____

**Strip 9-33.** Rhythm:_____  Rate:_____  P wave:_____

PR interval:_____  QRS:_____

Rhythm interpretation:_____

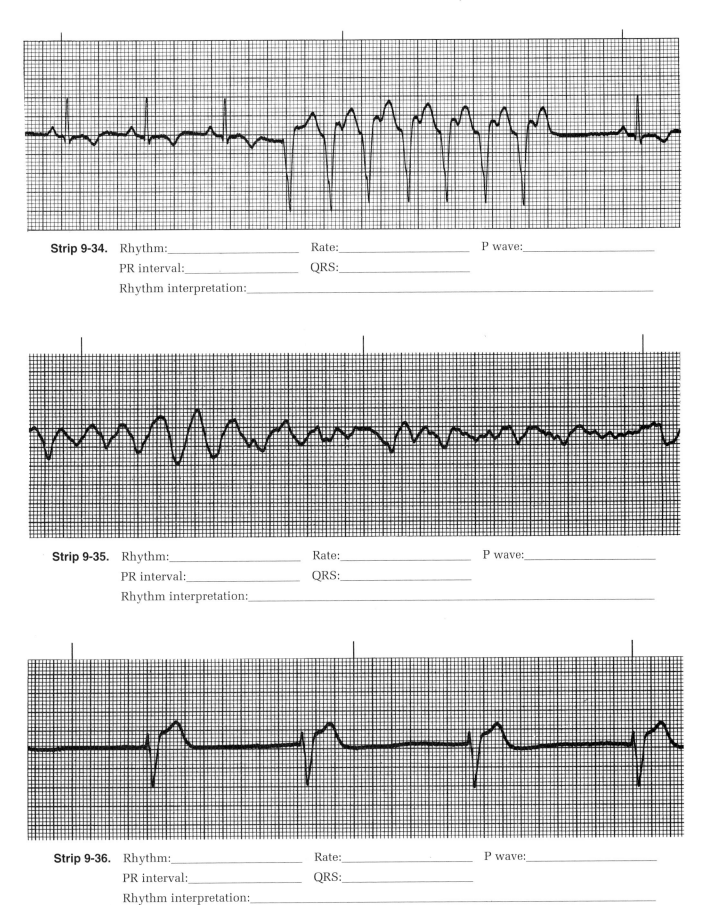

**Strip 9-34.** Rhythm:_____ Rate:_____ P wave:_____

PR interval:_____ QRS:_____

Rhythm interpretation:_____

**Strip 9-35.** Rhythm:_____ Rate:_____ P wave:_____

PR interval:_____ QRS:_____

Rhythm interpretation:_____

**Strip 9-36.** Rhythm:_____ Rate:_____ P wave:_____

PR interval:_____ QRS:_____

Rhythm interpretation:_____

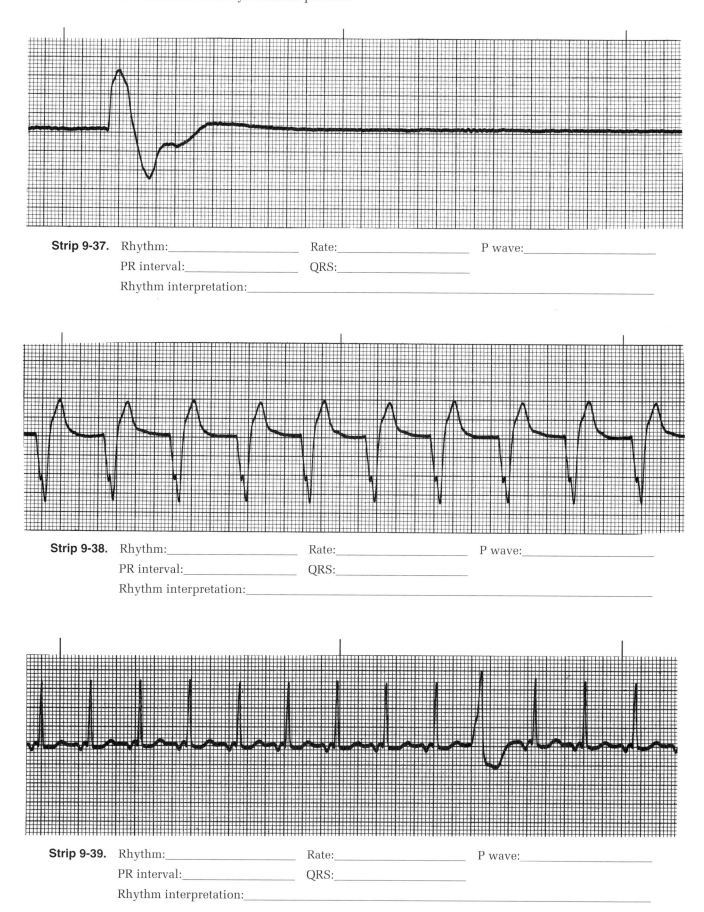

**Strip 9-37.** Rhythm:_____ Rate:_____ P wave:_____

PR interval:_____ QRS:_____

Rhythm interpretation:_____

**Strip 9-38.** Rhythm:_____ Rate:_____ P wave:_____

PR interval:_____ QRS:_____

Rhythm interpretation:_____

**Strip 9-39.** Rhythm:_____ Rate:_____ P wave:_____

PR interval:_____ QRS:_____

Rhythm interpretation:_____

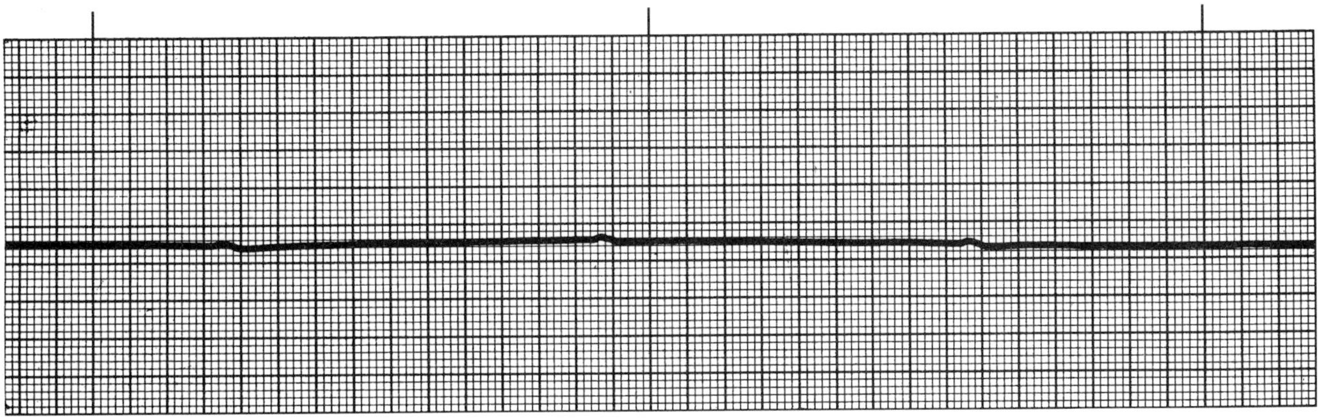

**Strip 9-40.** Rhythm:_____ Rate:_____ P wave:_____

PR interval:_____ QRS:_____

Rhythm interpretation:_____

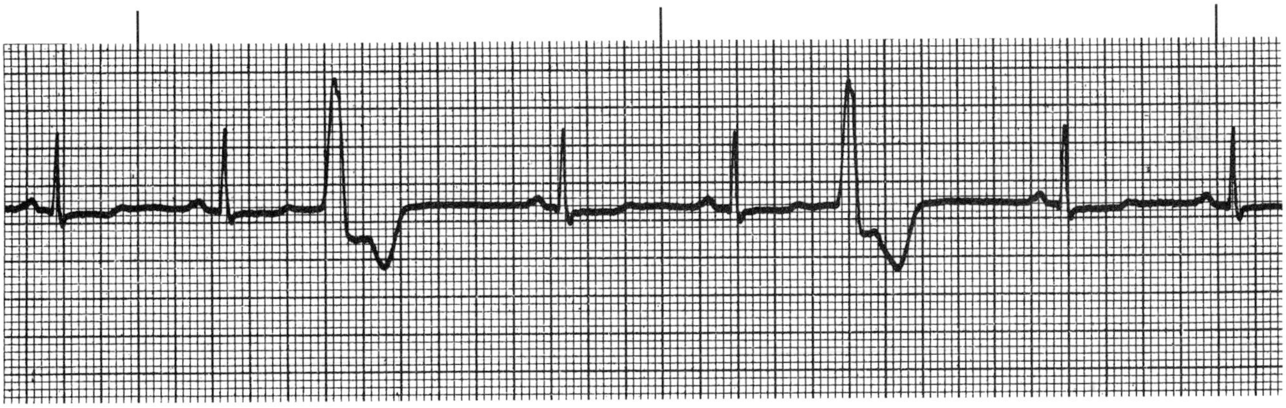

**Strip 9-41.** Rhythm:_____ Rate:_____ P wave:_____

PR interval:_____ QRS:_____

Rhythm interpretation:_____

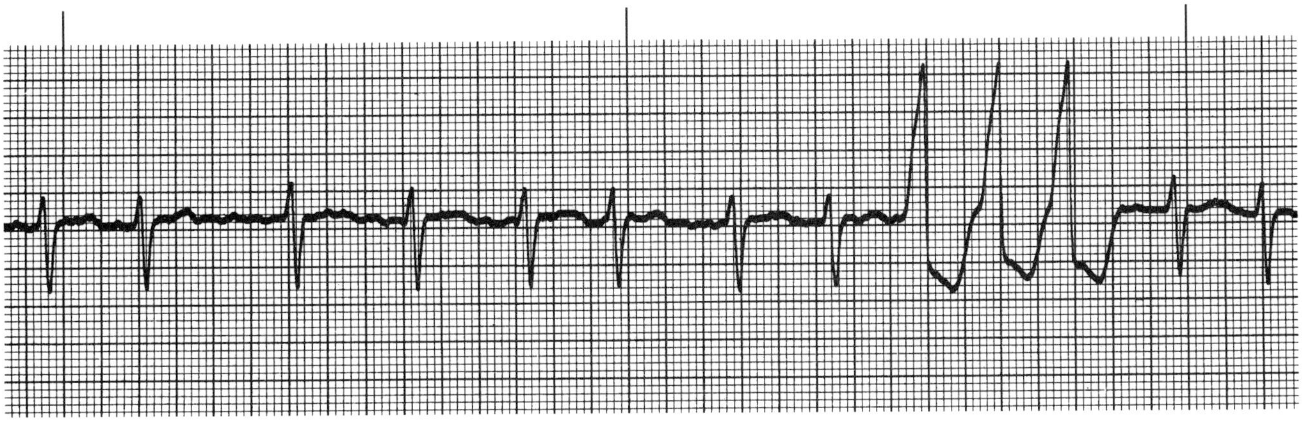

**Strip 9-42.** Rhythm:_____ Rate:_____ P wave:_____

PR interval:_____ QRS:_____

Rhythm interpretation:_____

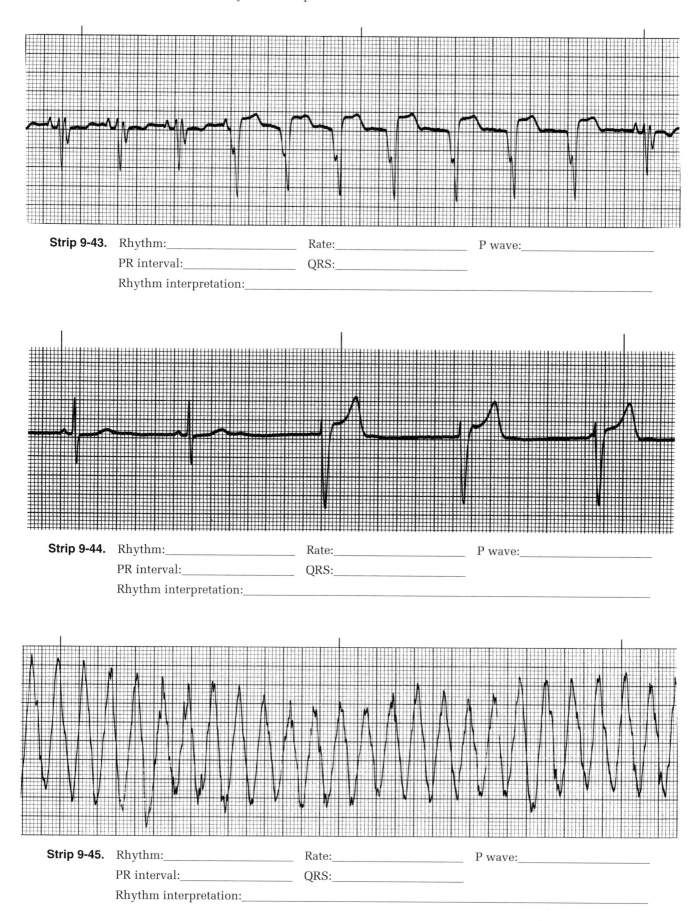

**Strip 9-43.** Rhythm:_____ Rate:_____ P wave:_____

PR interval:_____ QRS:_____

Rhythm interpretation:_____

**Strip 9-44.** Rhythm:_____ Rate:_____ P wave:_____

PR interval:_____ QRS:_____

Rhythm interpretation:_____

**Strip 9-45.** Rhythm:_____ Rate:_____ P wave:_____

PR interval:_____ QRS:_____

Rhythm interpretation:_____

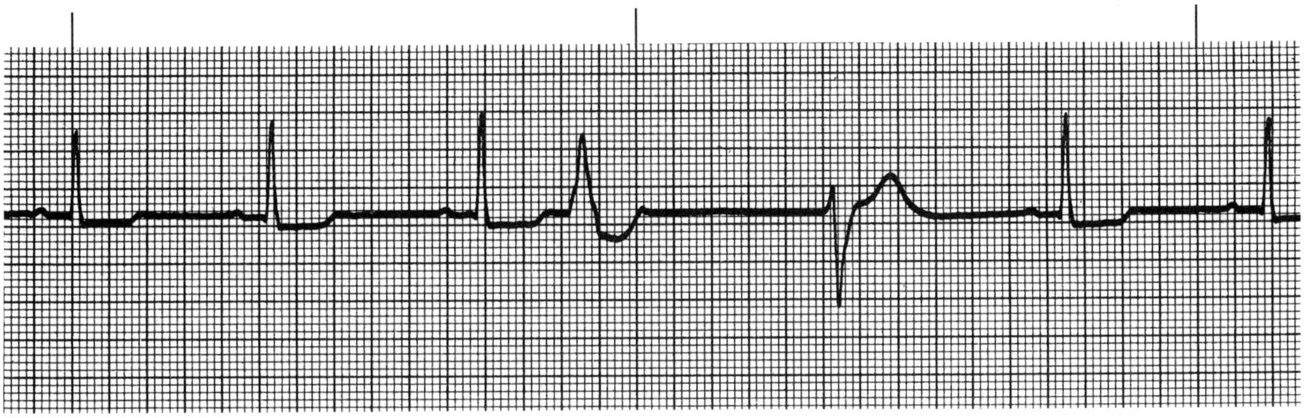

**Strip 9-46.** Rhythm:_____ Rate:_____ P wave:_____

PR interval:_____ QRS:_____

Rhythm interpretation:_____

Lead MCL₁

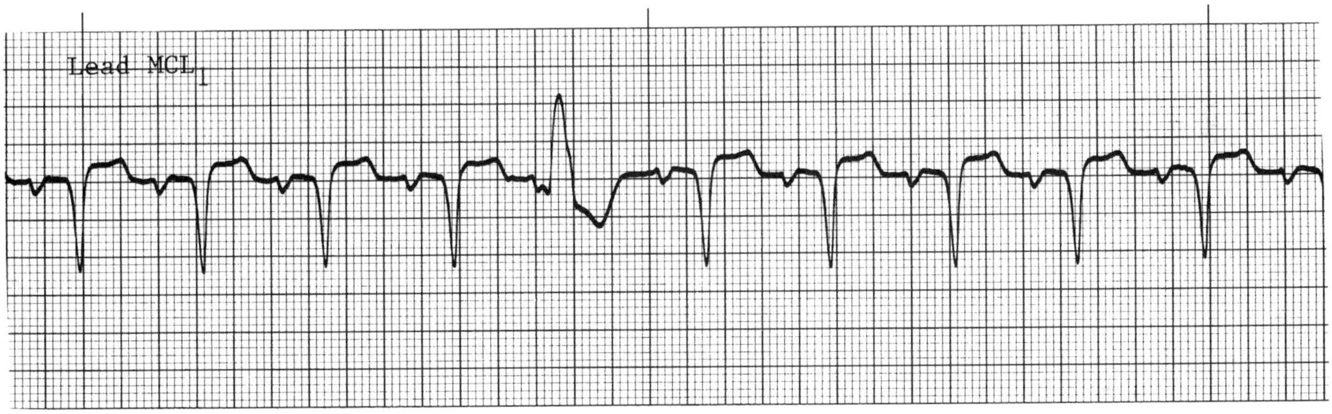

**Strip 9-47.** Rhythm:_____ Rate:_____ P wave:_____

PR interval:_____ QRS:_____

Rhythm interpretation:_____

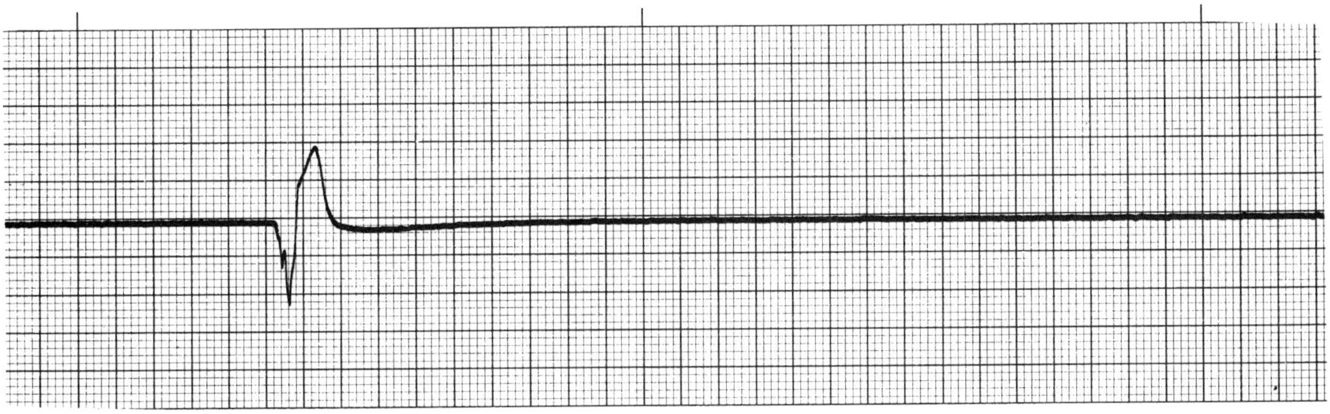

**Strip 9-48.** Rhythm:_____ Rate:_____ P wave:_____

PR interval:_____ QRS:_____

Rhythm interpretation:_____

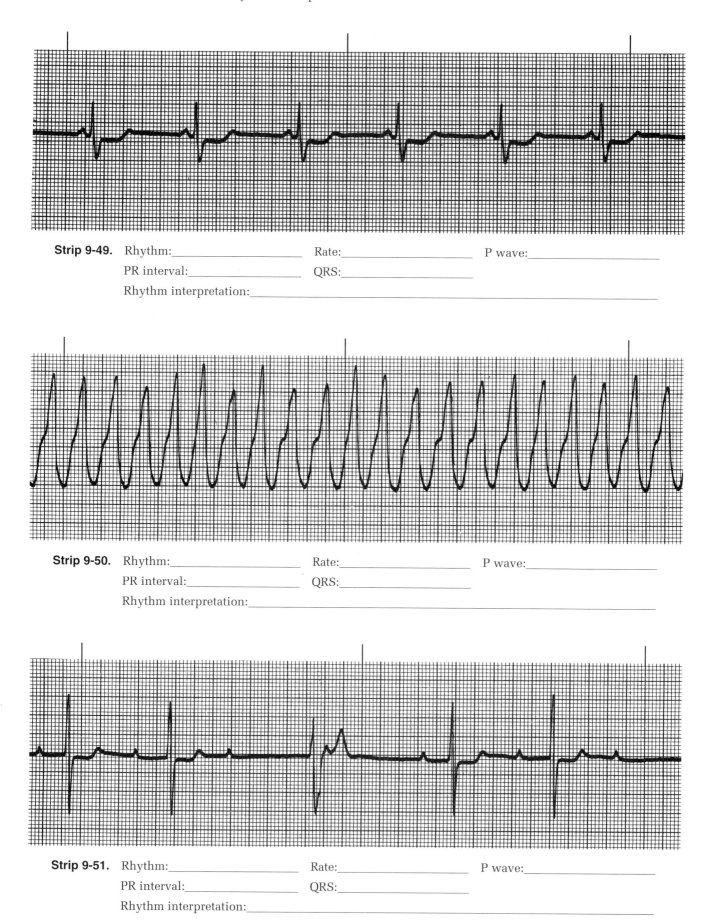

**Strip 9-49.** Rhythm:_____ Rate:_____ P wave:_____

PR interval:_____ QRS:_____

Rhythm interpretation:_____

**Strip 9-50.** Rhythm:_____ Rate:_____ P wave:_____

PR interval:_____ QRS:_____

Rhythm interpretation:_____

**Strip 9-51.** Rhythm:_____ Rate:_____ P wave:_____

PR interval:_____ QRS:_____

Rhythm interpretation:_____

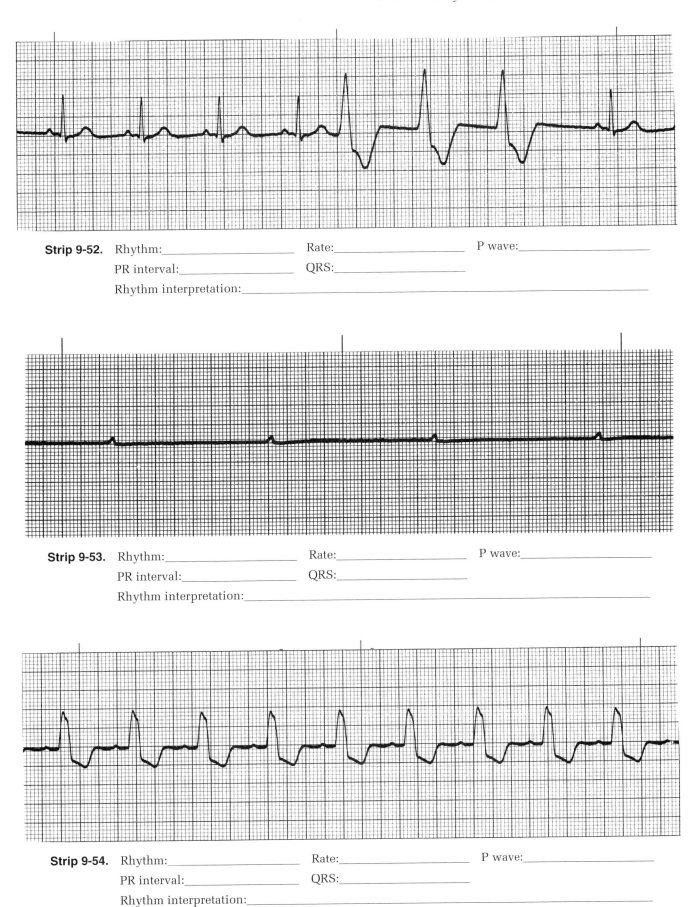

**Strip 9-52.** Rhythm:_____ Rate:_____ P wave:_____

PR interval:_____ QRS:_____

Rhythm interpretation:_____

**Strip 9-53.** Rhythm:_____ Rate:_____ P wave:_____

PR interval:_____ QRS:_____

Rhythm interpretation:_____

**Strip 9-54.** Rhythm:_____ Rate:_____ P wave:_____

PR interval:_____ QRS:_____

Rhythm interpretation:_____

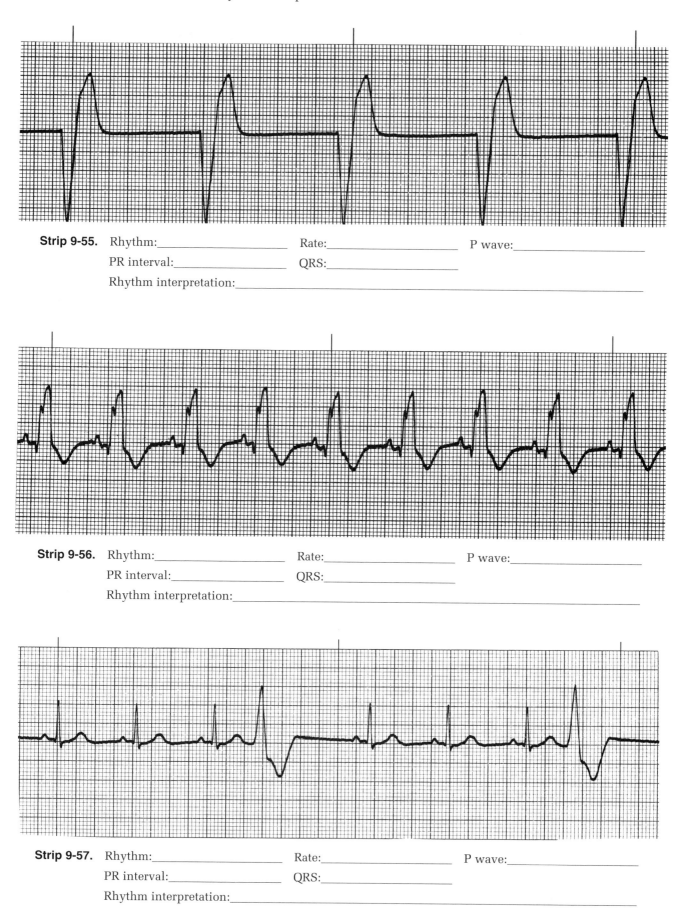

**Strip 9-55.** Rhythm:_____ Rate:_____ P wave:_____

PR interval:_____ QRS:_____

Rhythm interpretation:_____

**Strip 9-56.** Rhythm:_____ Rate:_____ P wave:_____

PR interval:_____ QRS:_____

Rhythm interpretation:_____

**Strip 9-57.** Rhythm:_____ Rate:_____ P wave:_____

PR interval:_____ QRS:_____

Rhythm interpretation:_____

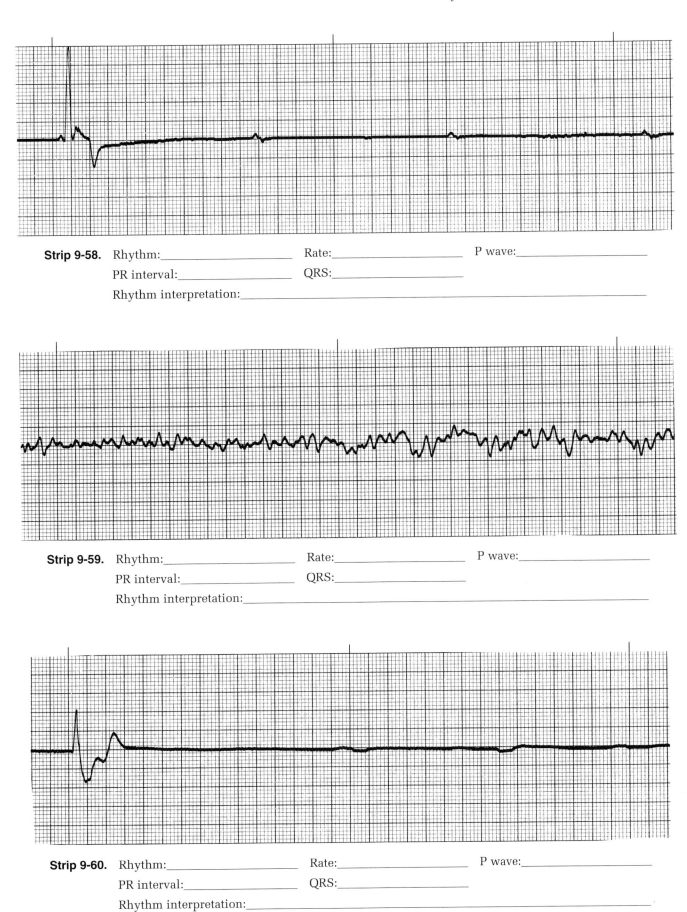

**Strip 9-58.** Rhythm:_____ Rate:_____ P wave:_____

PR interval:_____ QRS:_____

Rhythm interpretation:_____

**Strip 9-59.** Rhythm:_____ Rate:_____ P wave:_____

PR interval:_____ QRS:_____

Rhythm interpretation:_____

**Strip 9-60.** Rhythm:_____ Rate:_____ P wave:_____

PR interval:_____ QRS:_____

Rhythm interpretation:_____

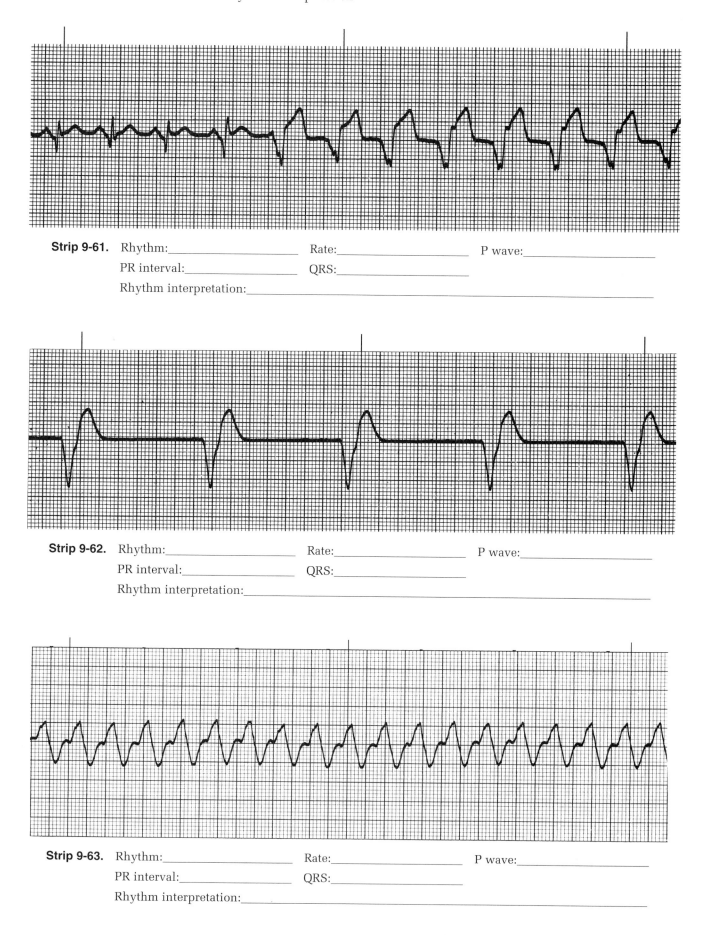

**Strip 9-61.** Rhythm:_____ Rate:_____ P wave:_____

PR interval:_____ QRS:_____

Rhythm interpretation:_____

**Strip 9-62.** Rhythm:_____ Rate:_____ P wave:_____

PR interval:_____ QRS:_____

Rhythm interpretation:_____

**Strip 9-63.** Rhythm:_____ Rate:_____ P wave:_____

PR interval:_____ QRS:_____

Rhythm interpretation:_____

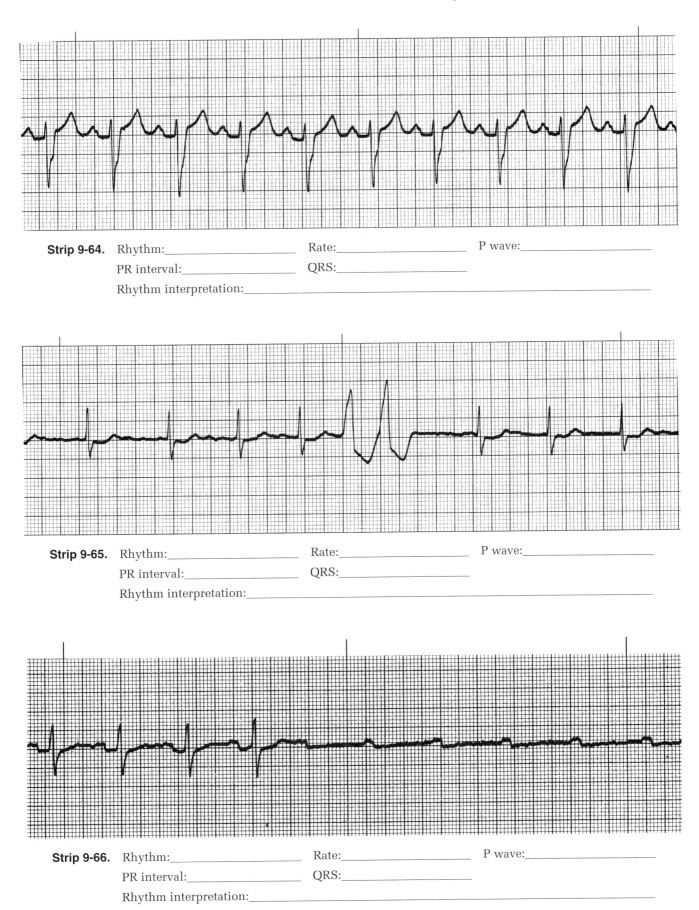

**Strip 9-64.** Rhythm:_____ Rate:_____ P wave:_____

PR interval:_____ QRS:_____

Rhythm interpretation:_____

**Strip 9-65.** Rhythm:_____ Rate:_____ P wave:_____

PR interval:_____ QRS:_____

Rhythm interpretation:_____

**Strip 9-66.** Rhythm:_____ Rate:_____ P wave:_____

PR interval:_____ QRS:_____

Rhythm interpretation:_____

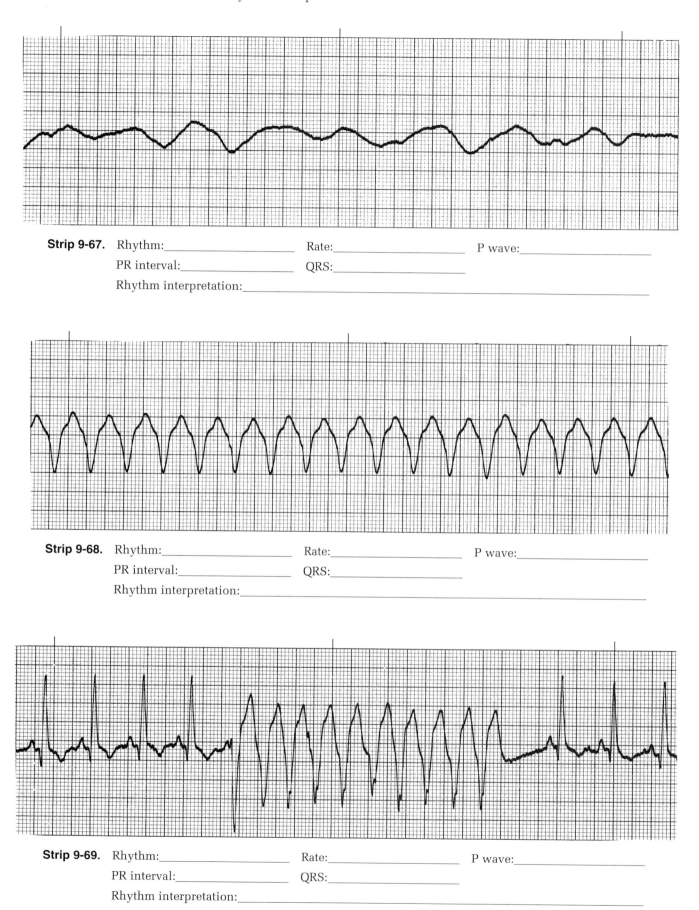

**Strip 9-67.** Rhythm:_____ Rate:_____ P wave:_____

PR interval:_____ QRS:_____

Rhythm interpretation:_____

**Strip 9-68.** Rhythm:_____ Rate:_____ P wave:_____

PR interval:_____ QRS:_____

Rhythm interpretation:_____

**Strip 9-69.** Rhythm:_____ Rate:_____ P wave:_____

PR interval:_____ QRS:_____

Rhythm interpretation:_____

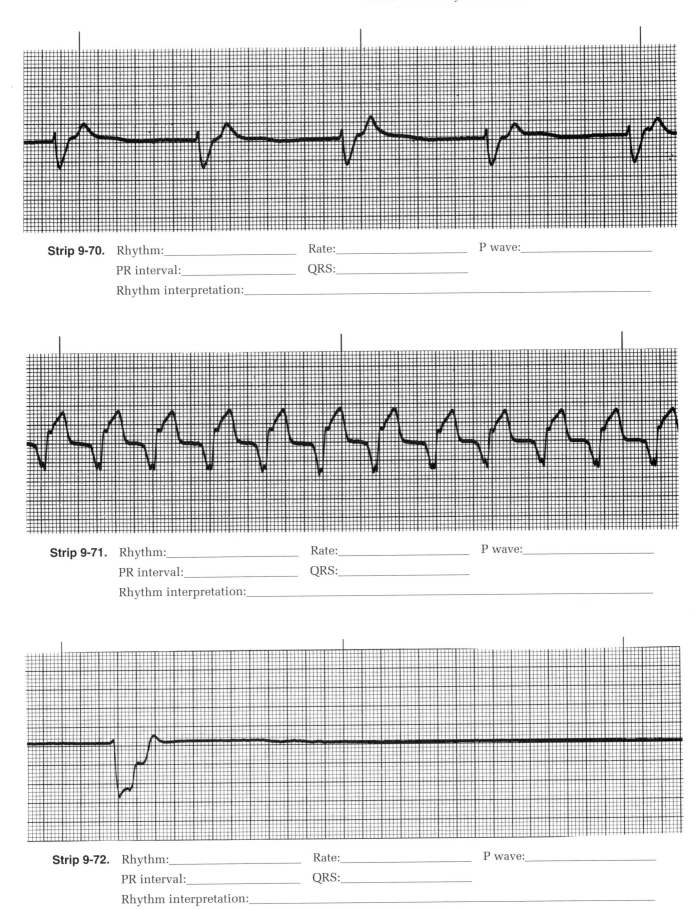

**Strip 9-70.** Rhythm:_____ Rate:_____ P wave:_____

PR interval:_____ QRS:_____

Rhythm interpretation:_____

**Strip 9-71.** Rhythm:_____ Rate:_____ P wave:_____

PR interval:_____ QRS:_____

Rhythm interpretation:_____

**Strip 9-72.** Rhythm:_____ Rate:_____ P wave:_____

PR interval:_____ QRS:_____

Rhythm interpretation:_____

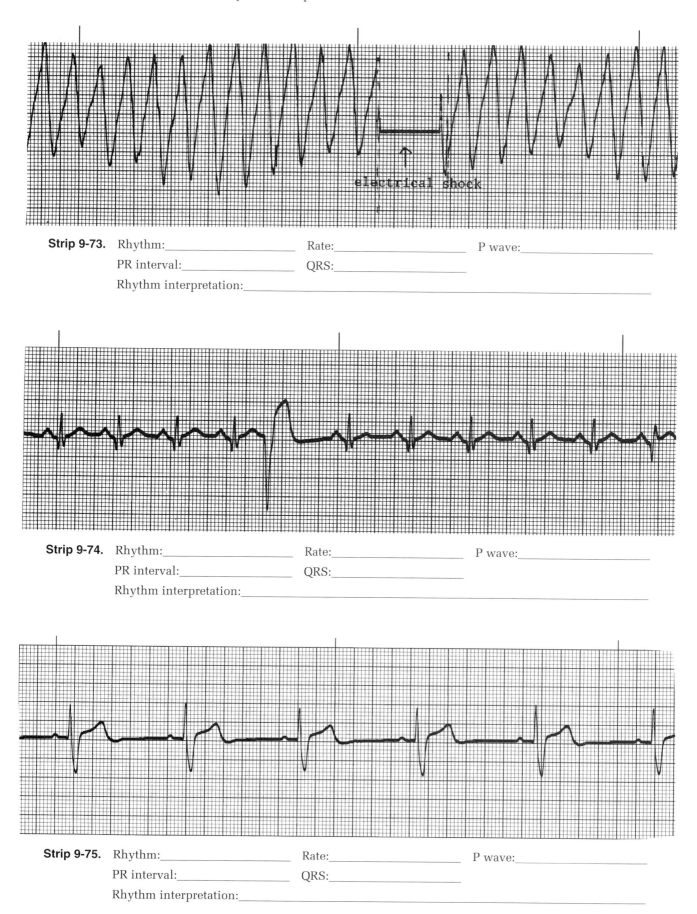

**Strip 9-73.** Rhythm:_____ Rate:_____ P wave:_____

PR interval:_____ QRS:_____

Rhythm interpretation:_____

**Strip 9-74.** Rhythm:_____ Rate:_____ P wave:_____

PR interval:_____ QRS:_____

Rhythm interpretation:_____

**Strip 9-75.** Rhythm:_____ Rate:_____ P wave:_____

PR interval:_____ QRS:_____

Rhythm interpretation:_____

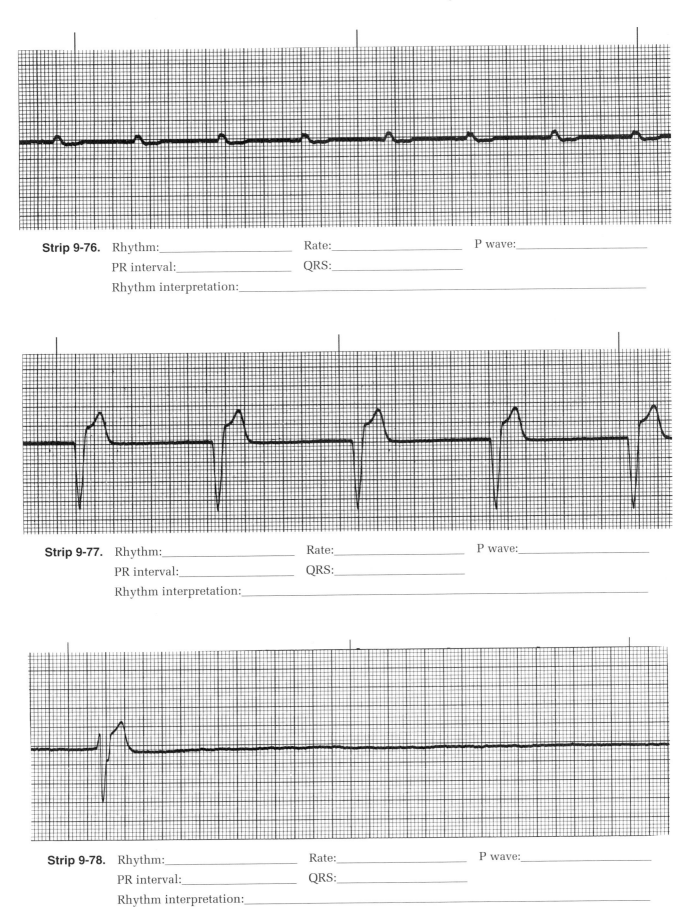

**Strip 9-76.** Rhythm:_____ Rate:_____ P wave:_____

PR interval:_____ QRS:_____

Rhythm interpretation:_____

**Strip 9-77.** Rhythm:_____ Rate:_____ P wave:_____

PR interval:_____ QRS:_____

Rhythm interpretation:_____

**Strip 9-78.** Rhythm:_____ Rate:_____ P wave:_____

PR interval:_____ QRS:_____

Rhythm interpretation:_____

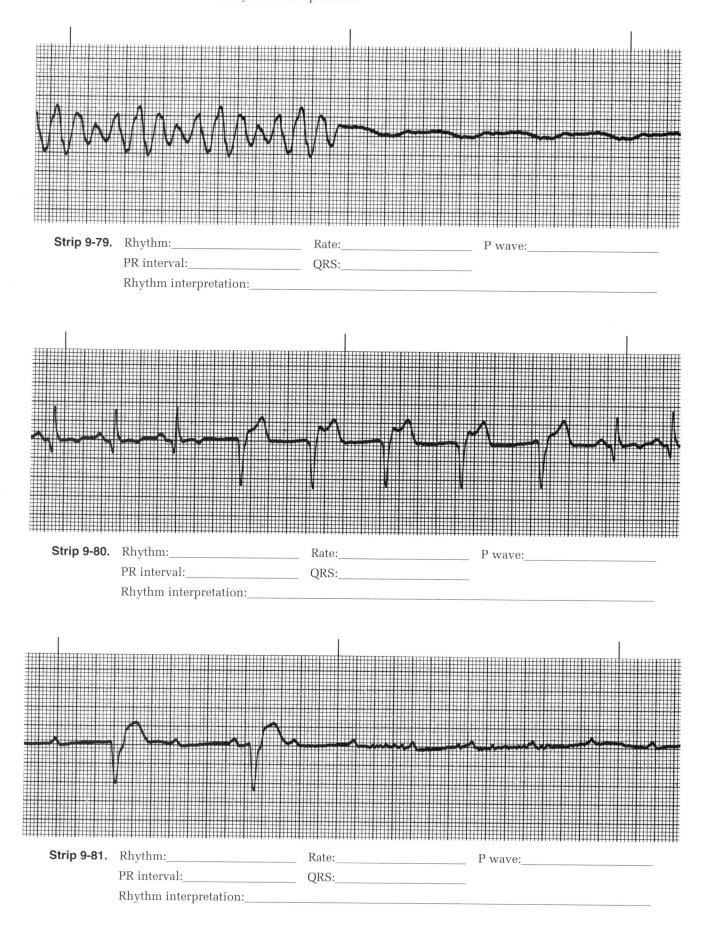

**Strip 9-79.** Rhythm:_____ Rate:_____ P wave:_____

PR interval:_____ QRS:_____

Rhythm interpretation:_____

**Strip 9-80.** Rhythm:_____ Rate:_____ P wave:_____

PR interval:_____ QRS:_____

Rhythm interpretation:_____

**Strip 9-81.** Rhythm:_____ Rate:_____ P wave:_____

PR interval:_____ QRS:_____

Rhythm interpretation:_____

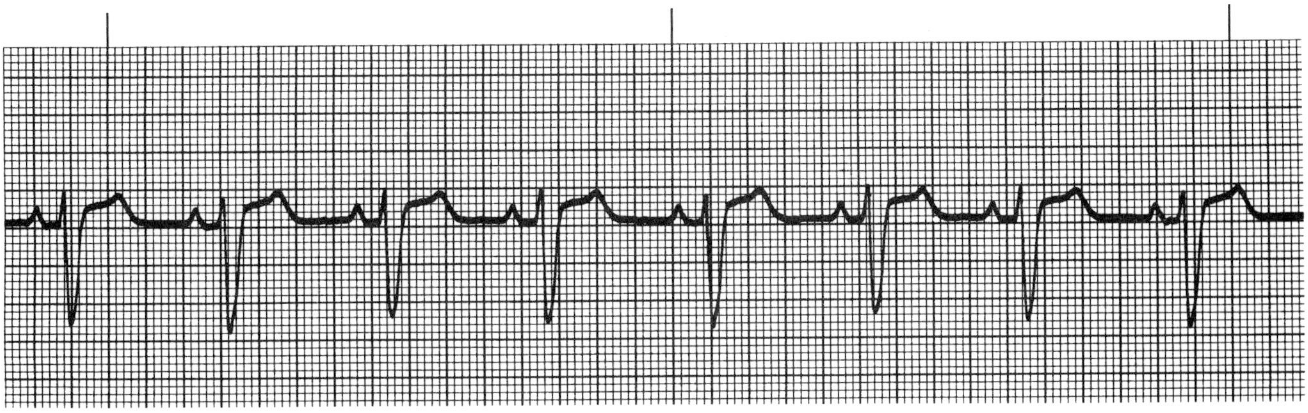

**Strip 9-82.** Rhythm:_____ Rate:_____ P wave:_____

PR interval:_____ QRS:_____

Rhythm interpretation:_____

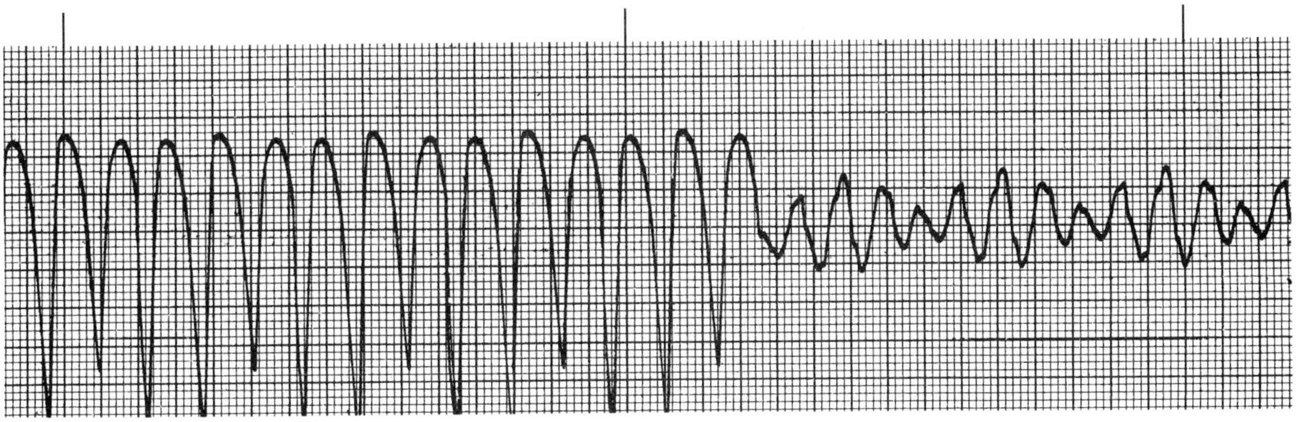

**Strip 9-83.** Rhythm:_____ Rate:_____ P wave:_____

PR interval:_____ QRS:_____

Rhythm interpretation:_____

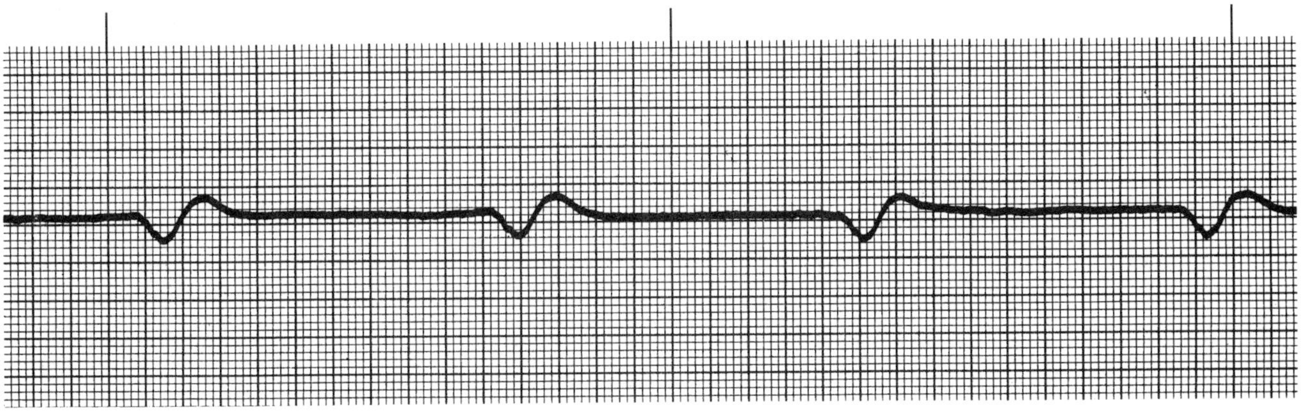

**Strip 9-84.** Rhythm:_____ Rate:_____ P wave:_____

PR interval:_____ QRS:_____

Rhythm interpretation:_____

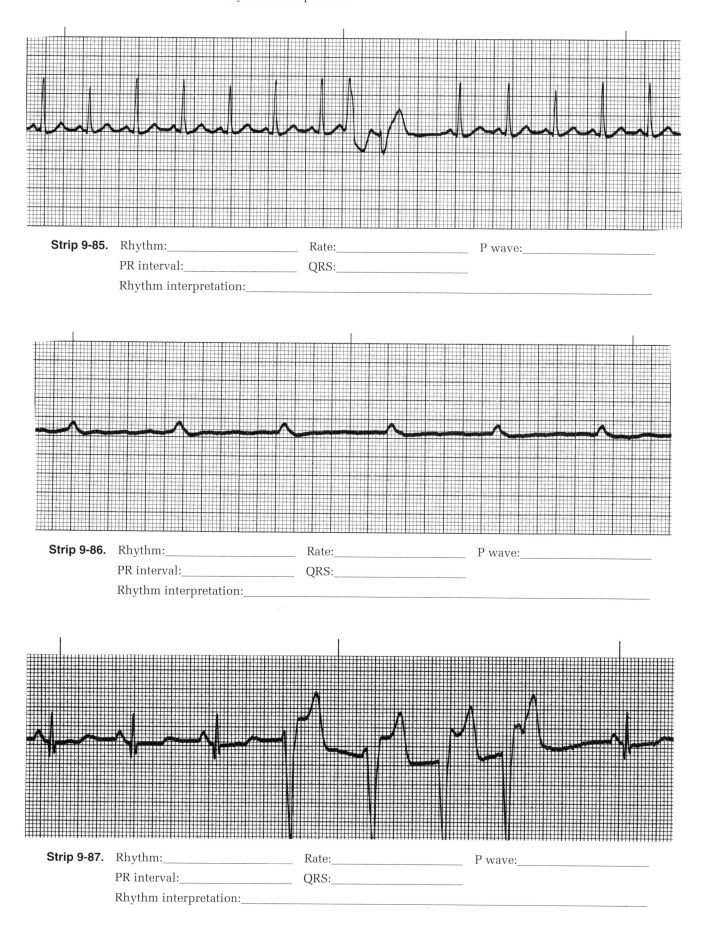

**Strip 9-85.** Rhythm:_____ Rate:_____ P wave:_____

PR interval:_____ QRS:_____

Rhythm interpretation:_____

**Strip 9-86.** Rhythm:_____ Rate:_____ P wave:_____

PR interval:_____ QRS:_____

Rhythm interpretation:_____

**Strip 9-87.** Rhythm:_____ Rate:_____ P wave:_____

PR interval:_____ QRS:_____

Rhythm interpretation:_____

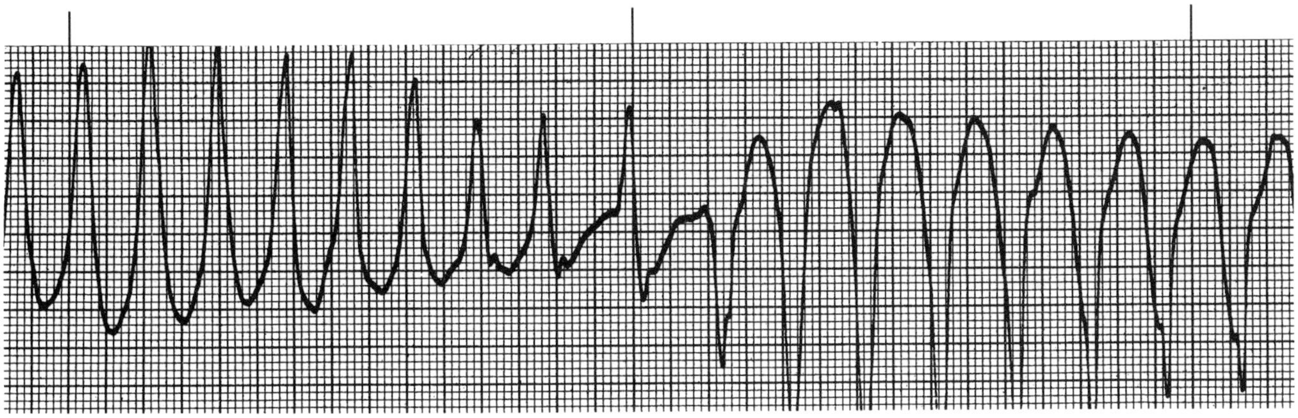

**Strip 9-88.** Rhythm:_____ Rate:_____ P wave:_____

PR interval:_____ QRS:_____

Rhythm interpretation:_____

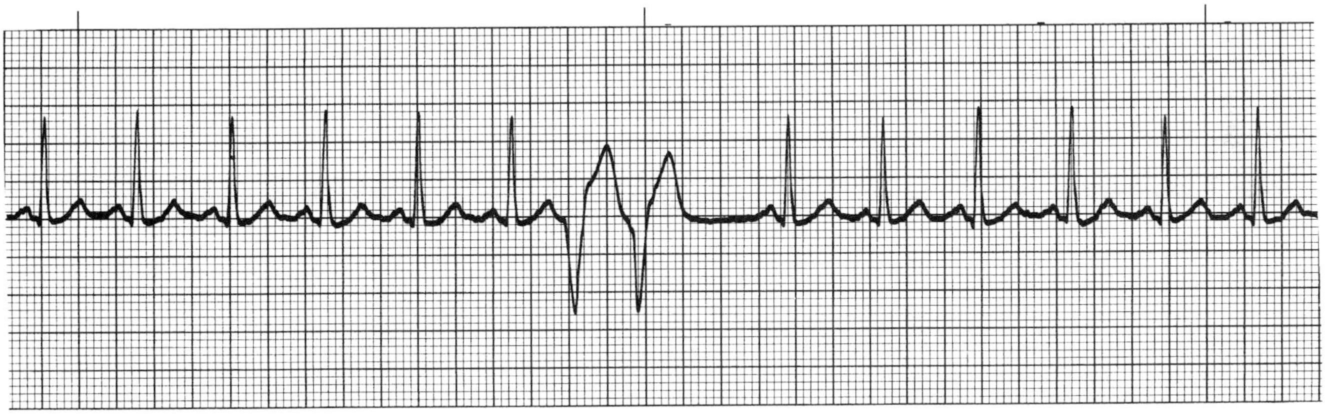

**Strip 9-89.** Rhythm:_____ Rate:_____ P wave:_____

PR interval:_____ QRS:_____

Rhythm interpretation:_____

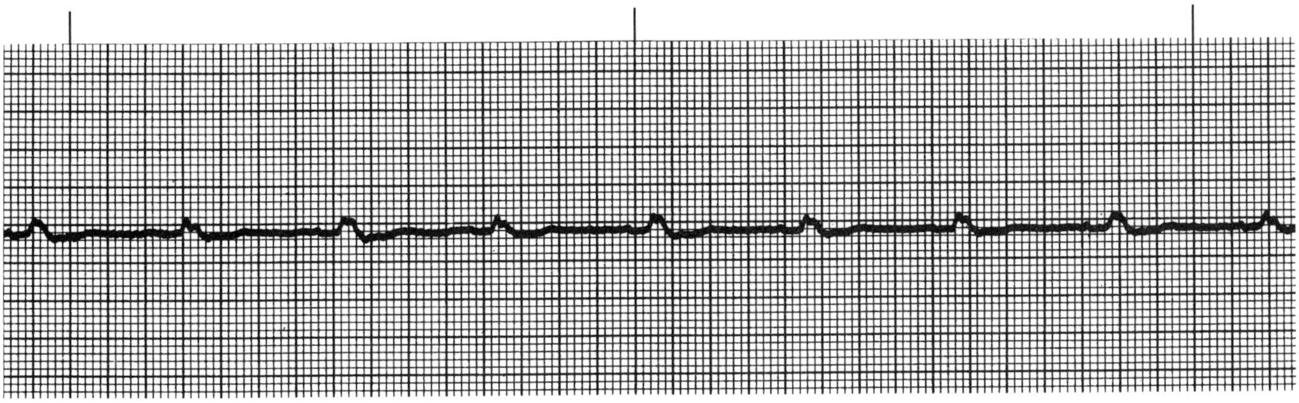

**Strip 9-90.** Rhythm:_____ Rate:_____ P wave:_____

PR interval:_____ QRS:_____

Rhythm interpretation:_____

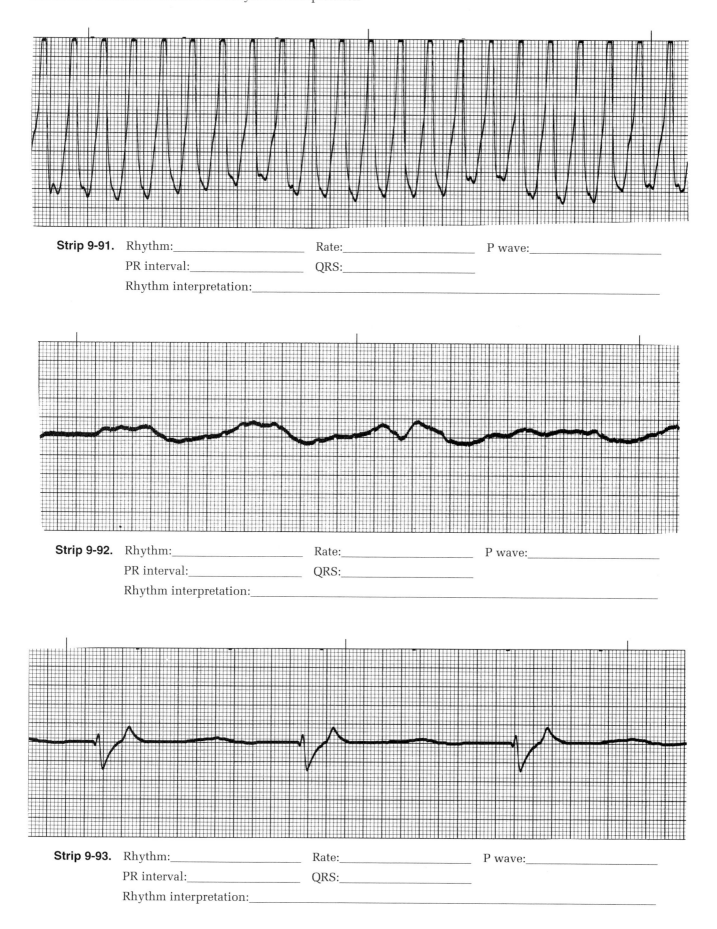

**Strip 9-91.** Rhythm:_____ Rate:_____ P wave:_____

PR interval:_____ QRS:_____

Rhythm interpretation:_____

**Strip 9-92.** Rhythm:_____ Rate:_____ P wave:_____

PR interval:_____ QRS:_____

Rhythm interpretation:_____

**Strip 9-93.** Rhythm:_____ Rate:_____ P wave:_____

PR interval:_____ QRS:_____

Rhythm interpretation:_____

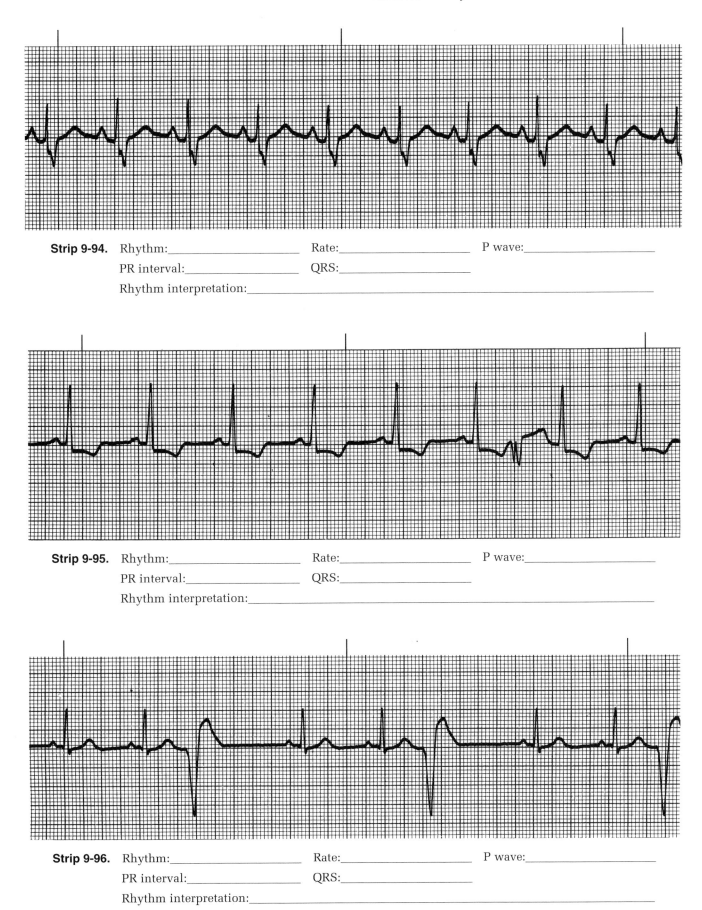

**Strip 9-94.** Rhythm:_____ Rate:_____ P wave:_____

PR interval:_____ QRS:_____

Rhythm interpretation:_____

**Strip 9-95.** Rhythm:_____ Rate:_____ P wave:_____

PR interval:_____ QRS:_____

Rhythm interpretation:_____

**Strip 9-96.** Rhythm:_____ Rate:_____ P wave:_____

PR interval:_____ QRS:_____

Rhythm interpretation:_____

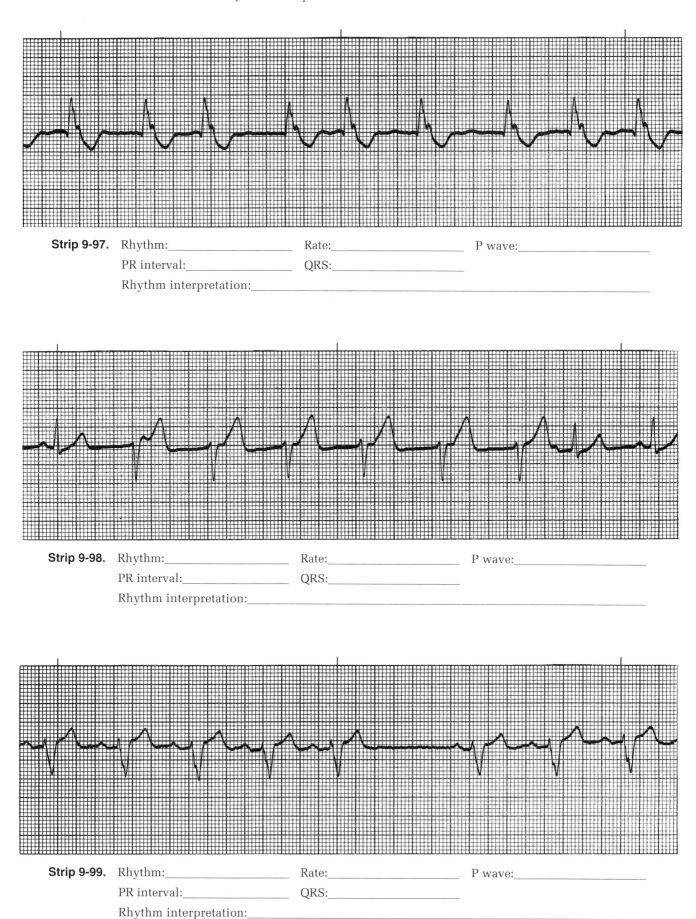

**Strip 9-97.** Rhythm:_____ Rate:_____ P wave:_____

PR interval:_____ QRS:_____

Rhythm interpretation:_____

**Strip 9-98.** Rhythm:_____ Rate:_____ P wave:_____

PR interval:_____ QRS:_____

Rhythm interpretation:_____

**Strip 9-99.** Rhythm:_____ Rate:_____ P wave:_____

PR interval:_____ QRS:_____

Rhythm interpretion:_____

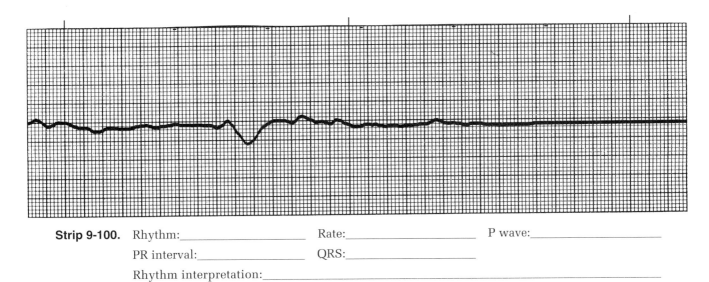

**Strip 9-100.** Rhythm:_____ Rate:_____ P wave:_____

PR interval:_____ QRS:_____

Rhythm interpretation:_____

# 10

## PACEMAKERS

A pacemaker is a battery-powered device that delivers an electrical stimulus to the myocardium, resulting in contraction. Pacemakers can be temporary or permanent and are used primarily when the patient's own heart rate is excessively slow, as in the following conditions: symptomatic sinus bradycardia, sinus arrest, sinus exit block, sick sinus syndrome (a degenerative process of the sinus node that produces alternating periods of bradycardia and tachycardia), slow atrial fibrillation; or when there is a potential for ventricular standstill to occur, as in second-degree AV block Mobitz II or third-degree AV block. Prophylactic temporary pacing is often done in the presence of a new right bundle branch block with either anterior or posterior fascicular block, in left bundle branch block with first-degree AV block, or when a bundle branch block is associated with second-degree or third-degree AV block, especially in the presence of an anterior MI.

A pacemaker functions in one of two ways: as a fixed-rate pacemaker or as a demand pacemaker. Fixed-rate pacemakers initiate impulses at a set rate regardless of the patient's intrinsic rate. The fixed-rate pacemaker competes with the patient's own heart rhythm and is potentially dangerous because the pacing stimulus may fall during the vulnerable period of the cardiac cycle and induce serious ventricular arrhythmias. This type pacemaker is used primarily when the patient has no intrinsic heart rate, such as during cardiac arrest. Demand pacemakers are designed with a sensing mechanism that inhibits discharge when the patient's heart rate is adequate and a pacing mechanism that triggers the pacemaker to fire when no intrinsic activity occurs within a predetermined period. Many different types of demand pacemakers are available:

**1.** Single-chamber pacemakers, which sense and pace either the atrium or the ventricle

**2.** Dual-chamber pacemakers, which sense and pace both the atrium and the ventricle

An advantage of the dual-chamber pacemakers is their ability to restore the AV synchronous sequence of the heart (atrial kick) that contributes 20% to 30% of cardiac output. An additional benefit of dual-chamber pacing is preservation of atrial electrical stability, which reduces the incidence of atrial fibrillation.

All pacemakers have some components in common—the pulse generator and the pacing catheter. The pulse generator houses the battery that creates the electrical signal, and contains the various controls or settings for pacemaker function (electrical output or milliamperes (mA), sensitivity or millivolts (mV), heart rate setting, mode of pacing, spe-

cialized settings, and so forth). The pacing catheter (often called the lead or electrode) serves as a transmission line between the pulse generator and the endocardium. Electrical impulses are conducted from the pulse generator to the endocardium while information about intrinsic electrical activity is relayed from the catheter tip back to the generator for processing.

## TEMPORARY PACEMAKERS

Temporary pacing can be accomplished with transvenous, epicardial, or transcutaneous (external) methods. With the external pacemaker system, large pacing pads are placed on the anterior and posterior chest (Figure 10-1). Placement of the pacing pads will affect the current required to obtain ventricular capture. The placement that offers the most direct current pathway to the heart will usually produce the lowest threshold. The pacing pads are attached to a pacing cable, which is then connected to a defibrillator/monitor. ECG leads are also attached to the patient. A pacing rate is set, and the mA dial is turned up until consistent capture is seen. The myocardium is stimulated indirectly by electric currents transmitted through the chest wall. Systems are also available that have the capability to monitor, externally pace, and defibrillate the patient through one set of chest pads.

External pacemakers are noninvasive, quick and easy to apply, and designed to function in the demand mode. Successful transcutaneous pacing requires a higher current output (mA) than conventional transvenous pacing. Delivery of this stronger current may cause chest wall pain and skin burns (although the larger pacing pad minimizes the risk of burns). Transcutaneous pacing is effective as a treatment when meaningful contractile activity is present (eg, in the hemodynamically significant bradycardias such as symptomatic sinus bradycardia, second-

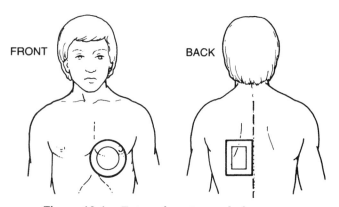

**Figure 10-1.** External pacing pad placement.

degree AV block Mobitz II, and third-degree AV block). External pacing is usually not effective for treatment of ventricular standstill or pulseless electrical activity (PEA) that occurs in the setting of cardiac arrest. This is because the primary problem in these situations is the inability of the myocardium to contract when appropriately stimulated. External pacemakers are used as a temporary measure in emergency situations when transvenous access is not readily available. Transvenous pacing is still the treatment of choice for patients requiring a temporary but longer period of pacemaker support.

With the temporary transvenous pacemaker (Figure 10-2), the pacing electrode is inserted by transvenous route (internal jugular, subclavian, antecubital, or femoral vein) into the apex of the right ventricle for ventricular pacing, the right atrium for atrial pacing, or both chambers for dual-chamber pacing. The electrode is then connected by way of a bridging cable to an external pulse generator. The endocardium is stimulated directly by electric currents transmitted from the pulse generator. Controls on the face of the pulse generator allow operator manipulation of pacing parameters. Removable batteries are contained within the generator housing. Although temporary transvenous atrial or dual-chamber pacing can be done, it is difficult to place temporary atrial wires and is not as reliable as single-chamber ventricular pacing.

Like transcutaneous pacing, the temporary transvenous pacemaker is also used to treat the hemodynamically significant bradycardias and is usually not effective when meaningful contractile activity is absent (ventricular standstill and PEA). For significant unresolved rhythm or conduction disorders, permanent pacing is required.

Epicardial pacing electrodes (epicardial wires) are placed on the atria or ventricles during cardiac surgery. The electrode end of the wire is looped through or loosely sutured to the epicardial surface of the atria or ventricles, and the other end is pulled through the chest wall, sutured to the skin, attached to a bridging cable, and connected to an external pulse generator. A ground wire is often attached to the chest wall and pulled through with the other pacing wires. The number of wires present varies with the surgeon. There may be one or two atrial wires, one or two ventricular wires, one or two ground wires, or no ground wire. Epicardial pacing is used after cardiac surgery to treat hemodynamically significant bradycardias.

## PERMANENT PACEMAKERS

Implantation of a permanent pacemaker (Figure 10-3) does not automatically follow temporary pacing. The procedure is performed only after careful

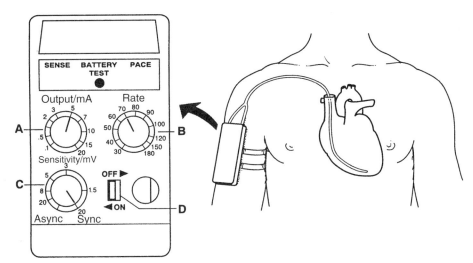

**Figure 10-2.** Temporary pacemaker.
**A. Output or mA Dial**
   Controls the amount of electrical energy delivered to the endocardium.
**B. Rate Dial**
   Determines the rate in beats per minute at which the stimulus is to be delivered.
**C. Sensitivity or mV Dial**
   Controls the ability of the generator to sense intrinsic activity.
   In maximum clockwise position, this provides demand (synchronous) pacing.
   In maximum counterclockwise position, this provides fixed rate (asynchronous) pacing.
**D. On/Off Control**
   Activates/inactivates the pulse generator.

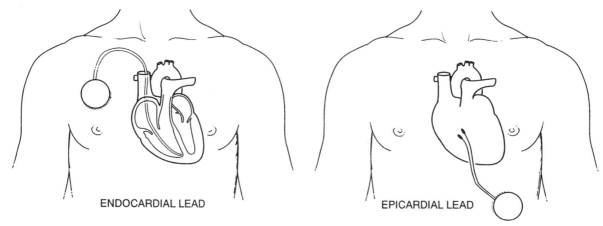

ENDOCARDIAL LEAD        EPICARDIAL LEAD

**Figure 10-3.** Permanent pacemaker.

analysis of each patient's clinical situation. Permanent pacemakers are usually implanted using intravenous (IV) conscious sedation and local anesthesia in the cardiac catheterization laboratory. The pulse generator is placed in a subcutaneous pocket in either the right or left pectoral area. The pacing lead is inserted through the cephalic vein or the subclavian vein into the right ventricular apex. For dual-chamber pacing, a second lead is placed in the right atrial appendage. Permanent pulse generators are powered by lithium batteries. Their life span is approximately 10 years, but this will depend on how the pacemaker is programmed and how often it paces. Many of the permanent pacemakers used today are multiprogrammable—some are capable of increasing the pacing rate in response to the body's need for increased cardiac output (rate-responsive capabilities), whereas others are programmed with antitachycardia features designed to terminate supraventricular and ventricular tachyarrhythmias using pacing techniques or shock. In situations where endocardial pacing cannot be achieved, the permanent pacemaker is inserted by a transthoracic approach in the operating room using general anesthesia. The pacing electrode is attached to the epicardial surface of the right or left ventricle, and the pulse generator is implanted in a subcutaneous pocket in the abdominal wall.

Basic functions of all pacemakers include the ability to sense, fire, and capture. Appropriate *sensing* implies that the pulse generator is able to "see" intrinsic patient beats. *Firing* means that the pulse generator has delivered a stimulus to the heart. *Capturing* means that the heart has responded to the stimulus. Most difficulties encountered with cardiac pacing result from abnormalities in sensing, firing, and/or capturing. Most of these difficulties can be traced to parameter settings, battery failure, problems at the interface of the catheter tip and endocardium, or problems with generator or lead integrity

(loose connections, break in pacing catheter, and so forth).

Single-chamber ventricular demand pacing is the most frequently used temporary transvenous type of pacing. This pacemaker paces and senses only in the ventricle and is inhibited only by ventricular activity. In other words, when ventricular activity is sensed, the pacemaker is inhibited (withholds a pacing stimulus), but, when ventricular activity is not sensed, the pacemaker will discharge impulses at a preset rate. Further discussion and ECG tracings will focus on the temporary transvenous ventricular demand pacemaker.

## PACEMAKER TERMS

### Ventricular Capture

Ventricular capture indicates that the ventricle has responded to a pacing stimulus (Figure 10-4, complex A). This is reflected on the ECG tracing by a stimulus artifact (a spike) followed by a wide QRS complex. Ventricular pacing causes sequential depolarization instead of synchronous depolarization. This means that one ventricle (usually the right) will be depolarized before the other. The prolonged depolarization time results in a wide QRS complex.

### Native Beat

A native beat (also called intrinsic beat) is produced by the patient's own electrical conduction system. This beat is shown in Figure 10-4, complex B.

### Fusion Beat

A fusion beat (see Figure 10-4, complex C) occurs when the pacemaker fires an electrical impulse at the

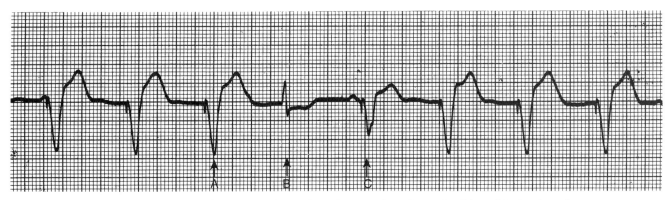

**Figure 10-4.** Ventricular capture (complex A), native beat (complex B), and fusion beat (complex C).

same time that the patient's normal electrical impulse has activated the ventricles. The two forces simultaneously depolarize the ventricles, resulting in a fusion beat. The fusion beat has the characteristics of both pacemaker and patient forces, although one usually dominates the other. The resulting complex is different in configuration and height from that caused by either of the forces alone. Fusion beats are normal.

### Pseudofusion Beat

A pseudofusion beat (Figure 10-5, complex D) occurs when a pacemaker spike falls within the QRS complex of a native beat but does not alter the height or configuration of the complex. The pacing stimulus had no effect on depolarization because the ventricle was already fully stimulated by the intrinsic beat. Pseudofusion beats are normal.

### Automatic Interval

The automatic interval (see Figure 10-5, complex E) refers to the heart rate at which the pacemaker is set. This interval is measured from one pacing spike to the next consecutive pacing spike.

### Pacemaker Rhythm

Pacemaker rhythm (Figure 10-6) occurs when the heart's rhythm is completely pacemaker induced. This is reflected by an ECG tracing in which no patient beats are seen and all QRS complexes are induced by the pacemaker.

## PACEMAKER MALFUNCTIONS

The most common malfunctions associated with the temporary transvenous ventricular demand pacemaker involve failure to capture and undersensing. These malfunctions are discussed below.

### Failure to Capture

Failure to capture (Figure 10-7) means that the ventricles failed to respond to a pacing stimulus. This is reflected on the ECG tracing by a pacing spike that occurs on time (at the automatic interval rate) but is not followed by a QRS complex. Failure to capture is common with temporary pacemakers and often results from the following:

**1.** *Problems with interface between catheter tip and endocardium.* Capture cannot occur if the lead is

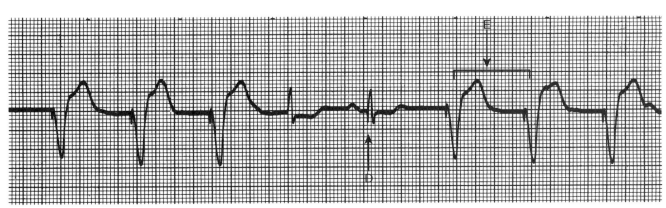

**Figure 10-5.** Pseudofusion beat (complex D) and automatic interval (complex E).

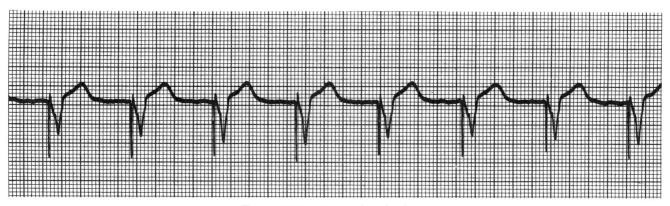

**Figure 10-6.** Pacemaker rhythm.

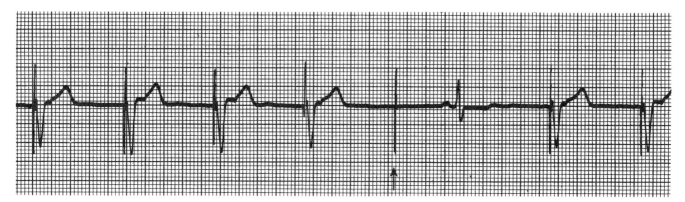

**Figure 10-7.** Loss of capture.

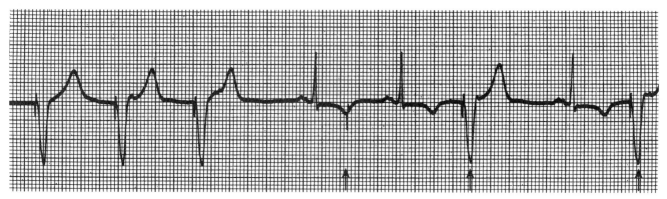

**Figure 10-8.** Undersensing.

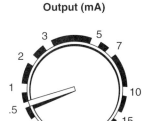

**Output (mA)**

The output (mA) dial controls the amount of electrical energy delivered to the myocardium. Turning the dial to a higher number increases the mA.

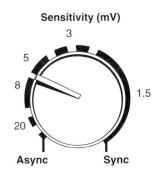

**Sensitivity (mV)**

The sensitivity (mV) dial controls the ability of the generator to sense intrinsic activity. Turning the dial to a low number increases the sensitivity. Turning the dial to a high number decreases the sensitivity.

**Figure 10-9.** Output (mA) and sensitivity (mV) dials on a temporary pulse generator.

dislodged. The electrode tip must be in contact with the endocardium for the electrical stimulus to cause depolarization. Also, capture usually cannot occur if the catheter tip lies in infarcted tissue. The electrode tip must be in contact with healthy endocardium that is capable of responding to the electrical stimulus.

**2.** *Increase in stimulation threshold.* The minimum amount of current required to cause a ventricular response is called *threshold* and is determined during pacemaker insertion. The milliamperes (mA) dial is usually set at two times the insertion threshold. Over a period of days, inflammation or fibrosis of tissue surrounding the catheter tip may raise the stimulation threshold, resulting in failure to capture. Effective capture is usually regained by simply increasing the milliamperes on the mA dial (see Figure 10-9). Table 10-1 summarizes the causes and appropriate interventions for failure to capture.

### Undersensing

Undersensing (Figure 10-8) occurs when the pulse generator does not sense the patient's intrinsic

beats. This problem is reflected on the ECG by a pacing spike that occurs earlier than it should after a native or paced beat. Ventricular capture may or may not occur. Under normal circumstances, the generator senses the beat before it and does not fire a stimulus until the time indicated by the automatic interval setting. Undersensing often results from:

**1.** *Problems with interface between catheter tip and endocardium.* The pacing catheter may be out of place or lying in infracted tissue.

**2.** *Sensitivity setting set too low* (Figure 10-9). High sensitivity settings (low number on sensitivity dial) instruct the pacemaker to sense virtually all intrinsic activity (even low-voltage signals), whereas low sensitivity settings (high number on sensitivity dial) instruct the pacemaker to virtually ignore all in-

**Table 10-1. Failure to Capture**

| Causes | Interventions |
| --- | --- |
| Electrical milliamperes (mA) set too low | Increase the mA setting on pulse generator until consistent capture is achieved. Increasing the mA is achieved by turning the mA dial clockwise to a higher number. |
| Dislodgement of lead or pacing lead positioned in infarcted tissue | Do overpenetrated chest x-ray to determine catheter position. |
| | If catheter is out of position, a temporary intervention is to place patient on left side (gravity may allow catheter to contact endocardium). |
| | Physician may need to reposition pacing catheter. |

**Table 10-2. Undersensing**

| Causes | Interventions |
| --- | --- |
| Sensitivity setting too low | Increase sensitivity on pulse generator by turning the sensitivity dial clockwise to a lower number. |
| Dislodgement of lead or pacing lead positioned in infarcted tissue | Do overpenetrated chest x-ray to determine catheter position. |
| | If catheter is out of position, a temporary intervention is to place patient on left side (gravity may allow catheter to contact endocardium). |
| | The pacemaker may be turned off until physician can assess the problem if: Initial interventions had no effect. Patient's heart rate is adequate. The pacing spike is falling in the T wave, and there is a great potential for lethal arrhythmias to be induced. |
| | Physician may need to reposition pacing catheter. |
| Pacer set on asynchronous (fixed-rate) mode | Turn sensitivity dial to synchronous (demand) mode. |

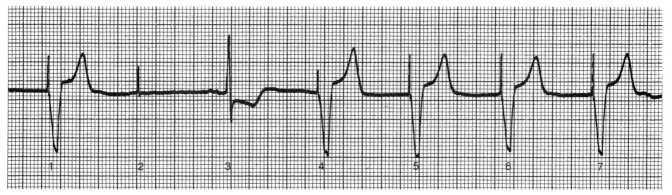

**Figure 10-10.** Pacemaker Analysis Strip #1.

1. The automatic interval can be measured from #4 to #5. Mark automatic interval on index card. The heart rate is 63.
2. #2 can be analyzed by placing left mark on index card on spike of beat just before it; #2 matches right mark on index card; #2 occurs on time but does not cause ventricular depolarization so it indicates failure to capture.
3. #3 is a native beat—it doesn't need analyzing.
4. #4 can be analyzed by placing left mark on R wave of native QRS just before it; #4 matches right mark on index card; #4 occurs on time and causes ventricular depolarization, indicating ventricular capture beat.
5. #5, #6, and #7 are all analyzed by placing left mark on spikes immediately preceding each beat to be analyzed—all occur on time and cause ventricular depolarization, indicating ventricular capture beats.

Interpretation: Failure to capture (one occurrence).

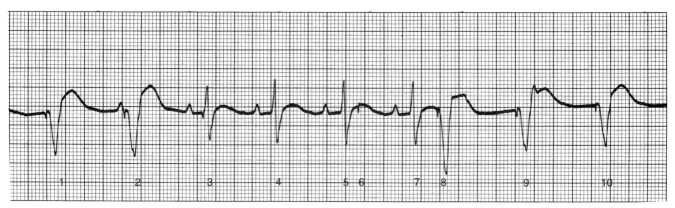

**Figure 10-11.** Pacemaker Analysis Strip #2.

1. The automatic interval can be measured from #1 to #2. Mark automatic interval on index card. The heart rate is 72.
2. #2 can be analyzed by placing left mark on index card on spike of beat immediately before it; #2 matches right mark on index card; #2 occurs on time and causes ventricular depolarization indicating ventricular capture beat.
3. #3 is a native beat (note spike at beginning of R wave); place left mark on spike of beat immediately before it; #3 matches right mark; #3 has a spike in it and is different from the other native beats (#4, #5, #7) in height so this represents a fusion beat.
4. #4 and #5 are native beats and do not need analyzing.
5. #6 can be analyzed by placing left mark on R wave of native beat just before it; #6 occurs much earlier than right mark; #6 indicates that generator did not sense preceding beat and represents undersensing problem.
6. #7 is a native beat.
7. #8 can be analyzed by placing left mark on R wave of native beat just before it; #8 occurs much earlier than right mark; #8 indicates the generator did not sense preceding beat and represents an undersensing problem. (Note: #6 represents an undersensing problem without capture while #8 represents an undersensing problem with capture.)
8. #9 can be analyzed by placing left mark on spike of beat just before it; #9 matches right mark; #9 occurs on time and causes ventricular depolarization indicating ventricular capture beat.
9. #10 can be analyzed by placing left mark on spike of beat just before it; #10 matches right mark; #10 occurs on time and causes ventricular depolarization indicating ventricular capture beat.

Interpretation: Undersensing malfunction (two occurrences).

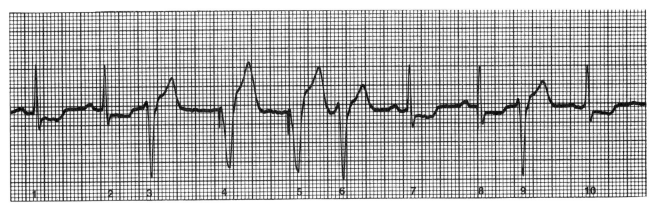

**Figure 10-12.** Pacemaker Analysis #3.

1. The automatic interval can be measured from #4 to #5. Mark automatic interval on index card. The pacing rate is 79.
2. The first 3 beats are patient produced (native beats or intrinsic beats) and don't need analyzing.
3. Beat #4 can be analyzed by placing left mark on index card on R wave of native QRS just before it; #4 matches right mark on index card; #5 occurs on time and causes ventricular depolarization, indicating ventricular capture beat.
4. Beat #5 can be analyzed by placing left mark on index card on spike of paced beat; #5 matches right mark on index card; #5 occurs on time and causes ventricular depolarization, indicating ventricular capture beat.
5. #6 through #10 are patient produced beats.
6. #8 has a pacing spike at the beginning of the QRS complex which doesn't alter the QRS configuration, indicating a pseudo fusion beat.
   Interpretation: Normal pacemaker function.

trinsic activity (even high-voltage signals). Increasing the pacemaker's sensitivity (by turning the sensitivity dial to a lower number) allows it to see smaller signals and may solve the problem.

**3.** *Pacemaker set on asynchronous (fixed-rate) mode.* In the asynchronous mode, the sensing circuit is off. This problem can be corrected by turning the sensitivity dial to synchronous (demand) mode.

Table 10-2 summarizes the causes and appropriate interventions for undersensing.

## ANALYZING PACEMAKER RHYTHM STRIPS (VENTRICULAR DEMAND TYPE)

When analyzing pacemaker rhythm strips, you will again need to use either calipers or an index card. The author has found the following steps to be helpful.

**Step 1.** Place an index card (or caliper) above two consecutive paced beats. Mark on index card the interval from one pacing spike to the next. This is called the *automatic interval* and indicates the heart rate at which the pacemaker is set. The automatic in-

terval measurement will assist you in determining if the pacemaker fired on time, too early, too late, or not at all.

**Step 2.** Start on left side of rhythm strip. Each pacing spike should be analyzed systematically to assess if the pacemaker is functioning appropriately.

**Step 3.** Identify pacing spike to be analyzed (only one spike should be analyzed at a time). Using marked index card (step 1), place left mark on spike of paced beat or R wave of native beat immediately preceding pacing spike being analyzed. Observe the relationship of the spike being analyzed to the right mark on index card.

    **a.** If spike being analyzed coincides with right mark, the possible answers include:
   Ventricular capture beat (normal)
   Fusion beat (normal)
   Pseudofusion beat (normal)
   Failure to capture (abnormal)

    **b.** If spike being analyzed occurs earlier than right mark, the answer is:
   Undersensing malfunction (abnormal)

Study Figures 10-10 through 10-12. These strips have been analyzed for you.

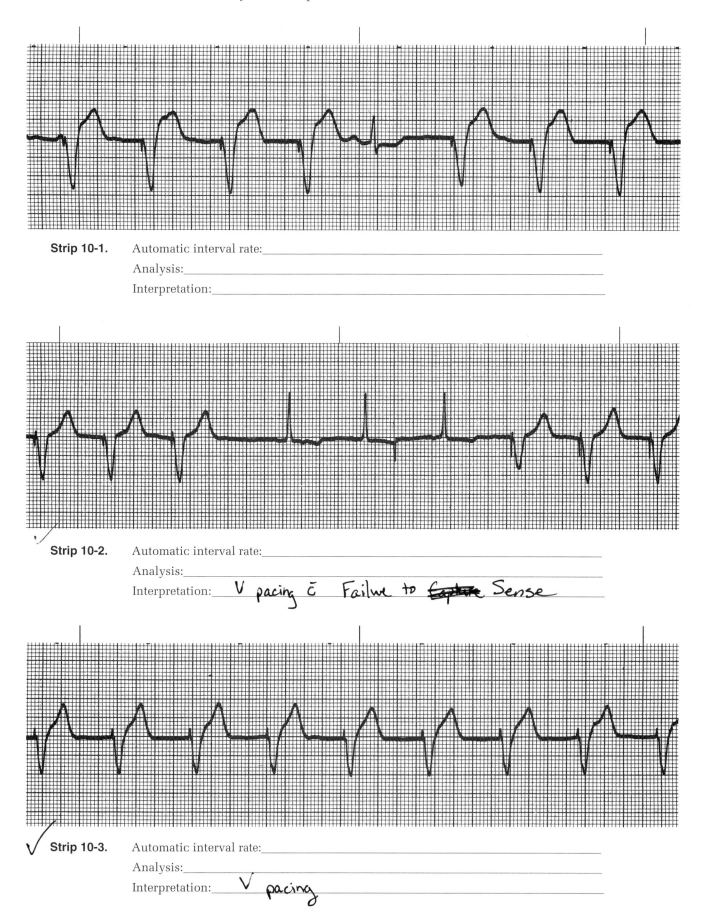

**Strip 10-1.**  Automatic interval rate:_____

Analysis:_____

Interpretation:_____

**Strip 10-2.**  Automatic interval rate:_____

Analysis:_____

Interpretation:___V pacing c̄ Failure to ~~Capture~~ Sense_____

**Strip 10-3.**  Automatic interval rate:_____

Analysis:_____

Interpretation:_____V pacing_____

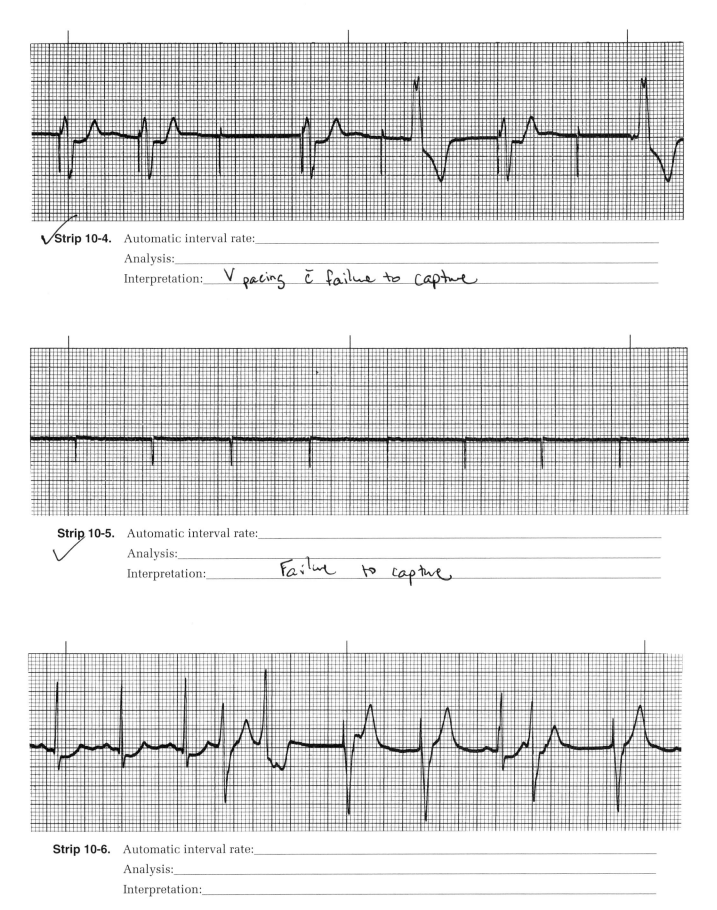

**Strip 10-4.** Automatic interval rate:_____

Analysis:_____

Interpretation:___V pacing c̄ failure to capture_____

**Strip 10-5.** Automatic interval rate:_____

Analysis:_____

Interpretation:_____Failure to capture_____

**Strip 10-6.** Automatic interval rate:_____

Analysis:_____

Interpretation:_____

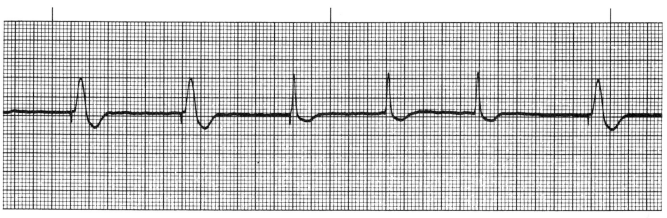

**Strip 10-7.**   Automatic interval rate:_____

Analysis:_____

Interpretation:_____

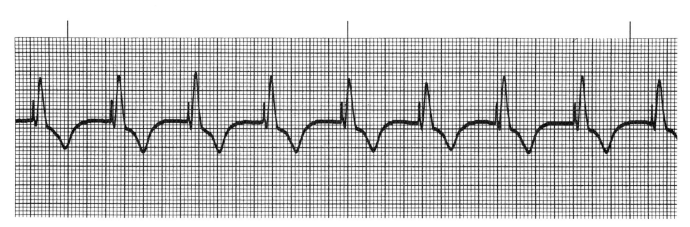

**Strip 10-8.**   Automatic interval rate:_____

Analysis:_____

Interpretation:_____

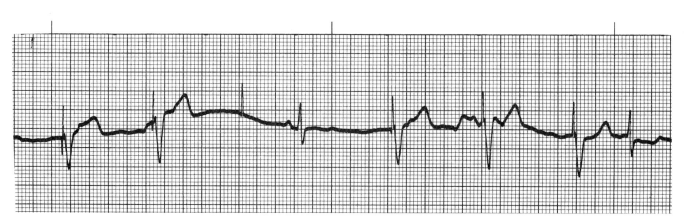

**Strip 10-9.**   Automatic interval rate:_____

Analysis:_____

Interpretation:_____

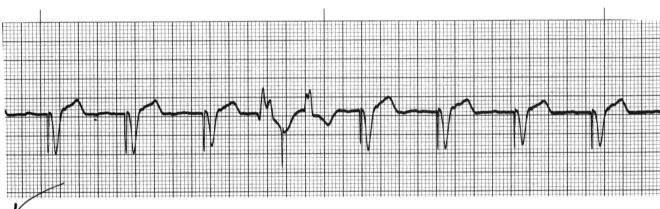

**Strip 10-10.** Automatic interval rate:_____

Analysis:_____

Interpretation:_____

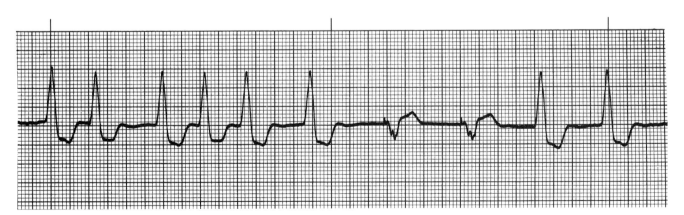

**Strip 10-11.** Automatic interval rate:_____

Analysis:_____

Interpretation:___V pacing c̄ Failure to Sense_____

**Strip 10-12.** Automatic interval rate:_____

Analysis:_____

Interpretation:_____

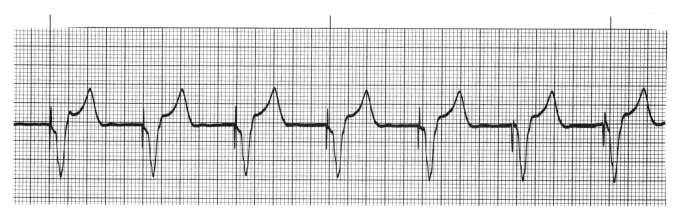

**Strip 10-13.** Automatic interval rate:_____

Analysis:_____

Interpretation:_____

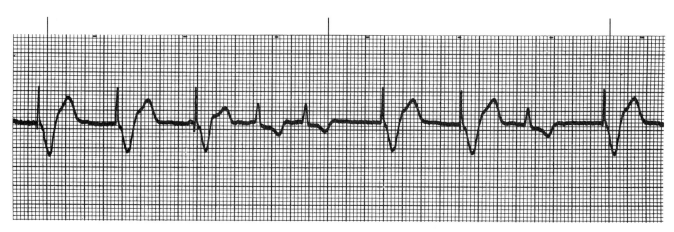

**Strip 10-14.** Automatic interval rate:_____

Analysis:_____

Interpretation:_____

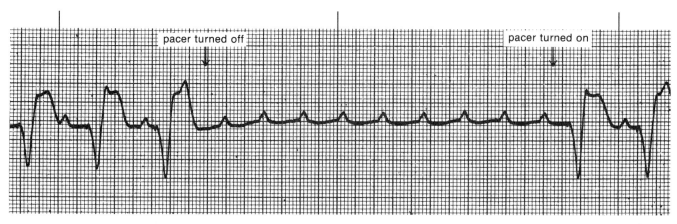

pacer turned off

pacer turned on

**Strip 10-15.** Automatic interval rate:_____

Analysis:_____

Interpretation:_____

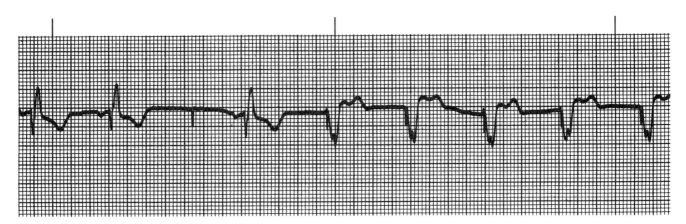

**Strip 10-16.** Automatic interval rate:_____

Analysis:_____

Interpretation:_____

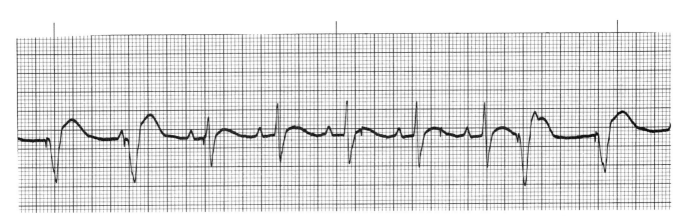

**Strip 10-17.** Automatic interval rate:_____

Analysis:_____

Interpretation:_____

**Strip 10-18.** Automatic interval rate:_____

Analysis:_____

Interpretation:_____

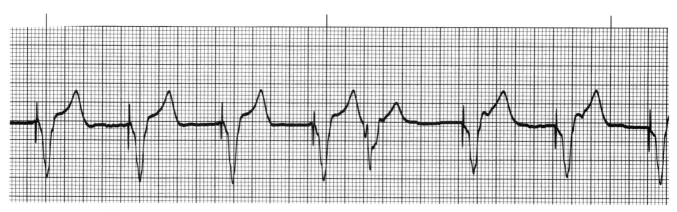

**Strip 10-19.** Automatic interval rate:_____

Analysis:_____

Interpretation:_____

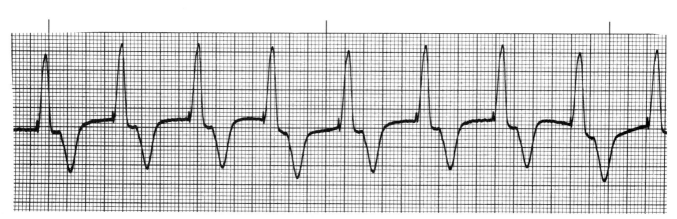

**Strip 10-20.** Automatic interval rate:_____

Analysis:_____

Interpretation:_____

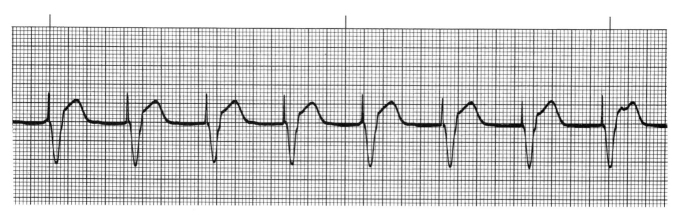

**Strip 10-21.** Automatic interval rate:_____

Analysis:_____

Interpretation:_____

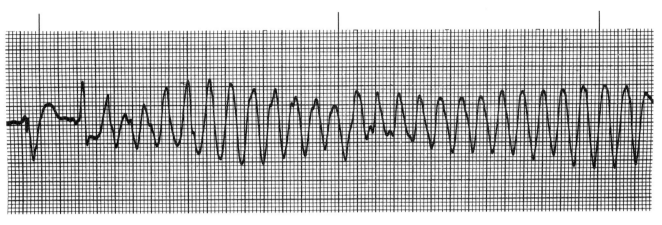

**Strip 10-22.** Automatic interval rate:_____

Analysis:_____

Interpretation:_____

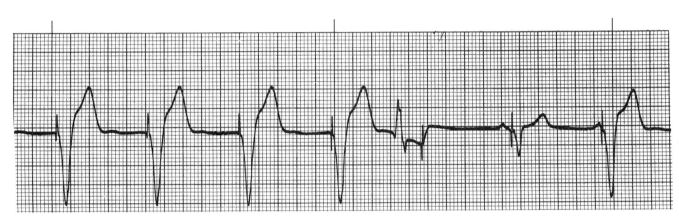

**Strip 10-23.** Automatic interval rate:_____

Analysis:_____

Interpretation:_____

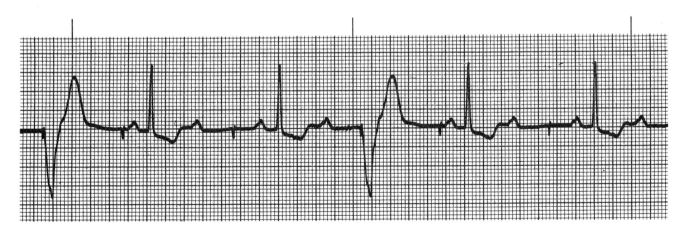

**Strip 10-24.** Automatic interval rate:_____

Analysis:_____

Interpretation:_____

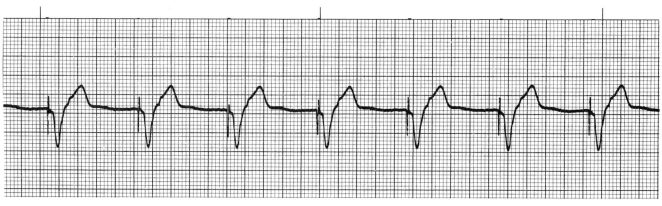

**Strip 10-25.** Automatic interval rate:_____

Analysis:_____

Interpretation:_____

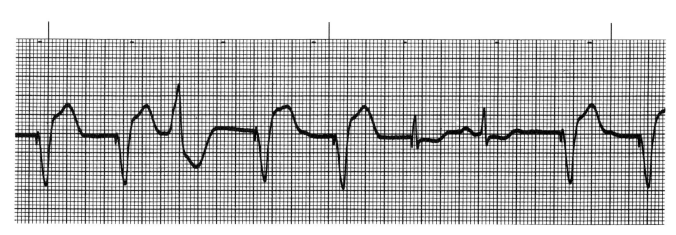

**Strip 10-26.** Automatic interval rate:_____

Analysis:_____

Interpretation:_____

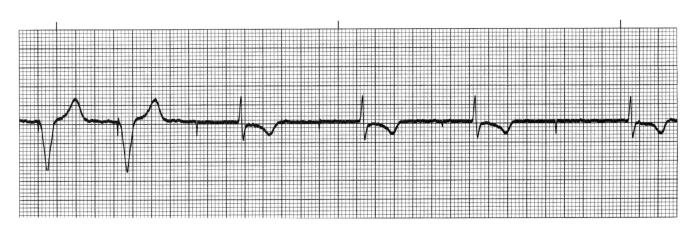

**Strip 10-27.** Automatic interval rate:_____

Analysis:_____

Interpretation:_____

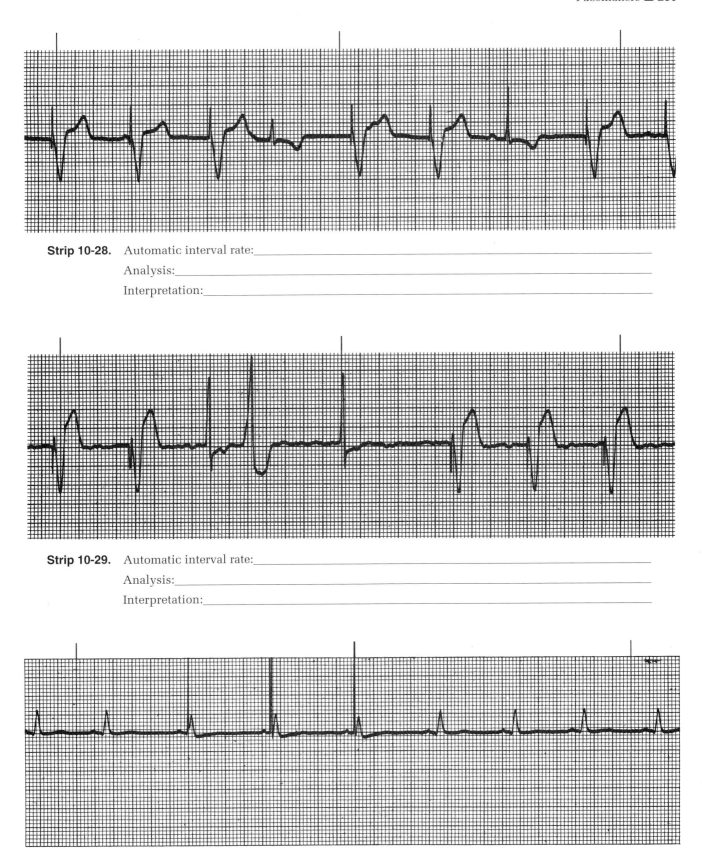

**Strip 10-28.** Automatic interval rate:_____

Analysis:_____

Interpretation:_____

**Strip 10-29.** Automatic interval rate:_____

Analysis:_____

Interpretation:_____

**Strip 10-30.** Automatic interval rate:_____

Analysis:_____

Interpretation:_____

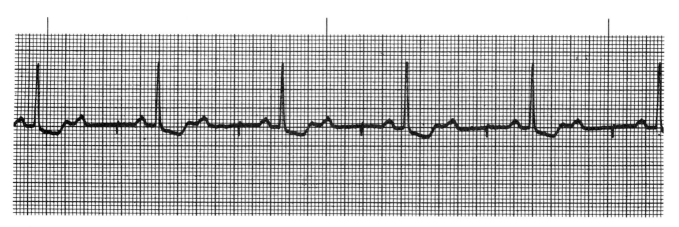

**Strip 10-31.** Automatic interval rate:_____

Analysis:_____

Interpretation:_____

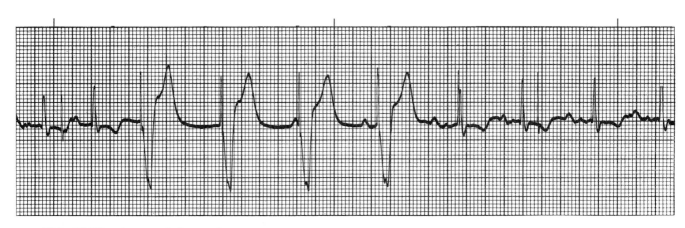

**Strip 10-32.** Automatic interval rate:_____

Analysis:_____

Interpretation:_____

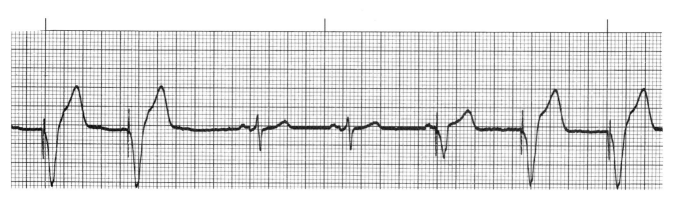

**Strip 10-33.** Automatic interval rate:_____

Analysis:_____

Interpretation:_____

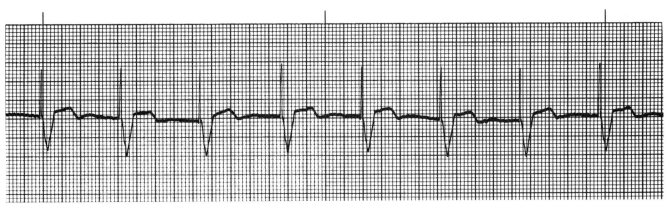

**Strip 10-34.** Automatic interval rate:_____

Analysis:_____

Interpretation:_____

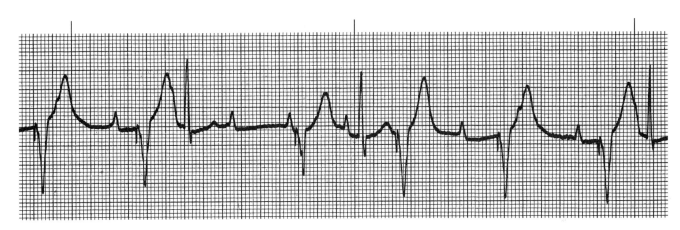

**Strip 10-35.** Automatic interval rate:_____

Analysis:_____

Interpretation:_____

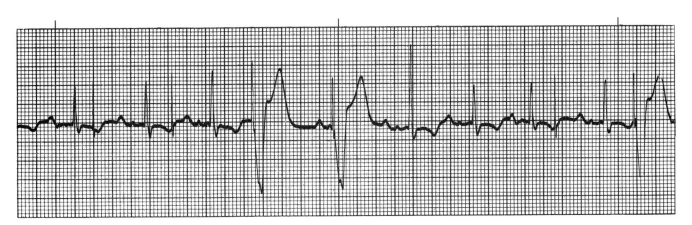

**Strip 10-36.** Automatic interval rate:_____

Analysis:_____

Interpretation:_____

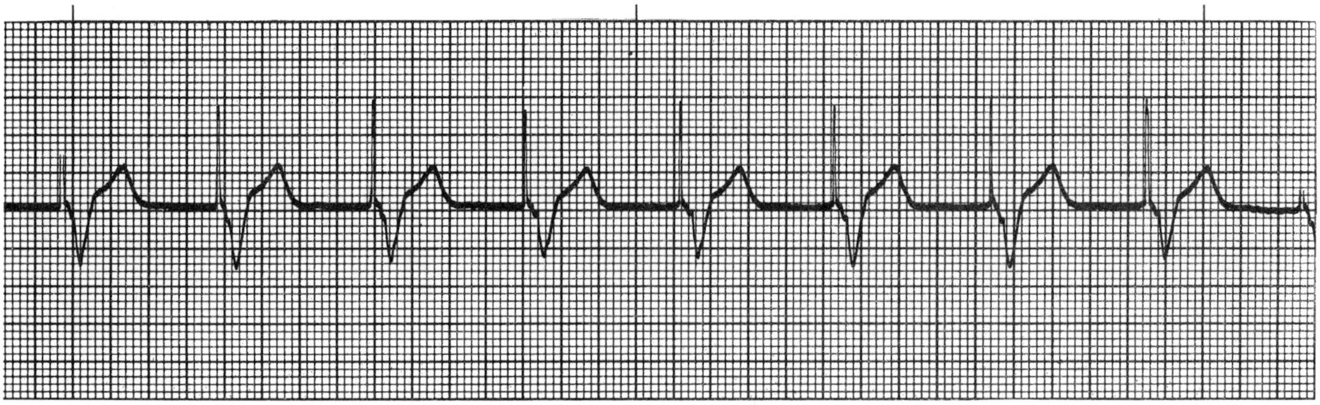

**Strip 10-37.** Automatic interval rate:_____

Analysis:_____

Interpretation:_____

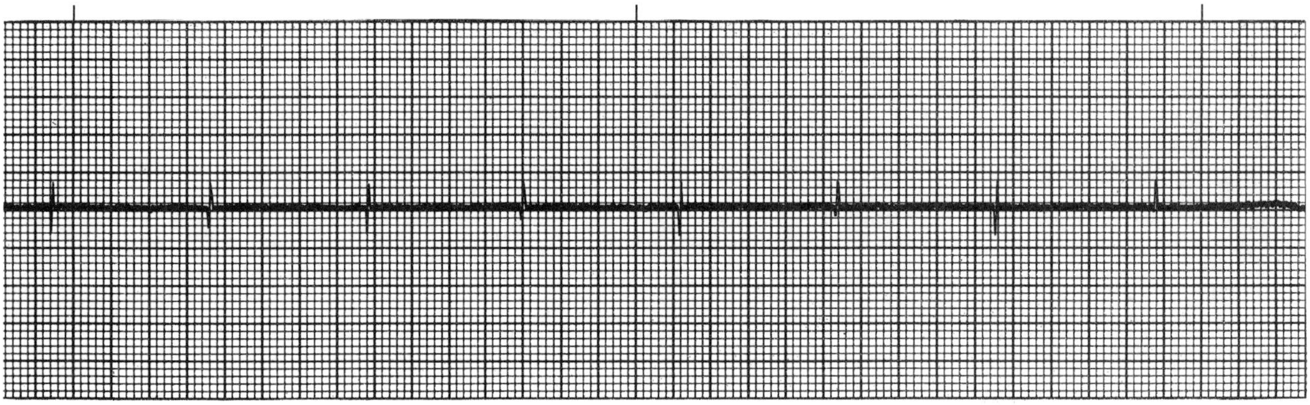

**Strip 10-38.** Automatic interval rate:_____

Analysis:_____

Interpretation:_____

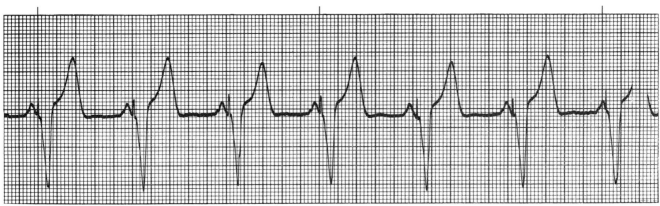

**Strip 10-39.** Automatic interval rate:_____

Analysis:_____

Interpretation:_____

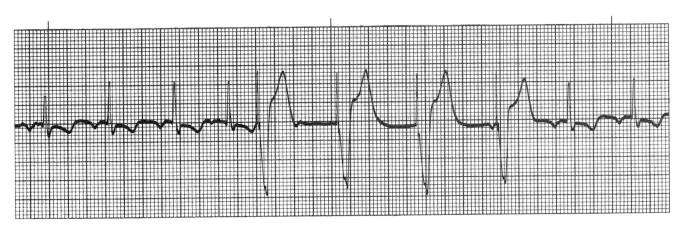

**Strip 10-40.** Automatic interval rate:_____

Analysis:_____

Interpretation:_____

# 11

# POST-TEST

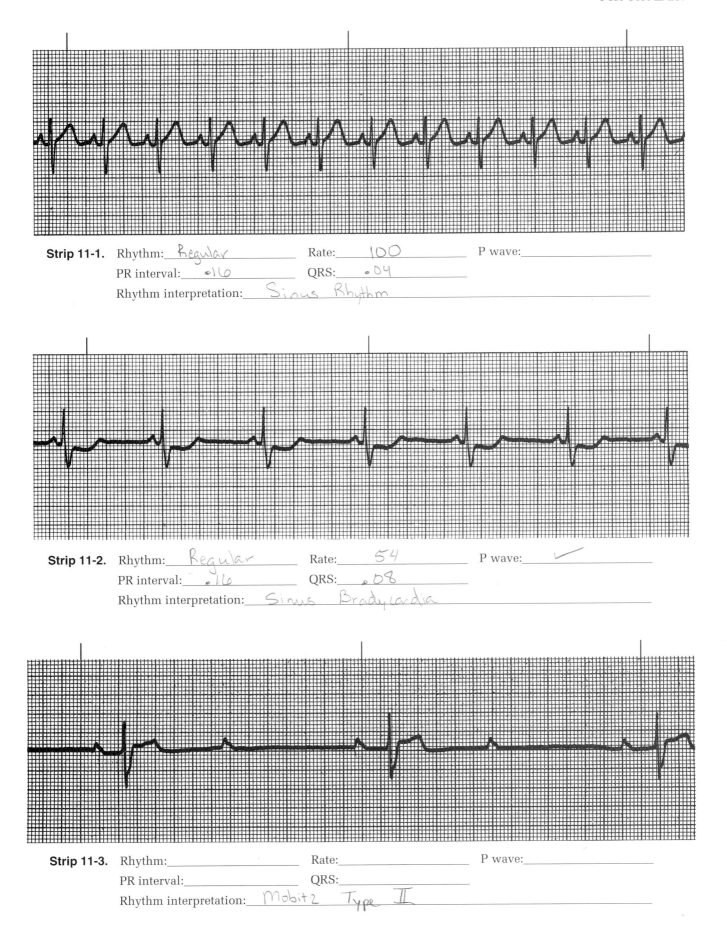

**Strip 11-1.** Rhythm: Regular    Rate: 100    P wave: _____
PR interval: .16    QRS: .04
Rhythm interpretation: Sinus Rhythm

**Strip 11-2.** Rhythm: Regular    Rate: 54    P wave: ✓
PR interval: .16    QRS: .08
Rhythm interpretation: Sinus Bradycardia

**Strip 11-3.** Rhythm: _____    Rate: _____    P wave: _____
PR interval: _____    QRS: _____
Rhythm interpretation: Mobitz Type II

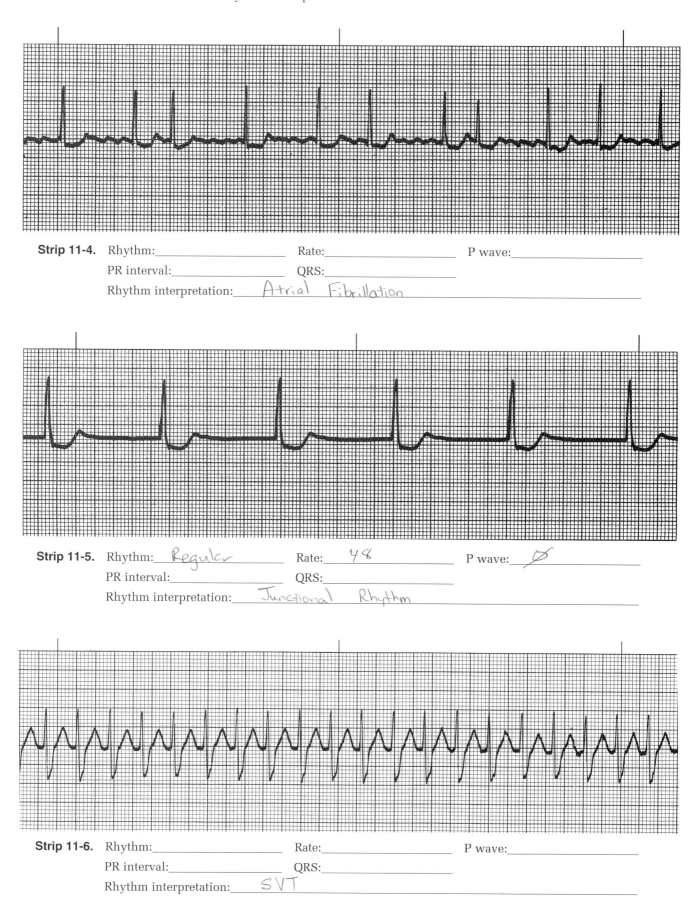

**Strip 11-4.** Rhythm:_____ Rate:_____ P wave:_____

PR interval:_____ QRS:_____

Rhythm interpretation:___Atrial Fibrillation_____

**Strip 11-5.** Rhythm:___Regular_____ Rate:___48_____ P wave:___Ø_____

PR interval:_____ QRS:_____

Rhythm interpretation:___Junctional Rhythm_____

**Strip 11-6.** Rhythm:_____ Rate:_____ P wave:_____

PR interval:_____ QRS:_____

Rhythm interpretation:___SVT_____

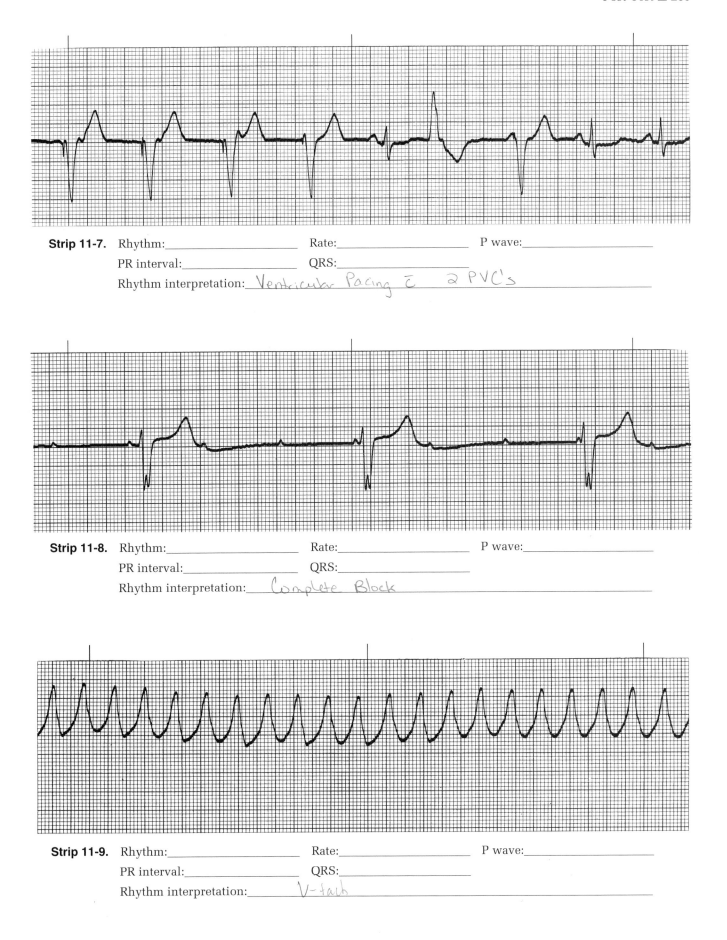

**Strip 11-7.** Rhythm:_____ Rate:_____ P wave:_____

PR interval:_____ QRS:_____

Rhythm interpretation: Ventricular Pacing c̄ 2 PVC's

**Strip 11-8.** Rhythm:_____ Rate:_____ P wave:_____

PR interval:_____ QRS:_____

Rhythm interpretation: Complete Block

**Strip 11-9.** Rhythm:_____ Rate:_____ P wave:_____

PR interval:_____ QRS:_____

Rhythm interpretation: V-tach

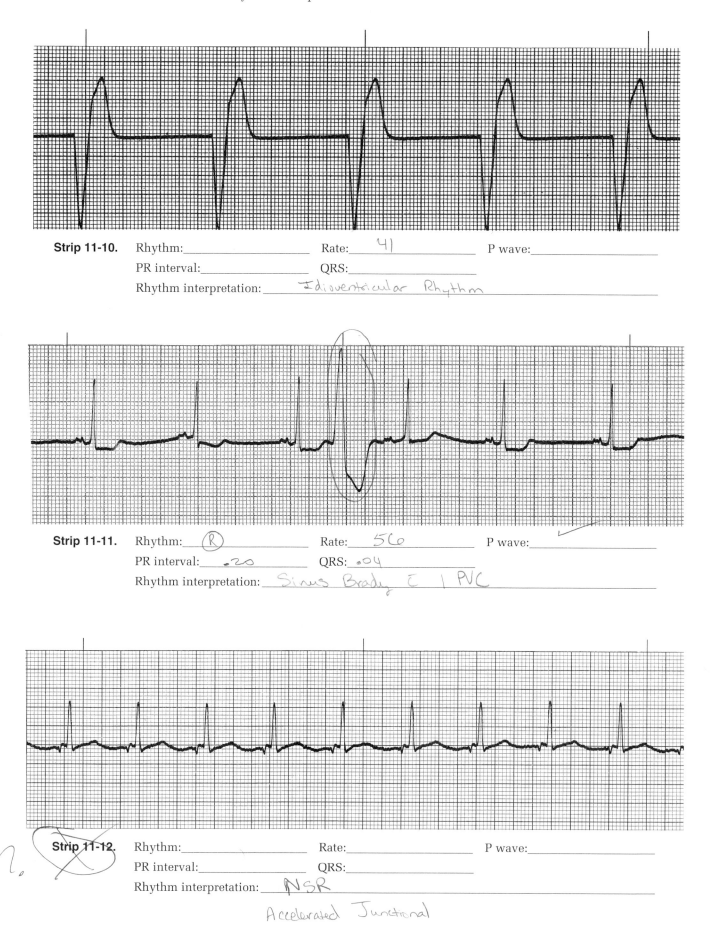

**Strip 11-10.** Rhythm:_____ Rate:___41_____ P wave:_____

PR interval:_____ QRS:_____

Rhythm interpretation:_____Idioventricular Rhythm_____

**Strip 11-11.** Rhythm:___Ⓡ_____ Rate:___56_____ P wave:_____

PR interval:___.20_____ QRS:__.04_____

Rhythm interpretation:___Sinus Brady c̄ 1 PVC_____

**Strip 11-12.** Rhythm:_____ Rate:_____ P wave:_____

PR interval:_____ QRS:_____

Rhythm interpretation:___NSR_____

Accelerated Junctional

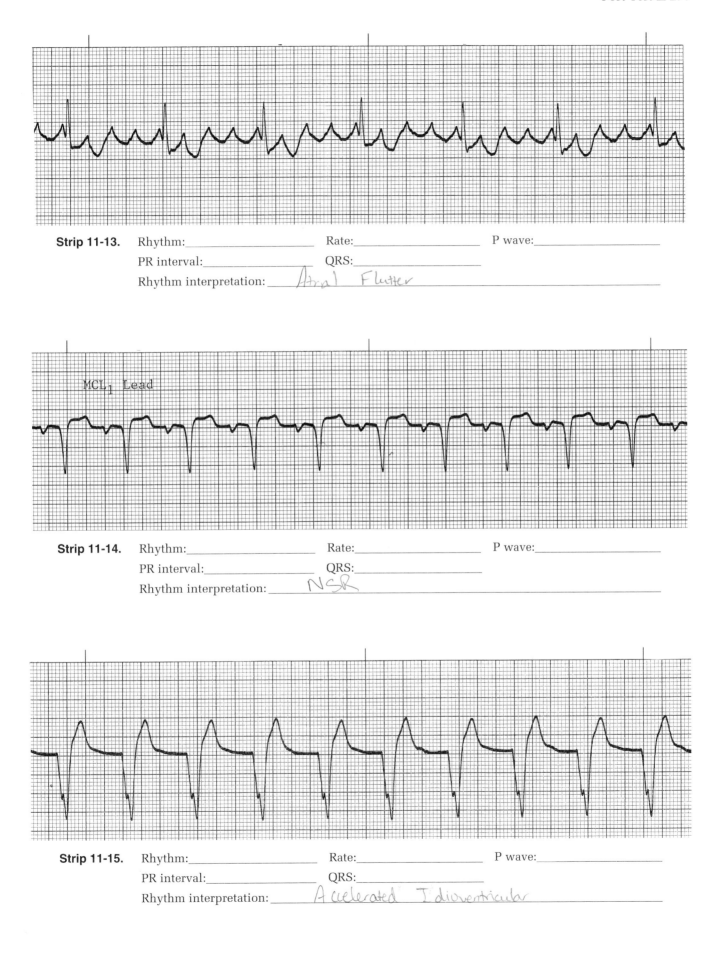

**Strip 11-13.** Rhythm:_____ Rate:_____ P wave:_____

PR interval:_____ QRS:_____

Rhythm interpretation:____Atrial Flutter_____

**Strip 11-14.** Rhythm:_____ Rate:_____ P wave:_____

PR interval:_____ QRS:_____

Rhythm interpretation:____NSR_____

**Strip 11-15.** Rhythm:_____ Rate:_____ P wave:_____

PR interval:_____ QRS:_____

Rhythm interpretation:____Accelerated Idioventricular_____

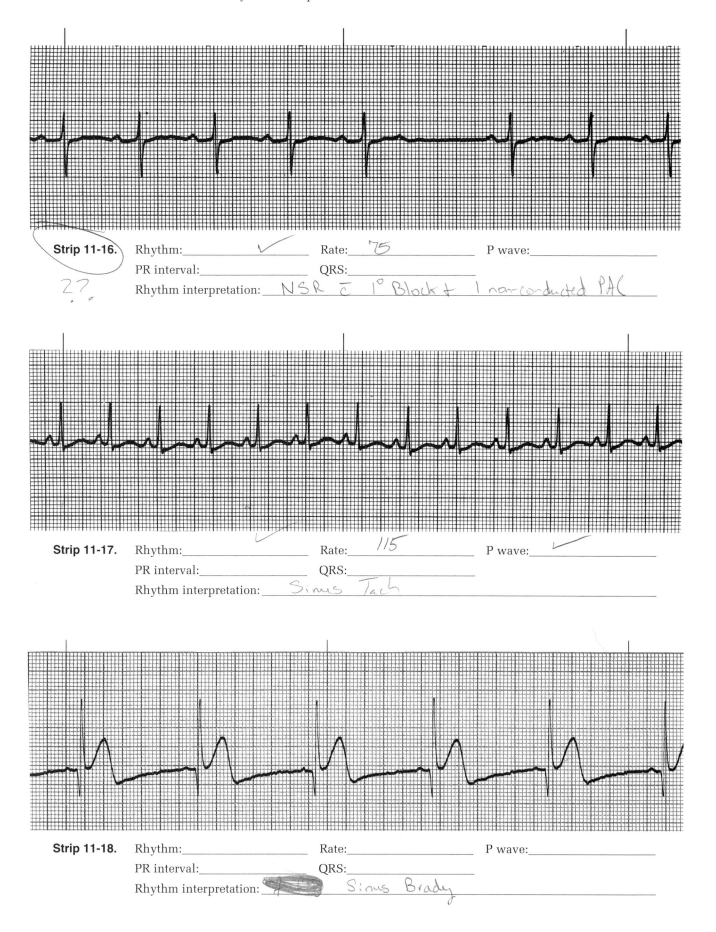

**Strip 11-16.**  Rhythm: ✓   Rate: 75   P wave: _____

2?.

PR interval: _____   QRS: _____

Rhythm interpretation: NSR c̄ 1° Block + 1 non-conducted PAC

**Strip 11-17.**  Rhythm: ✓   Rate: 115   P wave: ✓

PR interval: _____   QRS: _____

Rhythm interpretation: Sinus Tach

**Strip 11-18.**  Rhythm: _____   Rate: _____   P wave: _____

PR interval: _____   QRS: _____

Rhythm interpretation: Sinus Brady

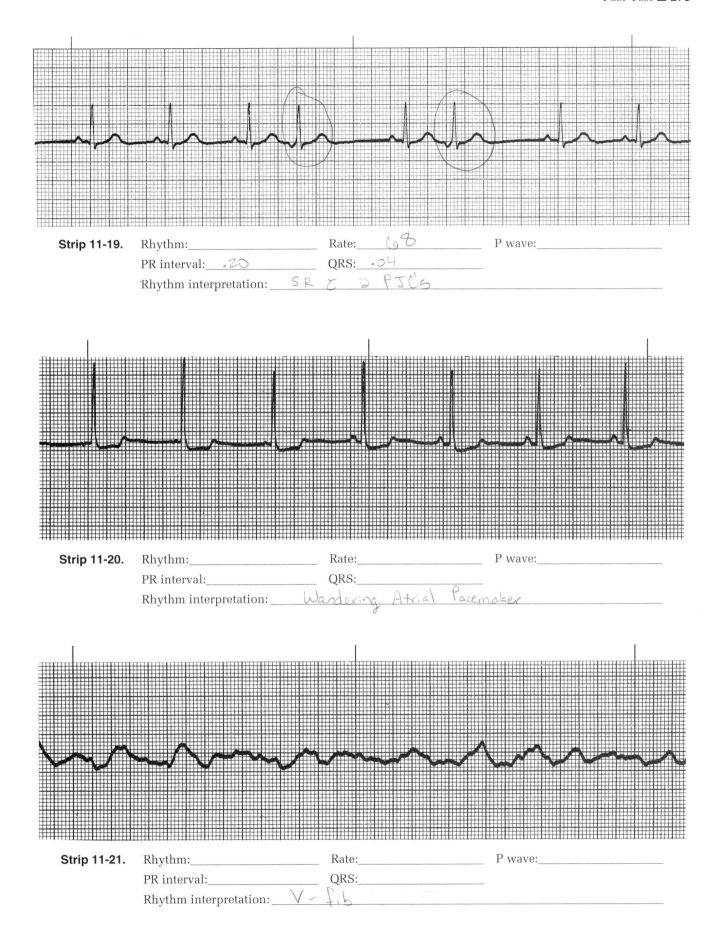

**Strip 11-19.** Rhythm:_____ Rate:____68____ P wave:_____

PR interval:____.20____ QRS:____.04____

Rhythm interpretation:____SR c̄ 2 PJC's____

**Strip 11-20.** Rhythm:_____ Rate:_____ P wave:_____

PR interval:_____ QRS:_____

Rhythm interpretation:____Wandering Atrial Pacemaker____

**Strip 11-21.** Rhythm:_____ Rate:_____ P wave:_____

PR interval:_____ QRS:_____

Rhythm interpretation:____V-fib____

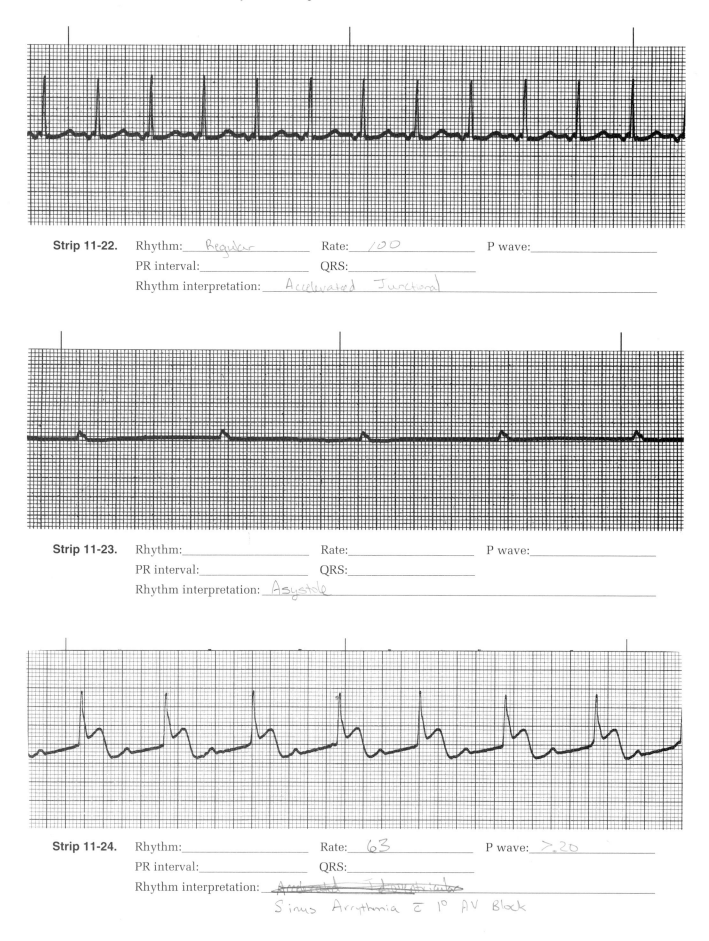

**Strip 11-22.** Rhythm: _Regular_  Rate: _100_  P wave: _____

PR interval: _____  QRS: _____

Rhythm interpretation: _Accelerated Junctional_

**Strip 11-23.** Rhythm: _____  Rate: _____  P wave: _____

PR interval: _____  QRS: _____

Rhythm interpretation: _Asystole_

**Strip 11-24.** Rhythm: _____  Rate: _63_  P wave: _>.20_

PR interval: _____  QRS: _____

Rhythm interpretation: _~~Accelerated Idioventricular~~_

_Sinus Arrythmia c̄ 1° AV Block_

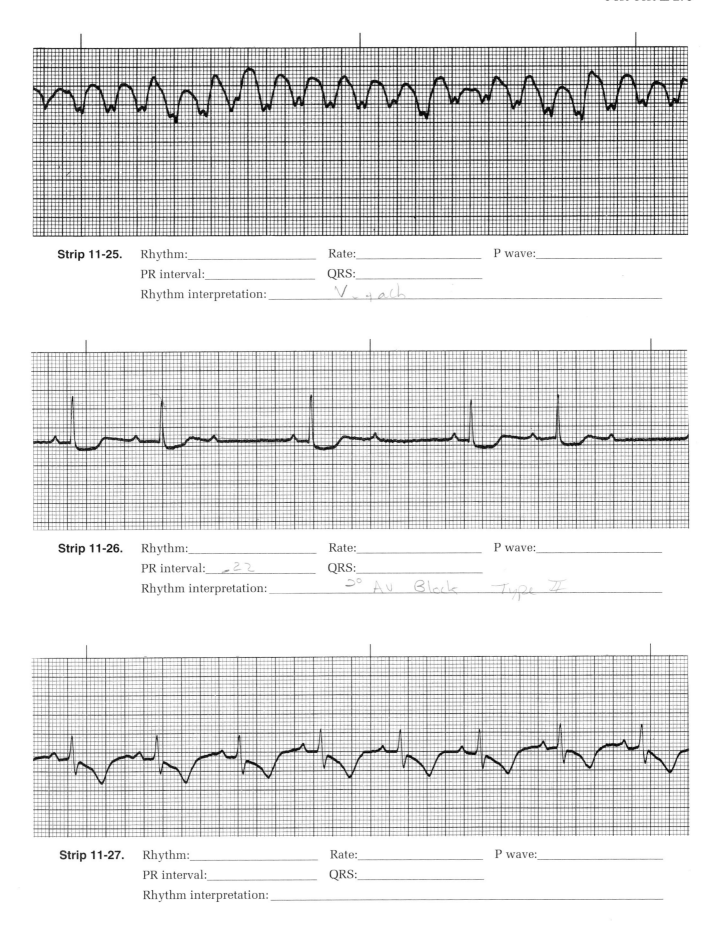

**Strip 11-25.** Rhythm:_____ Rate:_____ P wave:_____

PR interval:_____ QRS:_____

Rhythm interpretation:_____ V tach _____

**Strip 11-26.** Rhythm:_____ Rate:_____ P wave:_____

PR interval:___.22_____ QRS:_____

Rhythm interpretation:_____ 2° AV Block Type II _____

**Strip 11-27.** Rhythm:_____ Rate:_____ P wave:_____

PR interval:_____ QRS:_____

Rhythm interpretation:_____

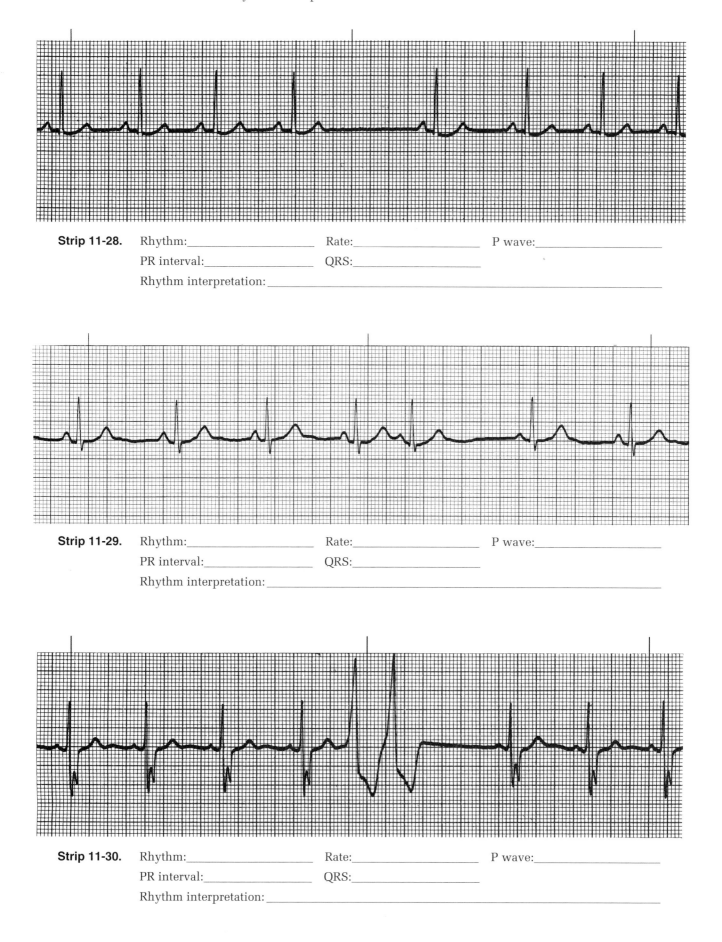

**Strip 11-28.** Rhythm:_____ Rate:_____ P wave:_____

PR interval:_____ QRS:_____

Rhythm interpretation:_____

**Strip 11-29.** Rhythm:_____ Rate:_____ P wave:_____

PR interval:_____ QRS:_____

Rhythm interpretation:_____

**Strip 11-30.** Rhythm:_____ Rate:_____ P wave:_____

PR interval:_____ QRS:_____

Rhythm interpretation:_____

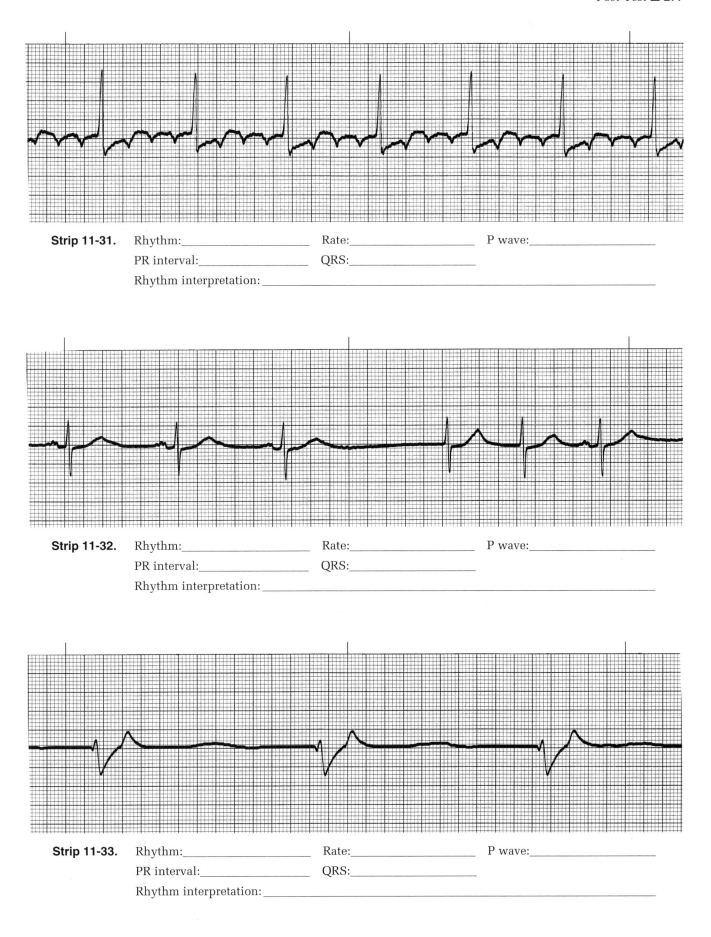

**Strip 11-31.** Rhythm:_____ Rate:_____ P wave:_____

PR interval:_____ QRS:_____

Rhythm interpretation: _____

**Strip 11-32.** Rhythm:_____ Rate:_____ P wave:_____

PR interval:_____ QRS:_____

Rhythm interpretation: _____

**Strip 11-33.** Rhythm:_____ Rate:_____ P wave:_____

PR interval:_____ QRS:_____

Rhythm interpretation: _____

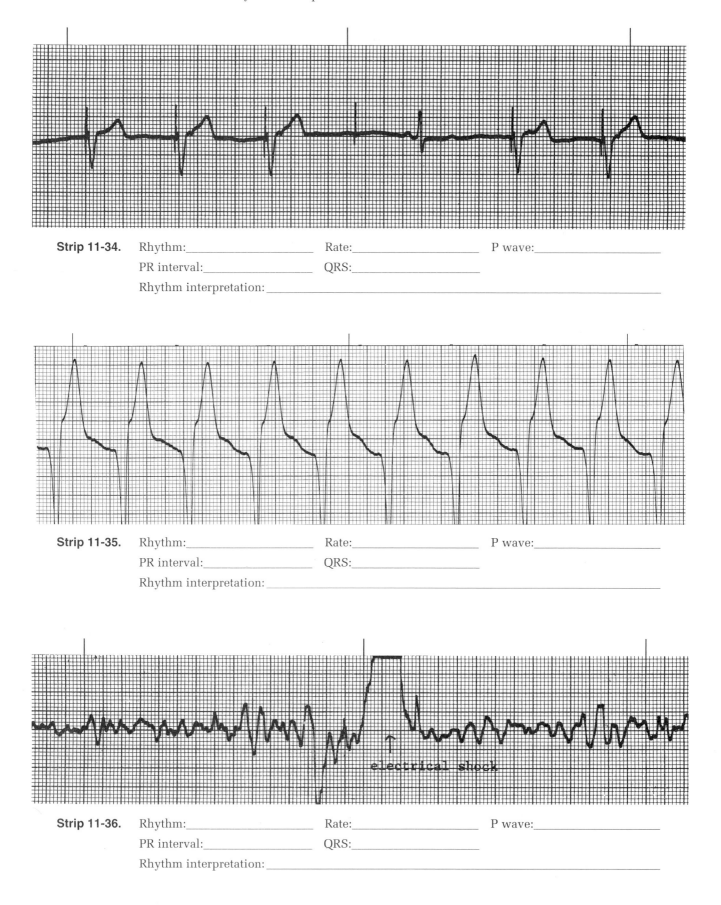

**Strip 11-34.** Rhythm:_____ Rate:_____ P wave:_____

PR interval:_____ QRS:_____

Rhythm interpretation: _____

**Strip 11-35.** Rhythm:_____ Rate:_____ P wave:_____

PR interval:_____ QRS:_____

Rhythm interpretation: _____

**Strip 11-36.** Rhythm:_____ Rate:_____ P wave:_____

PR interval:_____ QRS:_____

Rhythm interpretation: _____

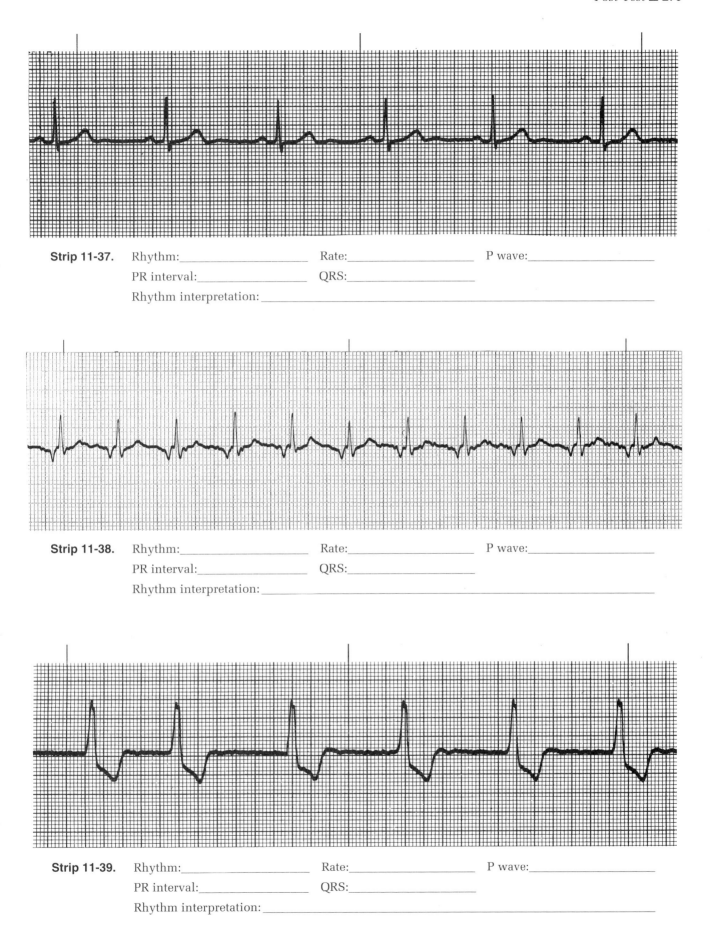

**Strip 11-37.** Rhythm:_____ Rate:_____ P wave:_____

PR interval:_____ QRS:_____

Rhythm interpretation:_____

**Strip 11-38.** Rhythm:_____ Rate:_____ P wave:_____

PR interval:_____ QRS:_____

Rhythm interpretation:_____

**Strip 11-39.** Rhythm:_____ Rate:_____ P wave:_____

PR interval:_____ QRS:_____

Rhythm interpretation:_____

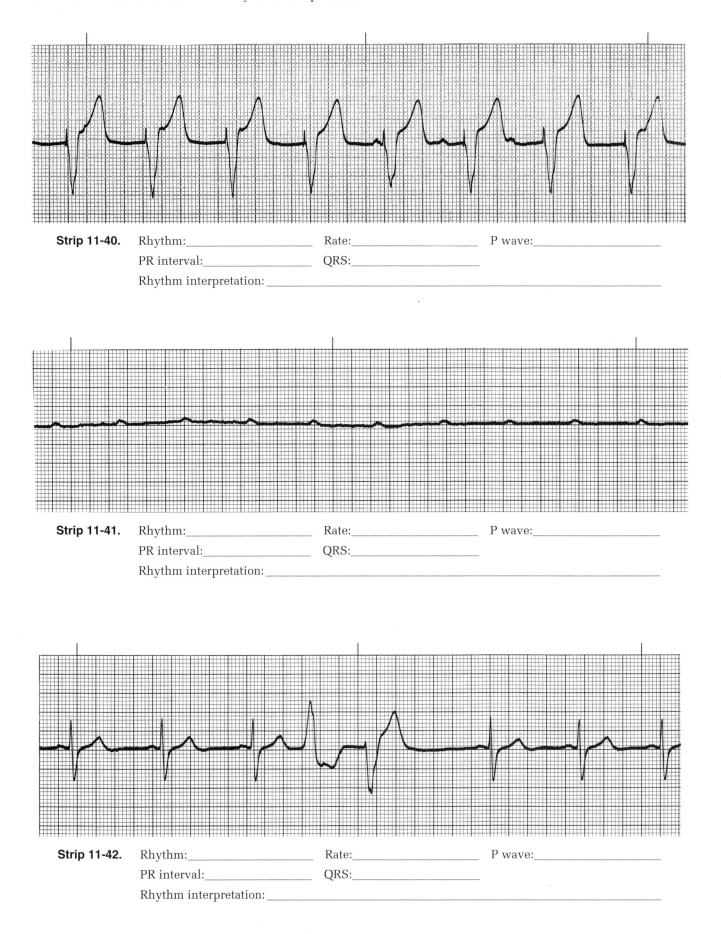

**Strip 11-40.** Rhythm:_____ Rate:_____ P wave:_____

PR interval:_____ QRS:_____

Rhythm interpretation: _____

**Strip 11-41.** Rhythm:_____ Rate:_____ P wave:_____

PR interval:_____ QRS:_____

Rhythm interpretation: _____

**Strip 11-42.** Rhythm:_____ Rate:_____ P wave:_____

PR interval:_____ QRS:_____

Rhythm interpretation: _____

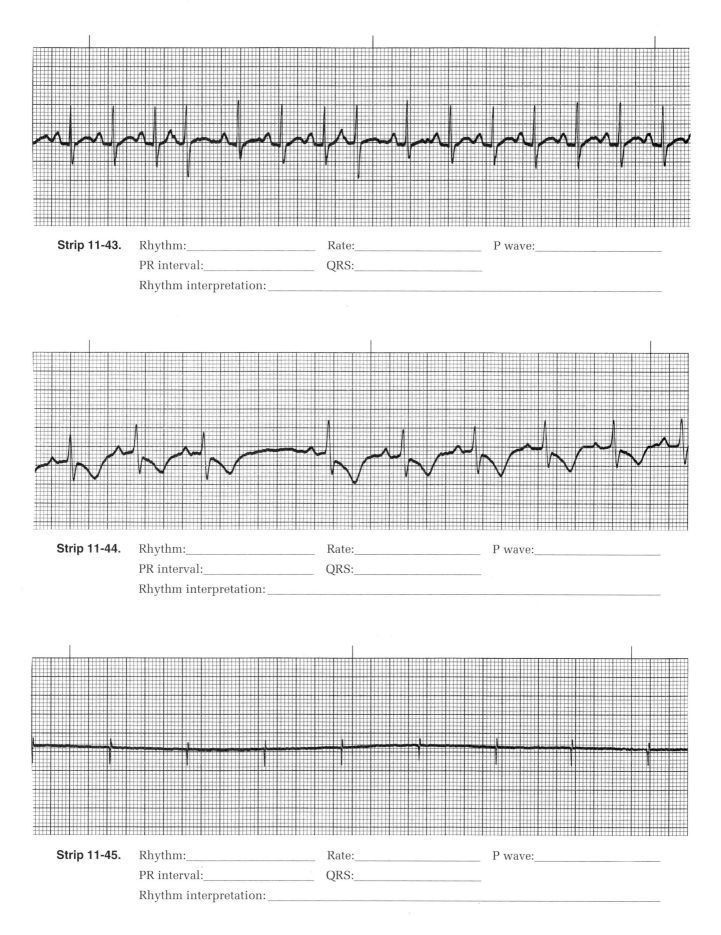

**Strip 11-43.** Rhythm:_____ Rate:_____ P wave:_____

PR interval:_____ QRS:_____

Rhythm interpretation:_____

**Strip 11-44.** Rhythm:_____ Rate:_____ P wave:_____

PR interval:_____ QRS:_____

Rhythm interpretation:_____

**Strip 11-45.** Rhythm:_____ Rate:_____ P wave:_____

PR interval:_____ QRS:_____

Rhythm interpretation:_____

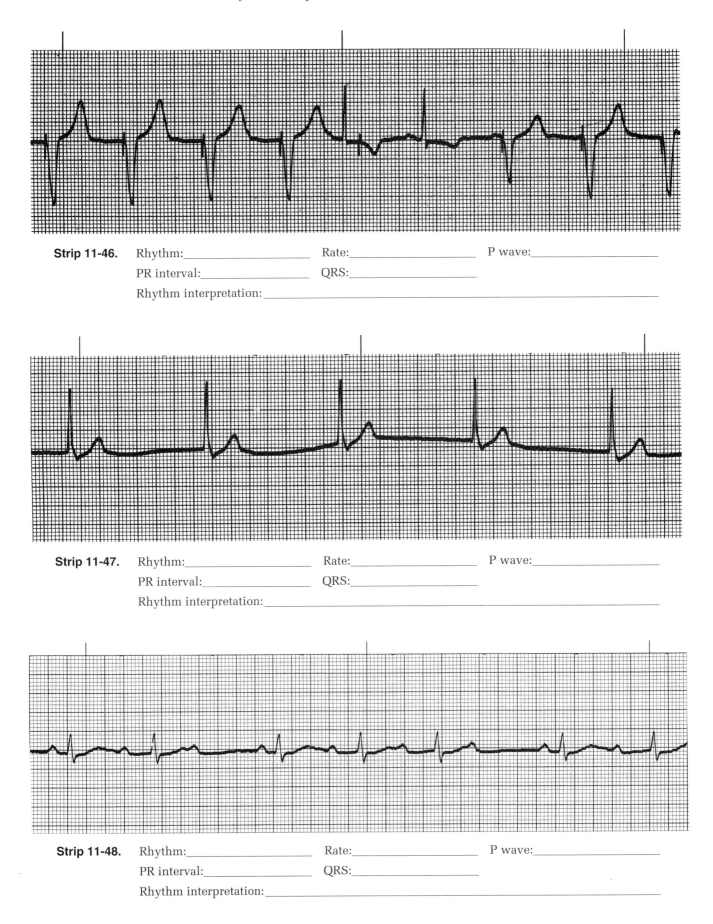

**Strip 11-46.** Rhythm:_____ Rate:_____ P wave:_____

PR interval:_____ QRS:_____

Rhythm interpretation: _____

**Strip 11-47.** Rhythm:_____ Rate:_____ P wave:_____

PR interval:_____ QRS:_____

Rhythm interpretation: _____

**Strip 11-48.** Rhythm:_____ Rate:_____ P wave:_____

PR interval:_____ QRS:_____

Rhythm interpretation: _____

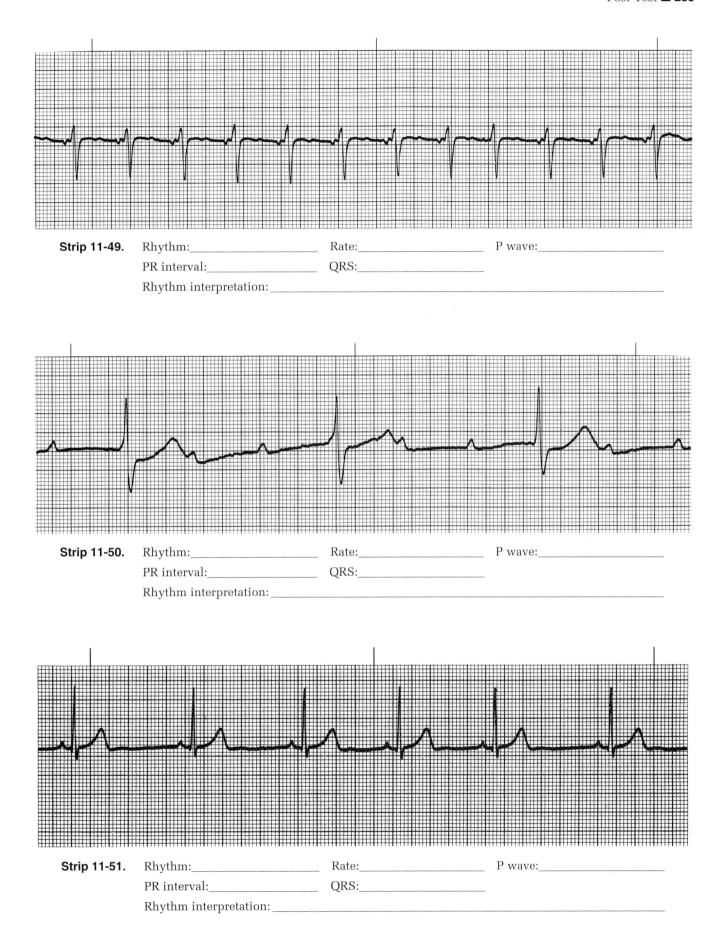

**Strip 11-49.** Rhythm:_____ Rate:_____ P wave:_____

PR interval:_____ QRS:_____

Rhythm interpretation: _____

**Strip 11-50.** Rhythm:_____ Rate:_____ P wave:_____

PR interval:_____ QRS:_____

Rhythm interpretation: _____

**Strip 11-51.** Rhythm:_____ Rate:_____ P wave:_____

PR interval:_____ QRS:_____

Rhythm interpretation: _____

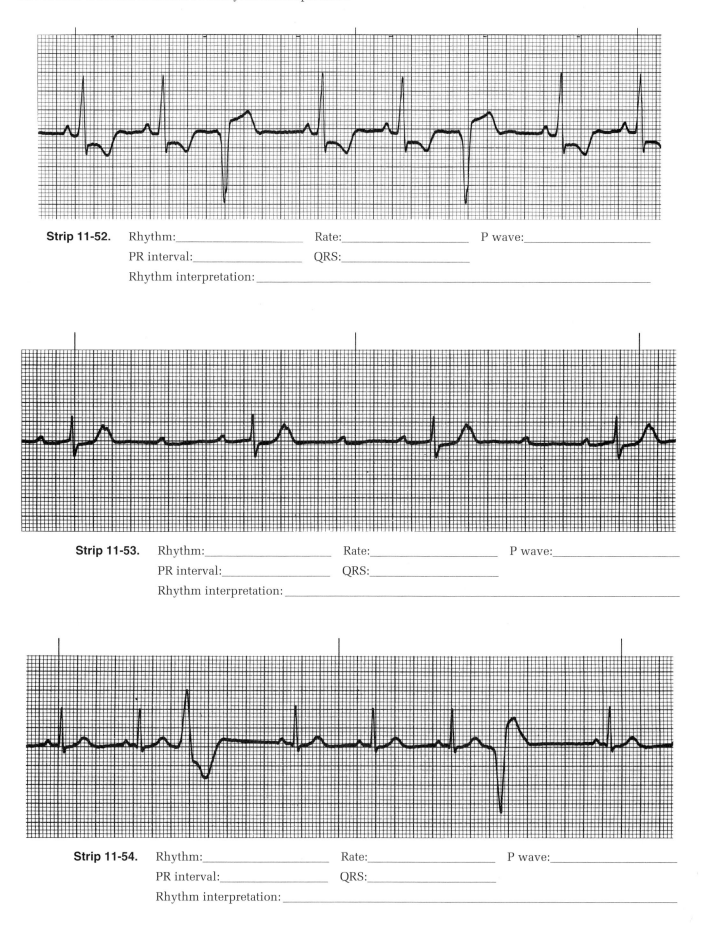

**Strip 11-52.** Rhythm:_____ Rate:_____ P wave:_____

PR interval:_____ QRS:_____

Rhythm interpretation: _____

**Strip 11-53.** Rhythm:_____ Rate:_____ P wave:_____

PR interval:_____ QRS:_____

Rhythm interpretation: _____

**Strip 11-54.** Rhythm:_____ Rate:_____ P wave:_____

PR interval:_____ QRS:_____

Rhythm interpretation: _____

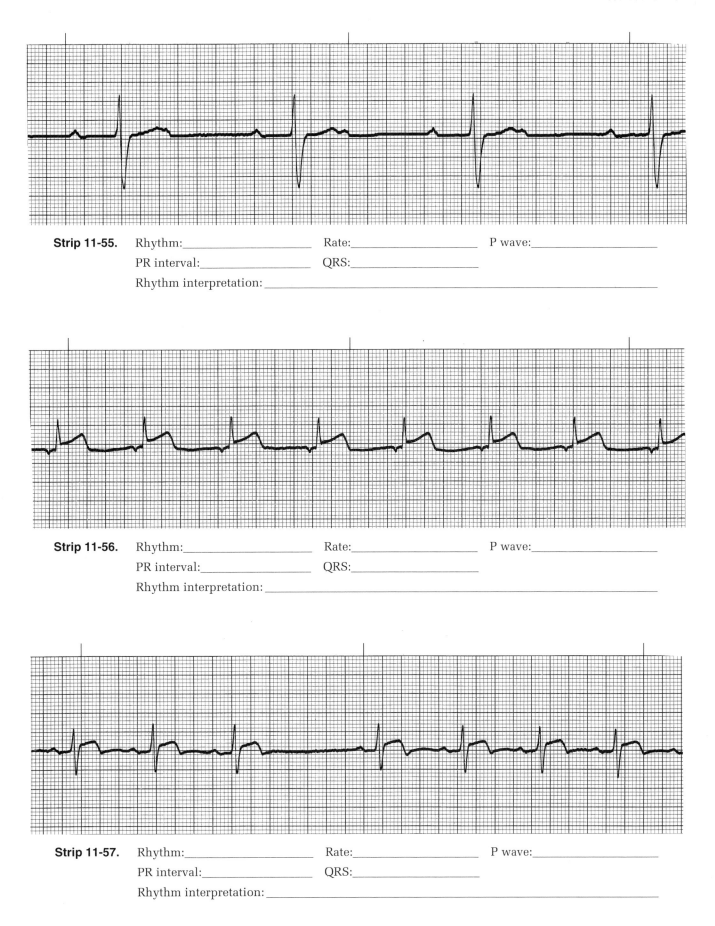

**Strip 11-55.** Rhythm:_____ Rate:_____ P wave:_____

PR interval:_____ QRS:_____

Rhythm interpretation:_____

**Strip 11-56.** Rhythm:_____ Rate:_____ P wave:_____

PR interval:_____ QRS:_____

Rhythm interpretation:_____

**Strip 11-57.** Rhythm:_____ Rate:_____ P wave:_____

PR interval:_____ QRS:_____

Rhythm interpretation:_____

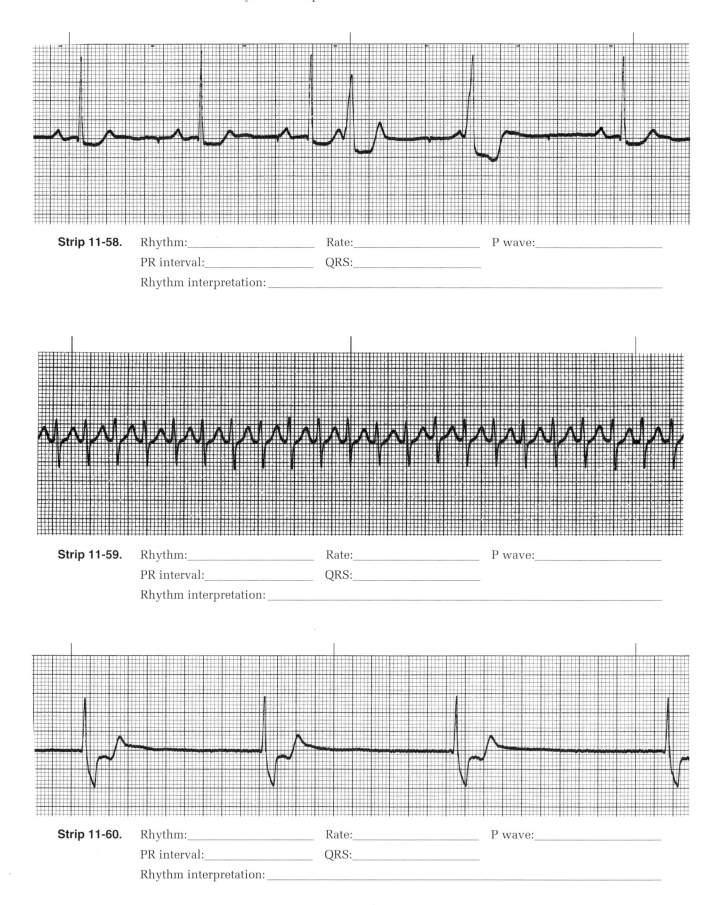

**Strip 11-58.** Rhythm:_____ Rate:_____ P wave:_____

PR interval:_____ QRS:_____

Rhythm interpretation:_____

**Strip 11-59.** Rhythm:_____ Rate:_____ P wave:_____

PR interval:_____ QRS:_____

Rhythm interpretation:_____

**Strip 11-60.** Rhythm:_____ Rate:_____ P wave:_____

PR interval:_____ QRS:_____

Rhythm interpretation:_____

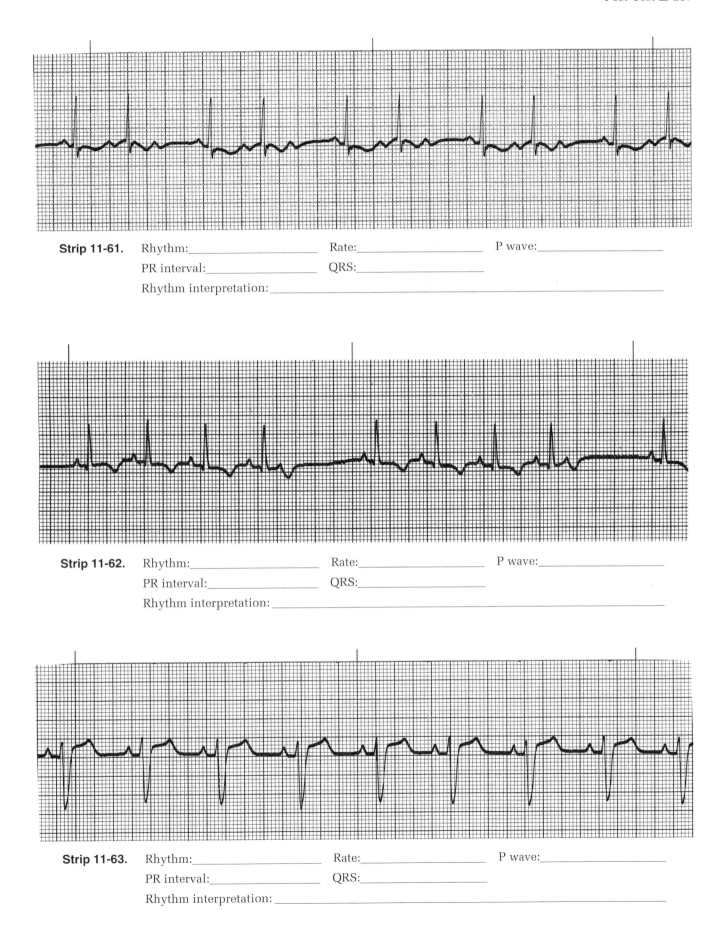

**Strip 11-61.** Rhythm:_____ Rate:_____ P wave:_____

PR interval:_____ QRS:_____

Rhythm interpretation: _____

**Strip 11-62.** Rhythm:_____ Rate:_____ P wave:_____

PR interval:_____ QRS:_____

Rhythm interpretation: _____

**Strip 11-63.** Rhythm:_____ Rate:_____ P wave:_____

PR interval:_____ QRS:_____

Rhythm interpretation: _____

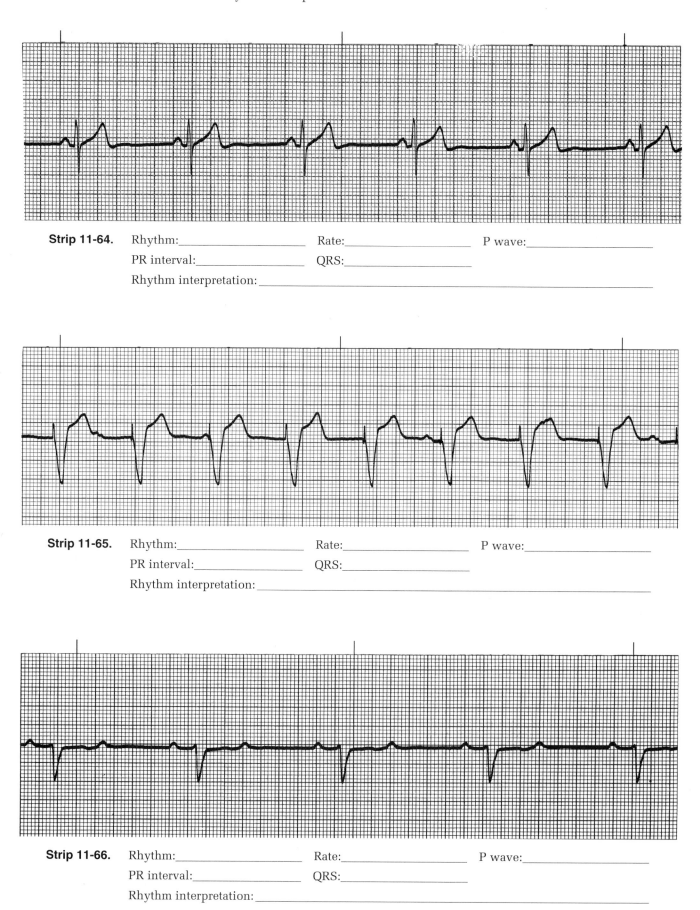

**Strip 11-64.** Rhythm:_____ Rate:_____ P wave:_____

PR interval:_____ QRS:_____

Rhythm interpretation:_____

**Strip 11-65.** Rhythm:_____ Rate:_____ P wave:_____

PR interval:_____ QRS:_____

Rhythm interpretation:_____

**Strip 11-66.** Rhythm:_____ Rate:_____ P wave:_____

PR interval:_____ QRS:_____

Rhythm interpretation:_____

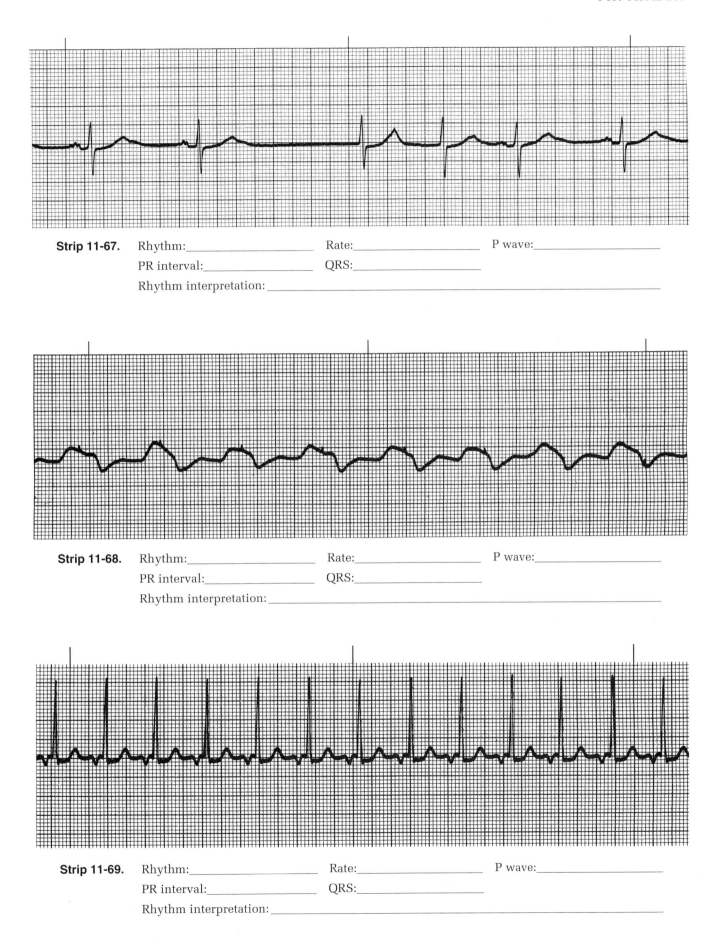

**Strip 11-67.** Rhythm:_____ Rate:_____ P wave:_____

PR interval:_____ QRS:_____

Rhythm interpretation: _____

**Strip 11-68.** Rhythm:_____ Rate:_____ P wave:_____

PR interval:_____ QRS:_____

Rhythm interpretation: _____

**Strip 11-69.** Rhythm:_____ Rate:_____ P wave:_____

PR interval:_____ QRS:_____

Rhythm interpretation: _____

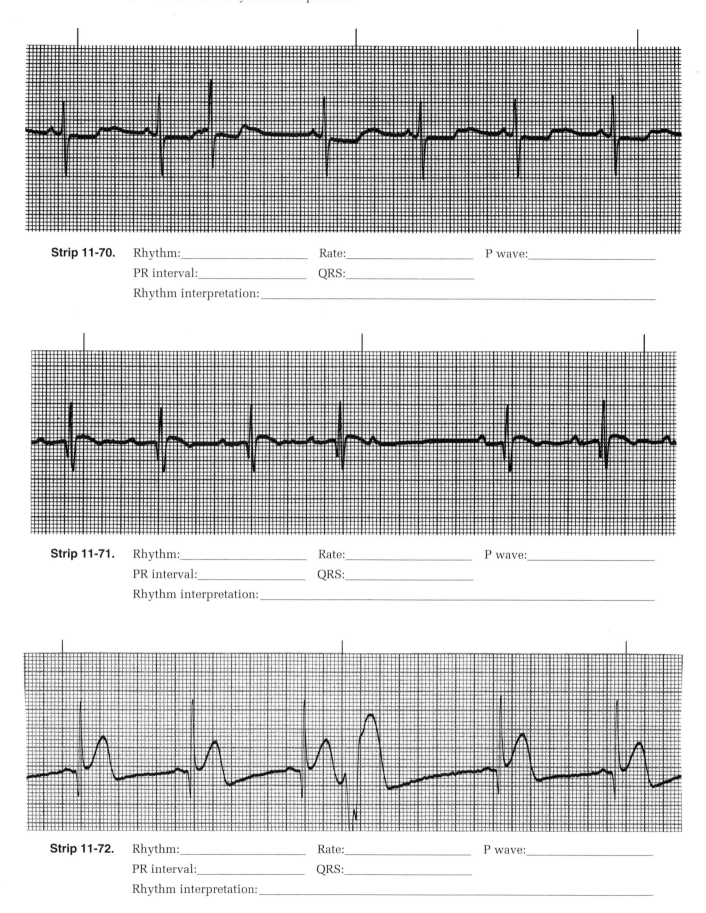

**Strip 11-70.** Rhythm:_____ Rate:_____ P wave:_____

PR interval:_____ QRS:_____

Rhythm interpretation:_____

**Strip 11-71.** Rhythm:_____ Rate:_____ P wave:_____

PR interval:_____ QRS:_____

Rhythm interpretation:_____

**Strip 11-72.** Rhythm:_____ Rate:_____ P wave:_____

PR interval:_____ QRS:_____

Rhythm interpretation:_____

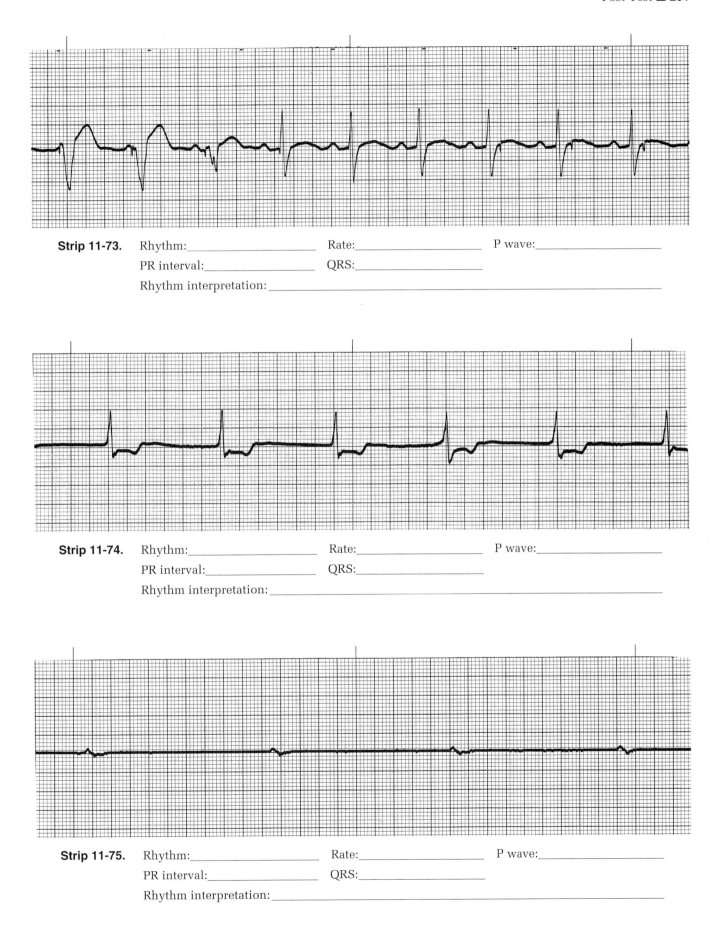

**Strip 11-73.** Rhythm:_____ Rate:_____ P wave:_____

PR interval:_____ QRS:_____

Rhythm interpretation: _____

**Strip 11-74.** Rhythm:_____ Rate:_____ P wave:_____

PR interval:_____ QRS:_____

Rhythm interpretation: _____

**Strip 11-75.** Rhythm:_____ Rate:_____ P wave:_____

PR interval:_____ QRS:_____

Rhythm interpretation: _____

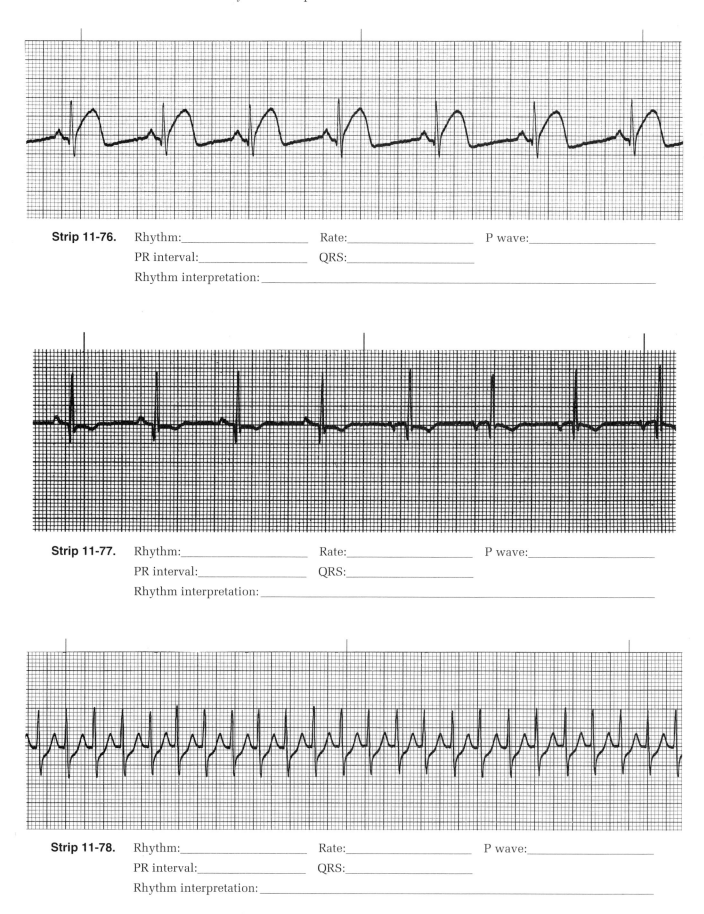

**Strip 11-76.** Rhythm:_____ Rate:_____ P wave:_____

PR interval:_____ QRS:_____

Rhythm interpretation: _____

**Strip 11-77.** Rhythm:_____ Rate:_____ P wave:_____

PR interval:_____ QRS:_____

Rhythm interpretation: _____

**Strip 11-78.** Rhythm:_____ Rate:_____ P wave:_____

PR interval:_____ QRS:_____

Rhythm interpretation: _____

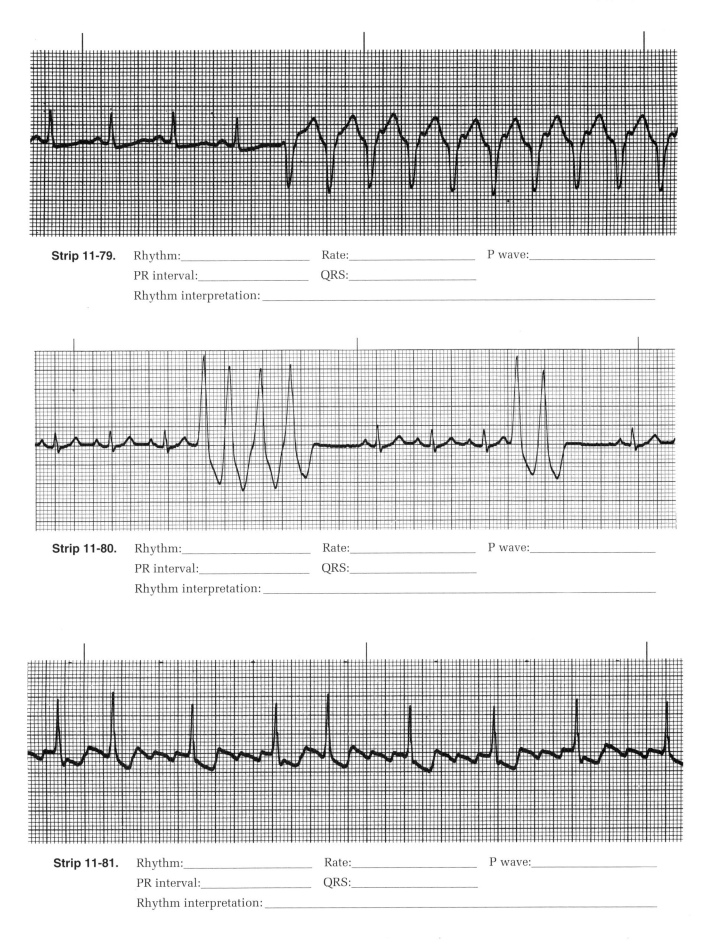

**Strip 11-79.** Rhythm:_____ Rate:_____ P wave:_____

PR interval:_____ QRS:_____

Rhythm interpretation: _____

**Strip 11-80.** Rhythm:_____ Rate:_____ P wave:_____

PR interval:_____ QRS:_____

Rhythm interpretation: _____

**Strip 11-81.** Rhythm:_____ Rate:_____ P wave:_____

PR interval:_____ QRS:_____

Rhythm interpretation: _____

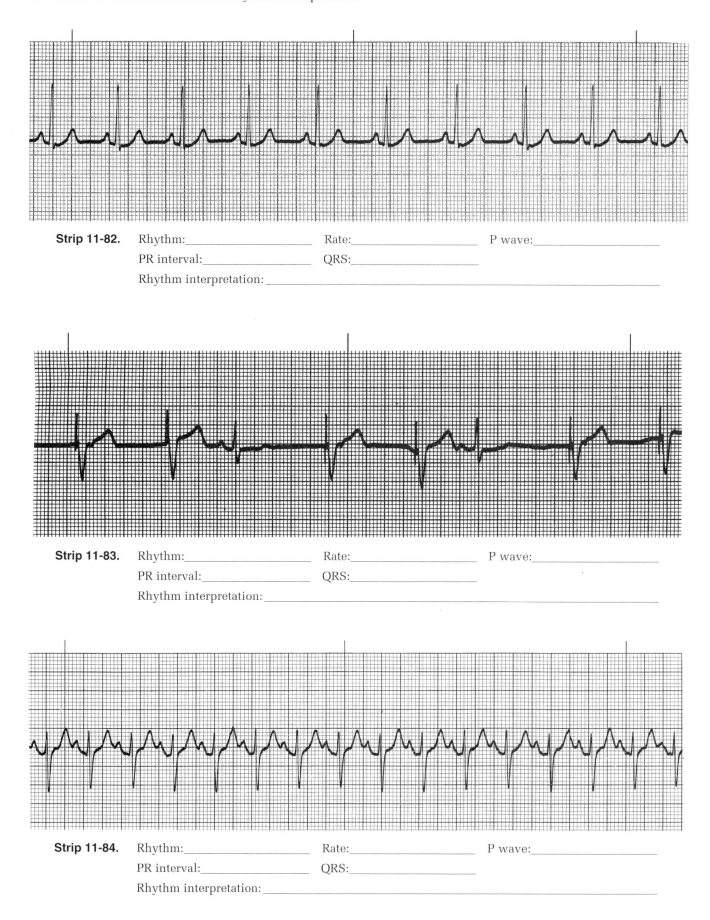

**Strip 11-82.** Rhythm:_____ Rate:_____ P wave:_____

PR interval:_____ QRS:_____

Rhythm interpretation: _____

**Strip 11-83.** Rhythm:_____ Rate:_____ P wave:_____

PR interval:_____ QRS:_____

Rhythm interpretation: _____

**Strip 11-84.** Rhythm:_____ Rate:_____ P wave:_____

PR interval:_____ QRS:_____

Rhythm interpretation: _____

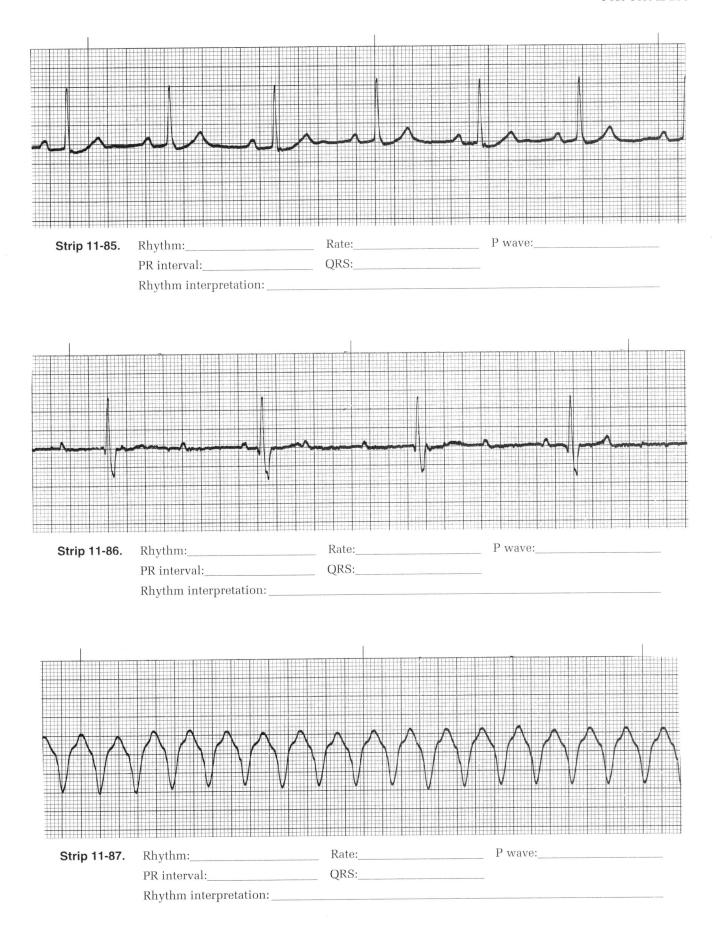

**Strip 11-85.** Rhythm:_____ Rate:_____ P wave:_____

PR interval:_____ QRS:_____

Rhythm interpretation: _____

**Strip 11-86.** Rhythm:_____ Rate:_____ P wave:_____

PR interval:_____ QRS:_____

Rhythm interpretation: _____

**Strip 11-87.** Rhythm:_____ Rate:_____ P wave:_____

PR interval:_____ QRS:_____

Rhythm interpretation: _____

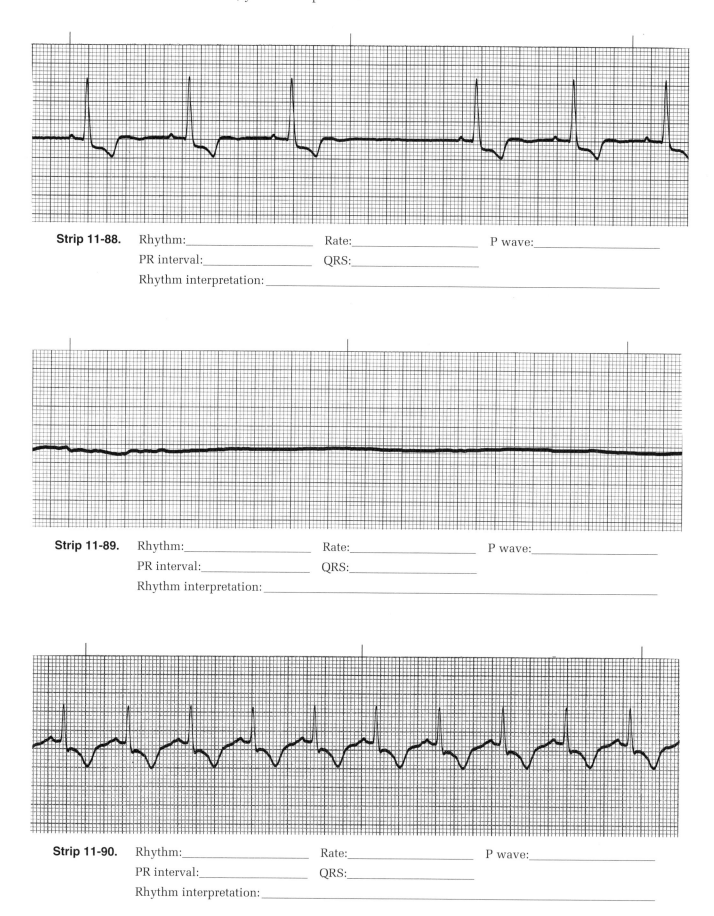

**Strip 11-88.**  Rhythm:_____  Rate:_____  P wave:_____

PR interval:_____  QRS:_____

Rhythm interpretation:_____

**Strip 11-89.**  Rhythm:_____  Rate:_____  P wave:_____

PR interval:_____  QRS:_____

Rhythm interpretation:_____

**Strip 11-90.**  Rhythm:_____  Rate:_____  P wave:_____

PR interval:_____  QRS:_____

Rhythm interpretation:_____

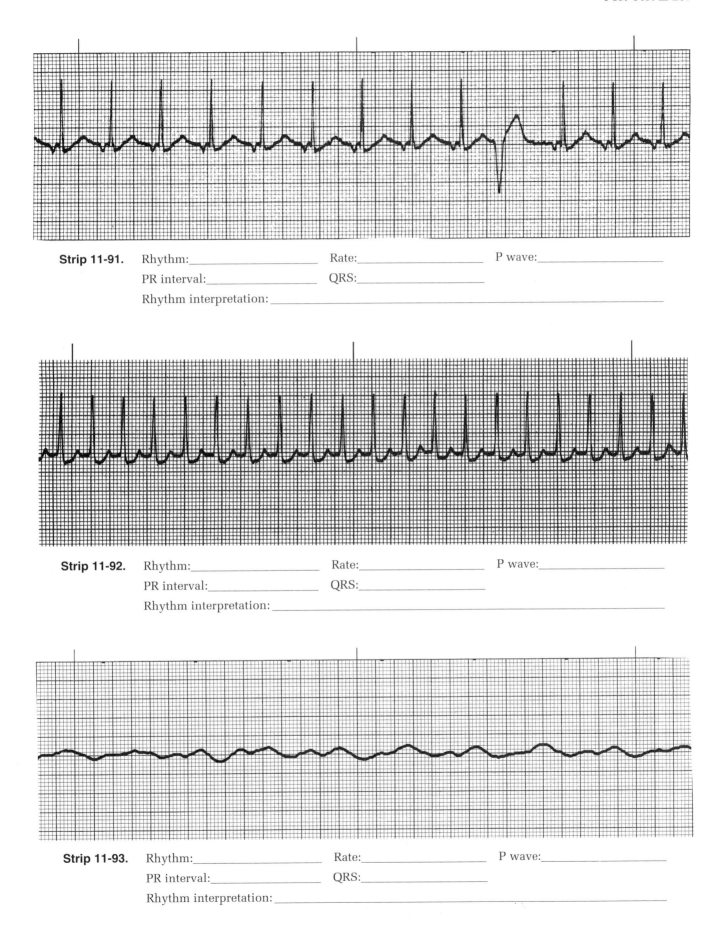

**Strip 11-91.** Rhythm:_____ Rate:_____ P wave:_____

PR interval:_____ QRS:_____

Rhythm interpretation: _____

**Strip 11-92.** Rhythm:_____ Rate:_____ P wave:_____

PR interval:_____ QRS:_____

Rhythm interpretation: _____

**Strip 11-93.** Rhythm:_____ Rate:_____ P wave:_____

PR interval:_____ QRS:_____

Rhythm interpretation: _____

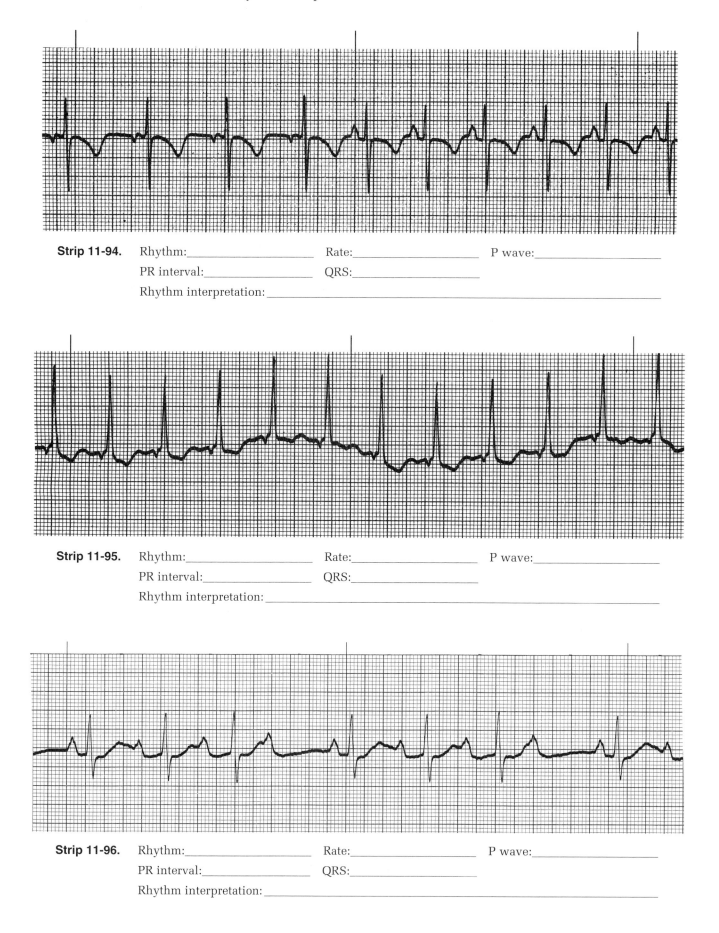

**Strip 11-94.** Rhythm:_____ Rate:_____ P wave:_____

PR interval:_____ QRS:_____

Rhythm interpretation:_____

**Strip 11-95.** Rhythm:_____ Rate:_____ P wave:_____

PR interval:_____ QRS:_____

Rhythm interpretation:_____

**Strip 11-96.** Rhythm:_____ Rate:_____ P wave:_____

PR interval:_____ QRS:_____

Rhythm interpretation:_____

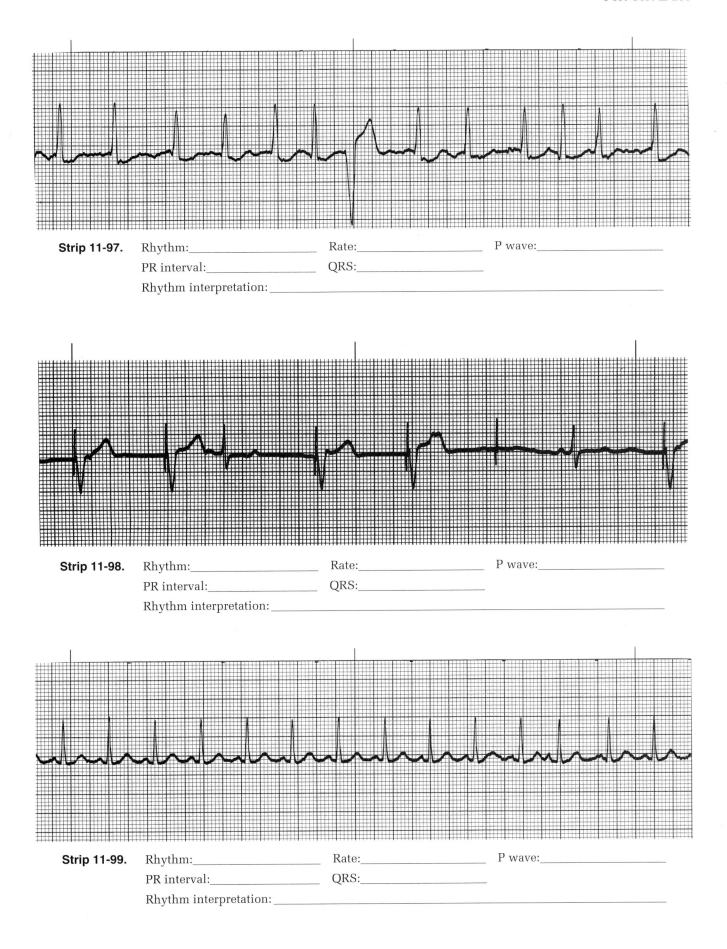

**Strip 11-97.** Rhythm:_____ Rate:_____ P wave:_____

PR interval:_____ QRS:_____

Rhythm interpretation:_____

**Strip 11-98.** Rhythm:_____ Rate:_____ P wave:_____

PR interval:_____ QRS:_____

Rhythm interpretation:_____

**Strip 11-99.** Rhythm:_____ Rate:_____ P wave:_____

PR interval:_____ QRS:_____

Rhythm interpretation:_____

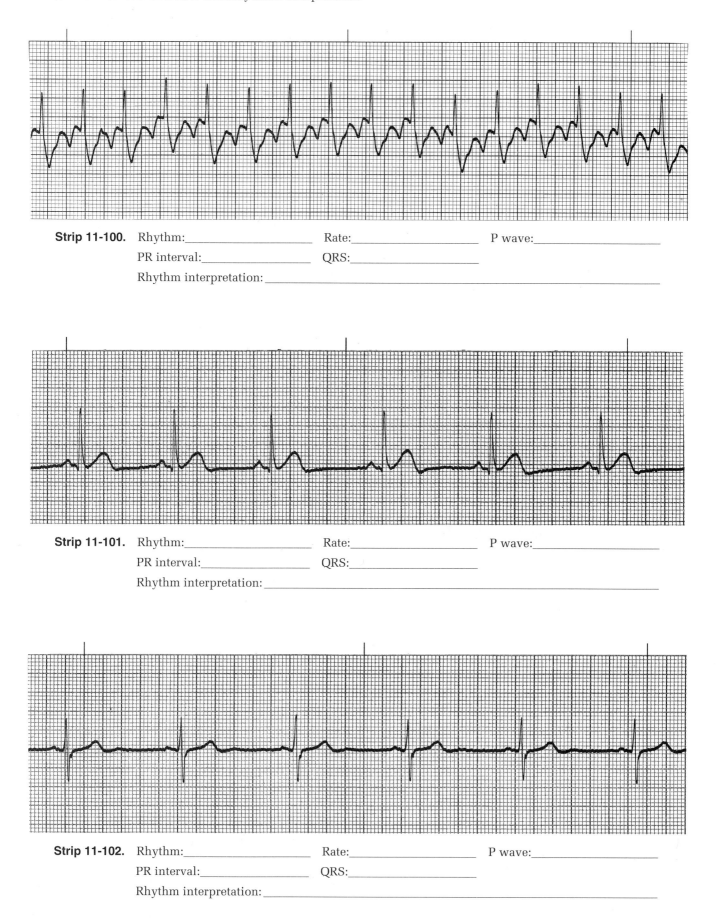

**Strip 11-100.** Rhythm:_____ Rate:_____ P wave:_____

PR interval:_____ QRS:_____

Rhythm interpretation: _____

**Strip 11-101.** Rhythm:_____ Rate:_____ P wave:_____

PR interval:_____ QRS:_____

Rhythm interpretation: _____

**Strip 11-102.** Rhythm:_____ Rate:_____ P wave:_____

PR interval:_____ QRS:_____

Rhythm interpretation: _____

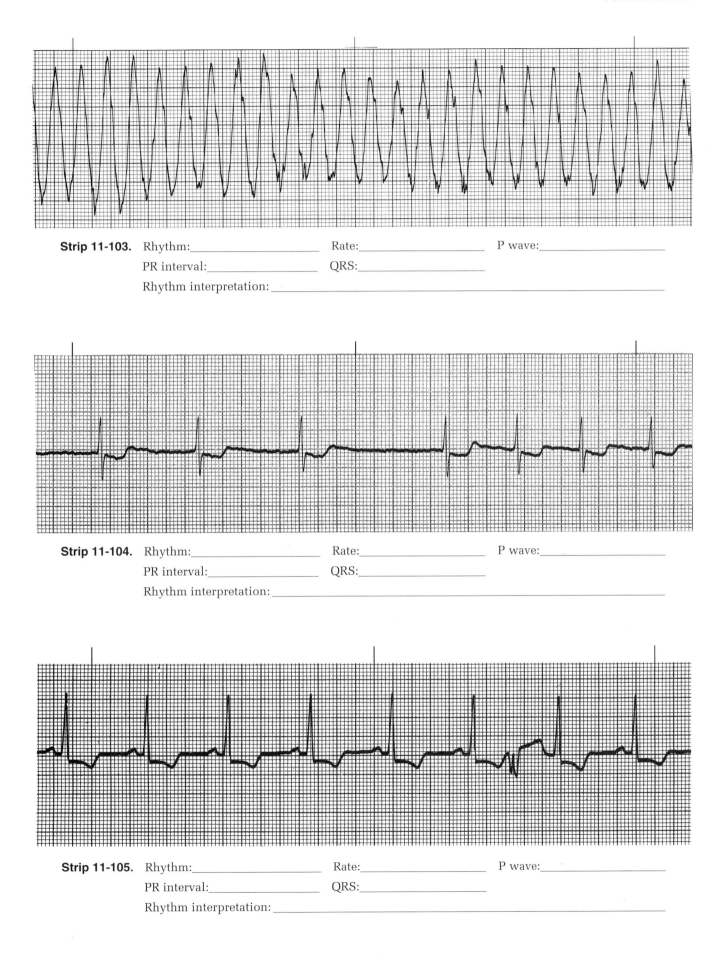

**Strip 11-103.** Rhythm:_____ Rate:_____ P wave:_____

PR interval:_____ QRS:_____

Rhythm interpretation: _____

**Strip 11-104.** Rhythm:_____ Rate:_____ P wave:_____

PR interval:_____ QRS:_____

Rhythm interpretation: _____

**Strip 11-105.** Rhythm:_____ Rate:_____ P wave:_____

PR interval:_____ QRS:_____

Rhythm interpretation: _____

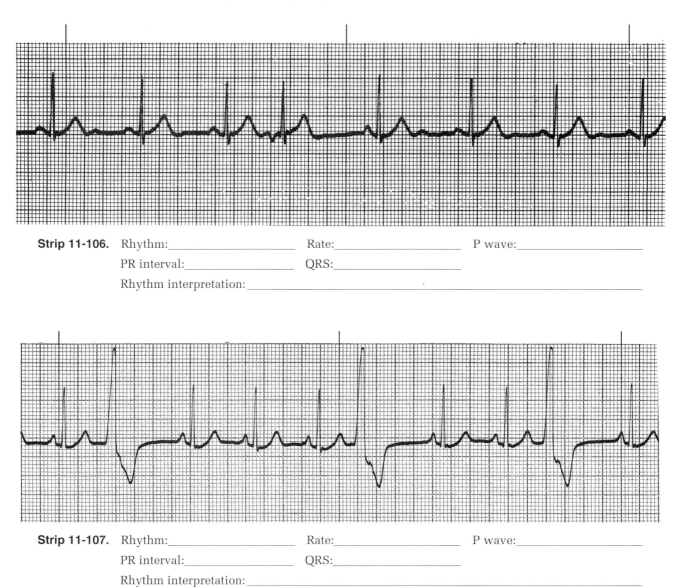

**Strip 11-106.** Rhythm:_____ Rate:_____ P wave:_____

PR interval:_____ QRS:_____

Rhythm interpretation:_____

**Strip 11-107.** Rhythm:_____ Rate:_____ P wave:_____

PR interval:_____ QRS:_____

Rhythm interpretation:_____

## Answer Keys to Chapter 3 and Chapters 5 through 11

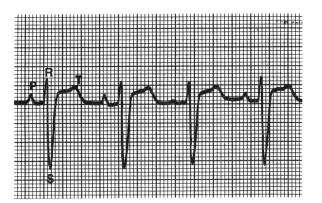

Strip 3-1.

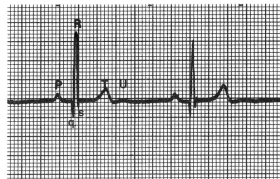

Strip 3-2.

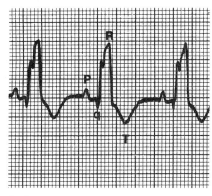

Strip 3-3.

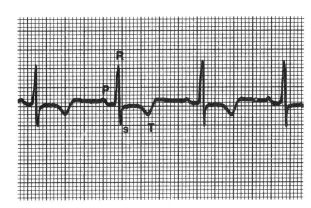

Strip 3-4.

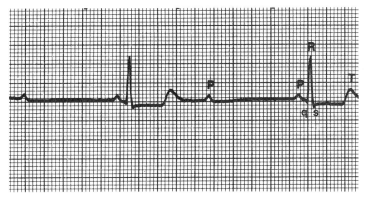

Strip 3-5.

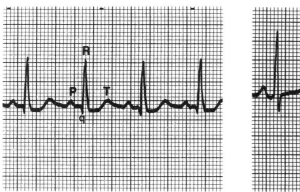

**Strip 3-6.**

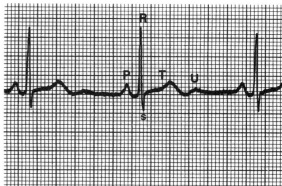

**Strip 3-7.**

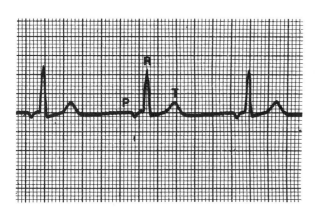

**Strip 3-8.**

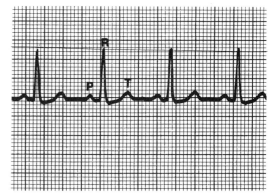

**Strip 3-9.**

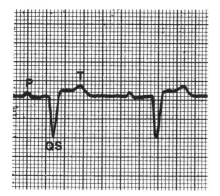

**Strip 3-10.**

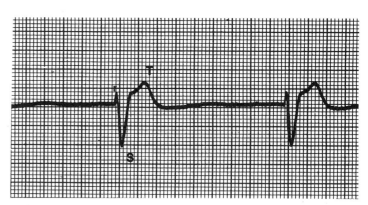

**Strip 3-11.**

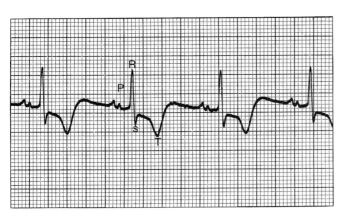

**Strip 3-12.**

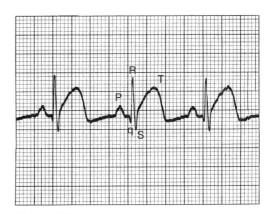

**Strip 3-13.**

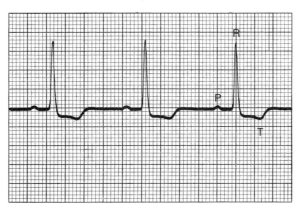

**Strip 3-14.**

**Strip 5-1**
Rhythm: Regular
Rate: 79
P waves: Sinus
PR interval: 0.14 to 0.16 seconds
QRS: 0.06 to 0.08 seconds
Comment: An inverted T wave is present

**Strip 5-2**
Rhythm: Regular
Rate: 45
P waves: Sinus
PR interval: 0.14 to 0.16 seconds
QRS: 0.08 seconds
Comment: A small U wave is seen after the T wave

**Strip 5-3**
Rhythm: Regular
Rate: 88
P waves: Sinus
PR interval: 0.20 seconds
QRS: 0.08–0.10 seconds
Comment: A depressed ST segment and biphasic
T wave is present

**Strip 5-4**
Rhythm: Irregular
Rate: 50
P waves: Sinus
PR interval: 0.16 to 0.18 seconds
QRS: 0.04 seconds

**Strip 5-5**
Rhythm: Regular
Rate: 50
P waves: Sinus
PR interval: 0.18–0.20 seconds
QRS: 0.06–0.08 seconds
Comment: An elevated ST segment is present

**Strip 5-6**
Rhythm: Regular
Rate: 136
P waves: Sinus
PR interval: 0.14 to 0.16 seconds
QRS: 0.06 to 0.08 seconds

**Strip 5-7**
Rhythm: Regular
Rate: 68
P waves: Sinus
PR interval: 0.16 to 0.18 seconds
QRS: 0.12 to 0.14 seconds
Comment: A U wave is present

**Strip 5-8**
Rhythm: Irregular
Rate: 50
P waves: Sinus
PR interval: 0.12 to 0.14 seconds
QRS: 0.06–0.08 seconds
Comment: An elevated ST segment and inverted
T wave are present

**Strip 5-9**
Rhythm: Regular
Rate: 94
P waves: Sinus
PR interval: 0.14 to 0.16 seconds
QRS: 0.06 to 0.08 seconds
Comment: A depressed ST segment is present

**Strip 5-10**
Rhythm: Regular
Rate: 58
P waves: Sinus
PR interval: 0.16–0.18 seconds
QRS: 0.14–0.16 seconds

**Strip 5-11**
Rhythm: Regular
Rate: 56
P waves: Sinus
PR interval: 0.24–0.26 seconds
QRS: 0.04–0.06 seconds

**Strip 6-1**
Rhythm: Regular
Rate: 44
P waves: Sinus
PR interval: 0.20 seconds
QRS: 0.10 seconds
Rhythm interpretation: Sinus bradycardia; an
elevated ST segment and U wave is present

**Strip 6-2**
Rhythm: Regular
Rate: 68
P waves: Sinus
PR interval: 0.16–0.18 seconds
QRS: 0.06–0.08 seconds
Rhythm interpretation: Normal sinus rhythm;
ST depression and T wave inversion is present

**Strip 6-3**
Rhythm: Regular
Rate: 79
P waves: Sinus
PR interval: 0.14–0.16 seconds
QRS: 0.06–0.08 seconds
Rhythm interpretation: Normal sinus rhythm

**Strip 6-4**
Rhythm: Regular
Rate: 107
P waves: Sinus
PR interval: 0.12–0.16 seconds
QRS: 0.06–0.08 seconds
Rhythm interpretation: Sinus tachycardia;
ST depression and T wave inversion is present

**Strip 6-5**
Rhythm: Regular
Rate: 58
P waves: Sinus
PR interval: 0.16–0.18 seconds
QRS: 0.06–0.08 seconds
Rhythm interpretation: Sinus bradycardia; a
U wave is present

**Strip 6-6**
Rhythm: Basic rhythm regular; irregular during
pause
Rate: Basic rhythm 100
P waves: Sinus in basic rhythm; absent during
pause
PR interval: 0.16 to 0.20 seconds
QRS: 0.08 to 0.10 seconds in basic rhythm
Rhythm interpretation: Normal sinus rhythm with
sinus block; ST depression and T wave inversion is
present

**Strip 6-7**
Rhythm: Regular
Rate: 54
P waves: Sinus (notched P waves usually indicate
left atrial hypertrophy)
PR interval: 0.14–0.16 seconds
QRS: 0.06–0.08 seconds
Rhythm interpretation: Sinus bradycardia; a
U wave is present

**Strip 6-8**
Rhythm: Irregular
Rate: 50
P waves: Sinus
PR interval: 0.20 seconds
QRS: 0.06–0.08 seconds
Rhythm interpretation: Sinus arrhythmia; sinus
bradycardia (can also be interpreted as sinus
arrhythmia with a bradycardic rate). A U wave is
present

**Strip 6-9**
Rhythm: Basic rhythm regular; irregular during
pause
Rate: Basic rhythm rate 58
P waves: Sinus in basic rhythm; absent during pause
PR interval: 0.14–0.18 seconds basic rhythm; absent
during pause
QRS: 0.08–0.10 seconds basic rhythm; absent
during pause
Rhythm interpretation: Sinus bradycardia with
sinus arrest; a depressed ST segment and inverted T
wave is present

**Strip 6-10**
Rhythm: Regular
Rate: 125
P waves: Sinus
PR interval: 0.12–0.14 seconds
QRS: 0.06–0.08 seconds
Rhythm interpretation: Sinus tachycardia

**Strip 6-11**
Rhythm: Regular
Rate: 63
P waves: Sinus
PR interval: 0.18–0.20 seconds
QRS: 0.08 seconds
Rhythm interpretation: Normal sinus rhythm; a
U wave is present

**Strip 6-12**
Rhythm: Regular
Rate: 47
P waves: Sinus
PR interval: 0.18–0.20 seconds
QRS: 0.08 seconds
Rhythm interpretation: Sinus bradycardia; an
elevated ST segment is present

**Strip 6-13**
Rhythm: Irregular
Rate: 80
P waves: Sinus
PR interval: 0.12–0.14 seconds
QRS: 0.08 seconds
Rhythm interpretation: Sinus arrhythmia

**Strip 6-14**
Rhythm: Regular
Rate: 63
P waves: Sinus
PR interval: 0.18–0.20 seconds
QRS: 0.08–0.10 seconds
Rhythm interpretation: Normal sinus rhythm; ST
segment depression and T wave inversion is present

**Strip 6-15**
Rhythm: Basic rhythm irregular
Rate: Basic rhythm rate 60
P waves: Sinus
PR interval: 0.16 to 0.18 seconds
QRS: 0.08 to 0.10 seconds
Rhythm interpretation: Sinus arrhythmia with sinus
arrest/block; ST segment depression and T wave
inversion is present

**Strip 6-16**
Rhythm: Regular
Rate: 115
P waves: Sinus
PR interval: 0.16 to 0.18 seconds
QRS: 0.06 to 0.08 seconds
Rhythm interpretation: Sinus tachycardia; a
depressed ST segment and an inverted T wave is
present

**Strip 6-17**
Rhythm: Regular
Rate: 52
P waves: Sinus
PR interval: 0.16–0.18 seconds
QRS: 0.08–0.10 seconds
Rhythm interpretation: Sinus bradycardia

**Strip 6-18**
Rhythm: Irregular
Rate: 60
P waves: Sinus
PR interval: 0.16–0.18 seconds
QRS: 0.08–0.10 seconds
Rhythm interpretation: Sinus arrhythmia

**Strip 6-19**
Rhythm: Regular
Rate: 79
P waves: Sinus
PR interval: 0.16 to 0.20 seconds
QRS: 0.06 seconds
Rhythm interpretation: Normal sinus rhythm

**Strip 6-20**
Rhythm: Basic rhythm regular; irregular during
pause
Rate: Basic rhythm rate 88
P waves: Sinus in basic rhythm; absent during
pause
PR interval: 0.14 to 0.16 seconds in basic rhythm
QRS: 0.08 seconds in basic rhythm
Rhythm interpretation: Normal sinus rhythm with
sinus block; a U wave is present

**Strip 6-21**
Rhythm: Regular
Rate: 150
P waves: Sinus
PR interval: 0.12 seconds
QRS: 0.06 seconds
Rhythm interpretation: Sinus tachycardia

**Strip 6-22**
Rhythm: Regular
Rate: 60
P waves: Sinus
PR interval: 0.12 seconds
QRS: 0.08 seconds
Rhythm interpretation: Normal sinus rhythm;
T wave inversion is present

**Strip 6-23**
Rhythm: Irregular
Rate: 60
P waves: Sinus
PR interval: 0.16 seconds
QRS: 0.08 seconds
Rhythm interpretation: Sinus arrhythmia

**Strip 6-24**
Rhythm: Basic rhythm regular; irregular during
pause
Rate: Basic rhythm rate 60—rate slows to 47
following pause (temporary rate suppression can
occur following a pause in the basic rhythm)
P waves: Sinus in basic rhythm; absent during
pause
PR interval: 0.16–0.18 seconds in basic rhythm;
absent during pause
QRS: 0.06–0.08 seconds in basic rhythm; absent
during pause
Rhythm interpretation: Normal sinus rhythm with
sinus arrest

**Strip 6-25**
Rhythm: Regular
Rate: 125
P waves: Sinus
PR interval: 0.12–0.14 seconds
QRS: 0.04–0.06 seconds
Rhythm interpretation: Sinus tachycardia

**Strip 6-26**
Rhythm: Regular
Rate: 35
P waves: Sinus
PR interval: 0.14–0.16 seconds
QRS: 0.10 seconds
Rhythm interpretation: Marked sinus bradycardia

**Strip 6-27**
Rhythm: Basic rhythm regular; irregular during pause
Rate: Basic rhythm rate 72
P waves: Sinus in basic rhythm; absent during pause
PR interval: 0.14–0.16 seconds basic rhythm; absent during pause
QRS: 0.08–0.10 seconds basic rhythm; absent during pause
Rhythm interpretation: Normal sinus rhythm with sinus block

**Strip 6-28**
Rhythm: Irregular
Rate: 60
P waves: Sinus
PR interval: 0.12–0.14 seconds
QRS: 0.10 seconds
Rhythm interpretation: Sinus arrhythmia; a U wave is present

**Strip 6-29**
Rhythm: Regular
Rate: 65
P waves: Sinus
PR interval: 0.20 seconds
QRS: 0.08–0.10 seconds
Rhythm interpretation: Normal sinus rhythm; ST segment depression and T wave inversion is present

**Strip 6-30**
Rhythm: Basic rhythm regular; irregular during pause
Rate: Basic rhythm rate 68; rate slows to 63 following pause; rate suppression can occur following a pause in the basic rhythm; after several cycles the rate returns to the basic rate
P waves: Sinus in basic rhythm; absent during pause
PR interval: 0.16 seconds in basic rhythm; absent during pause
QRS: 0.06 to 0.08 seconds in basic rhythm; absent during pause
Rhythm interpretation: Normal sinus rhythm with sinus arrest; a U wave is present

**Strip 6-31**
Rhythm: Regular
Rate: 56
P waves: Sinus
PR interval: 0.12 to 0.14 seconds
QRS: 0.08 to 0.10 seconds
Rhythm interpretation: Sinus bradycardia; T wave inversion is present

**Strip 6-32**
Rhythm: Irregular
Rate: 60
P waves: Sinus
PR interval: 0.14–0.16 seconds
QRS: 0.06–0.08 seconds
Rhythm interpretation: Sinus arrhythmia

**Strip 6-33**
Rhythm: Regular
Rate: 115
P waves: Sinus
PR interval: 0.16–0.18 seconds
QRS: 0.06–0.08 seconds
Rhythm interpretation: Sinus tachycardia

**Strip 6-34**
Rhythm: Regular
Rate: 88
P waves: Sinus
PR interval: 0.18–0.20 seconds
QRS: 0.08 seconds
Rhythm interpretation: Normal sinus rhythm; ST segment depression is present

**Strip 6-35**
Rhythm: Irregular
Rate: 60
P waves: Sinus
PR interval: 0.14–0.16 seconds
QRS: 0.06–0.08 seconds
Rhythm interpretation: Sinus arrhythmia

**Strip 6-36**
Rhythm: Regular
Rate: 41
P waves: Sinus
PR interval: 0.16–0.18 seconds
QRS: 0.06–0.08 seconds
Rhythm interpretation: Sinus bradycardia; ST segment depression is present

**Strip 6-37**
Rhythm: Basic rhythm regular; irregular during pause
Rate: Basic rhythm rate 88
P waves: Sinus
PR interval: 0.20 seconds
QRS: 0.06 to 0.08 seconds
Rhythm interpretation: Normal sinus rhythm with sinus arrest; ST segment depression is present

**Strip 6-38**
Rhythm: Regular
Rate: 107
P waves: Sinus
PR interval: 0.16–0.18 seconds
QRS: 0.06–0.08 seconds
Rhythm interpretation: Sinus tachycardia

**Strip 6-39**
Rhythm: Regular
Rate: 107
P waves: Sinus
PR interval: 0.16–0.18 seconds
QRS: 0.06–0.08 seconds
Rhythm interpretation: Sinus tachycardia;
ST segment elevation is present

**Strip 6-40**
Rhythm: Regular
Rate: 54
P waves: Sinus (notched P waves usually indicate
left atrial hypertrophy)
PR interval: 0.16–0.20 seconds
QRS: 0.06–0.08 seconds
Rhythm interpretation: Sinus bradycardia

**Strip 6-41**
Rhythm: Regular
Rate: 94
P waves: Sinus (negative P waves are normal in lead
$MCL_1$)
PR interval: 0.18–0.20 seconds
QRS: 0.08–0.10 seconds (negative QRS complexes
are normal in lead $MCL_1$)
Rhythm interpretation: Normal sinus rhythm

**Strip 6-42**
Rhythm: Irregular
Rate: 40
P waves: Sinus
PR interval: 0.18 to 0.20 seconds
QRS: 0.06 to 0.08 seconds
Rhythm interpretation: Sinus arrhythmia with sinus
bradycardia; (can also be interpreted as sinus
arrhythmia with a bradycardic rate); ST segment
elevation is present

**Strip 6-43**
Rhythm: Basic rhythm regular; irregular during pause
Rate: Basic rhythm rate 63
P waves: Sinus in basic rhythm; absent during pause
PR interval: 0.18 to 0.20 seconds in basic rhythm;
absent during pause
QRS: 0.04 to 0.06 seconds in basic rhythm; absent
during pause
Rhythm interpretation: Normal sinus rhythm with
sinus arrest; ST segment depression is present

**Strip 6-44**
Rhythm: Irregular
Rate: 60
P waves: Sinus
PR interval: 0.12–0.14 seconds
QRS: 0.08–0.10 seconds
Rhythm interpretation: Sinus arrhythmia;
ST segment elevation is present

**Strip 6-45**
Rhythm: Regular
Rate: 27
P waves: Sinus
PR interval: 0.14 to 0.16 seconds
QRS: 0.08 to 0.10 seconds
Rhythm interpretation: Sinus bradycardia with
extremely slow rate; ST segment depression is
present

**Strip 6-46**
Rhythm: Irregular
Rate: 50
P waves: Sinus
PR interval: 0.12–0.14 seconds
QRS: 0.06–0.08 seconds
Rhythm interpretation: Sinus arrhythmia; sinus
bradycardia (can also be interpreted as sinus
arrhythmia with a bradycardic rate)

**Strip 6-47**
Rhythm: Regular
Rate: 136
P waves: Sinus
PR interval: 0.12–0.14 seconds
QRS: 0.06–0.08 seconds
Rhythm interpretation: Sinus tachycardia

**Strip 6-48**
Rhythm: Irregular
Rate: 70
P waves: Sinus
PR interval: 0.16 to 0.20 seconds
QRS: 0.04 to 0.06 seconds
Rhythm interpretation: Sinus arrhythmia; a U wave
is present

**Strip 6-49**
Rhythm: Regular
Rate: 52
P waves: Sinus
PR interval: 0.12 seconds
QRS: 0.08 seconds
Rhythm interpretation: Sinus bradycardia

**Strip 6-50**
Rhythm: Regular
Rate: 60
P waves: Sinus
PR interval: 0.16–0.18 seconds
QRS: 0.08 seconds
Rhythm interpretation: Normal sinus rhythm; an elevated ST segment is present

**Strip 6-51**
Rhythm: Regular
Rate: 107
P waves: Sinus
PR interval: 0.12 to 0.14 seconds
QRS: 0.06 to 0.08 seconds
Rhythm interpretation: Sinus tachycardia

**Strip 6-52**
Rhythm: Basic rhythm regular; irregular during pause
Rate: Basic rhythm rate 60; rate slows to 31 following pause—temporary rate suppression is common following a pause in the basic rhythm
P waves: Sinus
PR interval: 0.16–0.20 seconds
QRS: 0.06–0.08 seconds
Rhythm interpretation: Normal sinus rhythm with sinus arrest; ST segment depression and T wave inversion is present

**Strip 6-53**
Rhythm: Irregular
Rate: 50
P waves: Sinus
PR interval: 0.14 to 0.16 seconds
QRS: 0.06 to 0.08 seconds
Rhythm interpretation: Sinus arrhythmia; sinus bradycardia; (can also be interpreted as sinus arrhythmia with a bradycardic rate) a U wave is present

**Strip 6-54**
Rhythm: Basic rhythm regular; irregular during pause
Rate: Basic rhythm rate 94—rate slows to 54 following pause (rate suppression can occur temporarily following a pause in the basic rhythm)
P waves: Sinus in basic rhythm; absent during pause
PR interval: 0.16–0.18 seconds in basic rhythm; absent during pause
QRS: 0.08–0.10 seconds
Rhythm interpretation: Normal sinus rhythm with sinus block

**Strip 6-55**
Rhythm: Regular
Rate: 65
P waves: Sinus
PR interval: 0.16–0.18 seconds
QRS: 0.06 seconds
Rhythm interpretation: Normal sinus rhythm

**Strip 6-56**
Rhythm: Regular
Rate: 125
P waves: Sinus
PR interval: 0.16 seconds
QRS: 0.08 seconds
Rhythm interpretation: Sinus tachycardia; ST segment depression is present

**Strip 6-57**
Rhythm: Irregular
Rate: 40
P waves: Sinus
PR interval: 0.16–0.18 seconds
QRS: 0.08 seconds
Rhythm interpretation: Sinus arrhythmia/sinus bradycardia (can also be interpreted as sinus arrhythmia with a bradycardic rate) a U wave is present

**Strip 6-58**
Rhythm: Regular
Rate: 72
P waves: Sinus
PR interval: 0.16 to 0.20 seconds
QRS: 0.06 to 0.08 seconds
Rhythm interpretation: Normal sinus rhythm; ST segment depression and T wave inversion are present

**Strip 6-59**
Rhythm: Regular
Rate: 50
P waves: Sinus
PR interval: 0.20 seconds
QRS: 0.06 to 0.08 seconds
Rhythm interpretation: Sinus bradycardia; ST segment depression and T wave inversion are present

**Strip 6-60**
Rhythm: Basic rhythm regular; irregular during pause
Rate: Basic rhythm rate 88
P waves: Sinus in basic rhythm; absent during pause
PR interval: 0.14 to 0.20 seconds in basic rhythm; absent during pause
QRS: 0.08 to 0.10 seconds in basic rhythm; absent during pause
Rhythm interpretation: Normal sinus rhythm with sinus block; ST segment depression is present

**Strip 6-61**
Rhythm: Regular
Rate: 72
P waves: Sinus
PR interval: 0.12–0.14 seconds
QRS: 0.06–0.08 seconds
Rhythm interpretation: Normal sinus rhythm; an inverted T wave is present

**Strip 6-62**
Rhythm: Regular
Rate: 125
P waves: Sinus
PR interval: 0.12 seconds
QRS: 0.04 seconds
Rhythm interpretation: Sinus tachycardia; ST segment depression is present

**Strip 6-63**
Rhythm: Regular
Rate: 44
P waves: Sinus
PR interval: 0.18–0.20 seconds
QRS: 0.06–0.08 seconds
Rhythm interpretation: Sinus bradycardia; a U wave is present

**Strip 6-64**
Rhythm: Regular
Rate: 79
P waves: Sinus
PR interval: 0.14 to 0.16 seconds
QRS: 0.04 to 0.06 seconds
Rhythm interpretation: Normal sinus rhythm; T wave inversion is present

**Strip 6-65**
Rhythm: Regular
Rate: 107
P waves: Sinus
PR interval: 0.18–0.20 seconds
QRS: 0.08–0.10 seconds
Rhythm interpretation: Sinus tachycardia; an elevated ST segment is present

**Strip 6-66**
Rhythm: Regular
Rate: 100
P waves: Sinus
PR interval: 0.20 seconds
QRS: 0.08 seconds
Rhythm interpretation: Normal sinus rhythm; an extremely elevated ST segment is present

**Strip 6-67**
Rhythm: Regular
Rate: 44
P waves: Sinus
PR interval: 0.14 to 0.16 seconds
QRS: 0.08 seconds
Rhythm interpretation: Sinus bradycardia; a U wave is present

**Strip 6-68**
Rhythm: Regular
Rate: 88
P waves: Sinus
PR interval: 0.18–0.20 seconds
QRS: 0.06–0.08 seconds
Rhythm interpretation: Normal sinus rhythm; a depressed ST segment is present

**Strip 6-69**
Rhythm: Regular
Rate: 136
P waves: Sinus
PR interval: 0.14–0.16 seconds
QRS: 0.08 seconds
Rhythm interpretation: Sinus tachycardia; an elevated ST segment is present

**Strip 6-70**
Rhythm: Basic rhythm regular; irregular during pause
Rate: Basic rhythm rate 56; rate slows to 50 after pause; rate suppression can occur following a pause in the basic rhythm; after several cycles the rate returns to the basic rate
P waves: Sinus in basic rhythm; absent during pause
PR interval: 0.14 to 0.16 in basic rhythm; absent during pause
QRS: 0.08 to 0.10 seconds in basic rhythm; absent during pause
Rhythm interpretation: Sinus bradycardia with sinus arrest

**Strip 6-71**
Rhythm: Regular
Rate: 115
P waves: Sinus
PR interval: 0.14–0.16 seconds
QRS: 0.08–0.10 seconds
Rhythm interpretation: Sinus tachycardia; ST segment depression is present

**Strip 6-72**
Rhythm: Regular
Rate: 79
P waves: Sinus
PR interval: 0.14–0.16 seconds
QRS: 0.06–0.08 seconds
Rhythm interpretation: Normal sinus rhythm; a depressed ST segment and a biphasic T wave is present

**Strip 6-73**
Rhythm: Regular
Rate: 54
P waves: Sinus
PR interval: 0.14–0.16 seconds
QRS: 0.06–0.08 seconds
Rhythm interpretation: Sinus bradycardia; an elevated ST segment is present

**Strip 6-74**
Rhythm: Regular
Rate: 94
P waves: Sinus
PR interval: 0.16 seconds
QRS: 0.08–0.10 seconds
Rhythm interpretation: Normal sinus rhythm; ST segment depression and a biphasic T wave is present

**Strip 6-75**
Rhythm: Regular
Rate: 94
P waves: Sinus
PR interval: 0.16 to 0.20 seconds
QRS: 0.06 to 0.08 seconds
Rhythm interpretation: Normal sinus rhythm

**Strip 6-76**
Rhythm: Regular
Rate: 125
P waves: Sinus
PR interval: 0.12 seconds
QRS: 0.06 to 0.08 seconds
Rhythm interpretation: Sinus tachycardia

**Strip 6-77**
Rhythm: Regular
Rate: 79
P waves: Sinus
PR interval: 0.18–0.20 seconds
QRS: 0.06–0.08 seconds
Rhythm interpretation: Normal sinus rhythm; an elevated ST segment is present

**Strip 6-78**
Rhythm: Regular
Rate: 58
P waves: Sinus
PR interval: 0.16–0.18 seconds
QRS: 0.06–0.08 seconds
Rhythm interpretation: Sinus bradycardia; an elevated ST segment and a U wave are present

**Strip 6-79**
Rhythm: Basic rhythm regular; irregular during pause
Rate: Basic rhythm rate 107—rate slows to 94 for 1 cycle following pause (temporary rate suppression can occur following a pause in the basic rhythm)
P waves: Sinus in basic rhythm; absent during pause
PR interval: 0.16–0.20 seconds in basic rhythm; absent during pause
QRS: 0.10 seconds in basic rhythm; absent during pause
Rhythm interpretation: Sinus tachycardia with sinus block; baseline artifact is present

**Strip 6-80**
Rhythm: Regular
Rate: 84
P waves: Sinus
PR interval: 0.16 seconds
QRS: 0.06 seconds
Rhythm interpretation: Normal sinus rhythm; T wave inversion is present

**Strip 6-81**
Rhythm: Regular
Rate: 56
P waves: Sinus
PR interval: 0.16–0.18 seconds
QRS: 0.06–0.08 seconds
Rhythm interpretation: Sinus bradycardia; T wave inversion is present

**Strip 6-82**
Rhythm: Regular
Rate: 125
P waves: Sinus
PR interval: 0.16–0.18 seconds
QRS: 0.04–0.06 seconds
Rhythm interpretation: Sinus tachycardia

**Strip 6-83**
Rhythm: Basic rhythm irregular
Rate: Basic rhythm rate 60
P waves: Sinus
PR interval: 0.20 seconds in basic rhythm; absent during pause
QRS: 0.06 to 0.08 seconds in basic rhythm; absent during pause
Rhythm interpretation: Sinus arrhythmia with sinus arrest/block; ST segment depression is present

**Strip 6-84**
Rhythm: Regular
Rate: 79
P waves: Sinus
PR interval: 0.12 seconds
QRS: 0.06–0.08 seconds
Rhythm interpretation: Normal sinus rhythm; an elevated ST segment is present

**Strip 6-85**
Rhythm: Regular
Rate: 136
P waves: Sinus
PR interval: 0.14–0.16 seconds
QRS: 0.06–0.08 seconds
Rhythm interpretation: Sinus tachycardia

**Strip 6-86**
Rhythm: Regular
Rate: 54
P waves: Sinus
PR interval: 0.16 seconds
QRS: 0.06–0.08 seconds
Rhythm interpretation: Sinus bradycardia

**Strip 6-87**
Rhythm: Basic rhythm regular; irregular during pause
Rate: Basic rhythm rate 84; rate slows to 75 for one cycle following the pause—rate suppression is common following pauses in the basic rhythm
P waves: Sinus in basic rhythm; absent during pause
PR interval: 0.16 to 0.18 seconds in basic rhythm; absent during pause
QRS: 0.06 to 0.08 seconds in basic rhythm; absent during pause
Rhythm interpretation: Normal sinus rhythm with sinus arrest

**Strip 6-88**
Rhythm: Regular
Rate: 100
P waves: Sinus
PR interval: 0.12–0.14 seconds
QRS: 0.08–0.10 seconds
Rhythm interpretation: Normal sinus rhythm; an elevated ST segment is present

**Strip 6-89**
Rhythm: Regular
Rate: 54
P waves: Sinus
PR interval: 0.18–0.20 seconds
QRS: 0.06–0.08 seconds
Rhythm interpretation: Sinus bradycardia; an elevated ST segment and T wave inversion is present

**Strip 6-90**
Rhythm: Basic rhythm regular; irregular during pause
Rate: Basic rhythm rate 72- rate slows to 68 for two cycles following pause (temporary rate suppression can occur following a pause in the basic rhythm)
P waves: Sinus in basic rhythm; absent during pause
PR interval: 0.12–0.14 seconds in basic rhythm; absent during pause
QRS: 0.06–0.08 seconds in basic rhythm; absent during pause
Rhythm interpretation: Normal sinus rhythm with sinus arrest; T wave inversion is present

**Strip 6-91**
Rhythm: Regular
Rate: 65
P waves: Sinus
PR interval: 0.14–0.16 seconds
QRS: 0.06–0.08 seconds
Rhythm interpretation: Normal sinus rhythm; a U wave is present

**Strip 6-92**
Rhythm: Regular
Rate: 63
P waves: Sinus
PR interval: 0.18–0.20 seconds
QRS: 0.08–0.10 seconds
Rhythm interpretation: Normal sinus rhythm; ST segment depression and T wave inversion is present

**Strip 6-93**
Rhythm: Basic rhythm regular; irregular during pause
Rate: Basic rhythm rate 79- rate slows to 72 following pause (temporary rate suppression can occur following a pause in the basic rhythm)
P waves: Sinus in basic rhythm; absent during pause
PR interval: 0.20 seconds in basic rhythm; absent during pause
QRS: 0.08–0.10 seconds in basic rhythm; absent during pause
Rhythm interpretation: Normal sinus rhythm with sinus arrest; ST segment depression and T wave inversion is present

**Strip 6-94**
Rhythm: Regular
Rate: 150
P waves: Sinus
PR interval: 0.12 seconds
QRS: 0.04 to 0.06 seconds
Rhythm interpretation: Sinus tachycardia

**Strip 6-95**
Rhythm: Regular
Rate: 136
P waves: Sinus
PR interval: 0.12 seconds
QRS: 0.06–0.08 seconds
Rhythm interpretation: Sinus tachycardia

**Strip 6-96**
Rhythm: Irregular
Rate: 50
P waves: Sinus
PR interval: 0.14–0.16 seconds
QRS: 0.08 seconds
Rhythm interpretation: Sinus bradycardia; sinus arrhythmia

**Strip 6-97**
Rhythm: Irregular
Rate: 40
P waves: Sinus
PR interval: 0.18–0.20 seconds
QRS: 0.06–0.08 seconds
Rhythm interpretation: Sinus bradycardia; sinus arrhythmia with sinus arrest/block

**Strip 6-98**
Rhythm: Regular
Rate: 136
P waves: Sinus
PR interval: 0.14–0.16 seconds
QRS: 0.08–0.10 seconds
Rhythm interpretation: Sinus tachycardia; ST segment elevation is present

**Strip 6-99**
Rhythm: Irregular
Rate: 50
P waves: Sinus
PR interval: 0.14–0.16 seconds
QRS: 0.08–0.10 seconds
Rhythm interpretation: Sinus arrhythmia; sinus bradycardia

**Strip 7-1**
Rhythm: Irregular
Rate: Ventricular rate 60; atrial rate not measurable
P waves: fibrillation waves present
PR interval: not measurable
QRS: 0.06–0.08 seconds
Rhythm interpretation: Atrial fibrillation; ST segment depression is present

**Strip 7-2**
Rhythm: Regular
Rate: 188
P waves: Hidden in T waves
PR interval: Not measurable
QRS: 0.06–0.08 seconds
Rhythm interpretation: Paroxysmal atrial tachycardia

**Strip 7-3**
Rhythm: Basic rhythm regular; irregular with PACs
Rate: Basic rhythm rate 94
P waves: Sinus P waves with basic rhythm; Premature, abnormal P waves with PACs
PR interval: 0.12 seconds (basic rhythm)
0.14 seconds (PACs)
QRS: 0.08–0.10 seconds (basic rhythm and PACs)
Rhythm interpretation: Normal sinus rhythm with 2 PACs (4th and 8th complex) ST segment depression is present

**Strip 7-4**
Rhythm: Irregular
Rate: 100
P waves: Vary in size, shape, position
PR interval: 0.12 seconds
QRS: 0.06 to 0.08 seconds
Rhythm interpretation: Wandering atrial pacemaker

**Strip 7-5**
Rhythm: Basic rhythm regular; irregular with PAC
Rate: Basic rhythm rate 125
P waves: Sinus P waves with basic rhythm; premature, pointed P wave with PAC
PR interval: 0.12 seconds (basic rhythm)
QRS: 0.04–0.06 seconds (basic rhythm)
Rhythm interpretation: Sinus tachycardia with one PAC (8th complex)

## Strip 7-6

Rhythm: Regular
Rate: 167
P waves: Pointed, abnormal
PR interval: 0.14 to 0.16 seconds
QRS: 0.06 to 0.08 seconds
Rhythm interpretation: Paroxysmal atrial tachycardia; ST segment depression is present

## Strip 7-7

Rhythm: Basic rhythm regular; irregular with nonconducted PAC
Rate: Basic rhythm rate 88
P waves: Sinus P waves with basic rhythm; premature, abnormal P wave with nonconducted PAC
PR interval: 0.16 seconds
QRS: 0.06 to 0.08 seconds
Rhythm interpretation: Normal sinus rhythm with nonconducted PAC (following 7th QRS) ST segment depression is present

## Strip 7-8

Rhythm: Irregular
Rate: Atrial, 320; ventricular, 80
P waves: Flutter waves are present (varying ratios)
PR interval: Not measurable
QRS: 0.06–0.08 seconds
Rhythm interpretation: Atrial flutter with variable block

## Strip 7-9

Rhythm: Irregular
Rate: 70
P waves: vary in size, shape, direction
PR interval: 0.12–0.14 seconds
QRS: 0.06–0.08 seconds
Rhythm interpretation: Wandering atrial pacemaker

## Strip 7-10

Rhythm: Irregular
Rate: Ventricular rate 60; Atrial rate not measurable
P waves: fibrillatory waves are present
PR interval: not measurable
QRS: 0.04–0.06 seconds
Rhythm interpretation: Atrial fibrillation

## Strip 7-11

Rhythm: Basic rhythm regular; irregular with PAC
Rate: Basic rate 72
P waves: Sinus with basic rhythm; premature, pointed with PAC
PR interval: 0.18–0.20 seconds (basic rhythm)
QRS: 0.06–0.08 seconds (basic rhythm)
Rhythm interpretation: Normal sinus rhythm with 1 PAC (6th complex)

## Strip 7-12

Rhythm: Regular
Rate: Atrial: 237 Ventricular: 79
P waves: 3 flutter waves to each QRS
PR interval: not necessary to measure
QRS: 0.04 seconds
Rhythm interpretation: Atrial flutter with 3:1 AV conduction

## Strip 7-13

Rhythm: Basic rhythm regular; irregular with PAC
Rate: Basic rate 107
P waves: Sinus with basic rhythm; premature, pointed P wave without QRS complex follows 5th QRS
PR interval: 0.18–0.20 seconds
QRS: 0.04–0.06 seconds
Rhythm interpretation: Sinus tachycardia with 1 non-conducted PAC (following 5th QRS)

## Strip 7-14

Rhythm: Irregular
Rate: Ventricular rate 110; atrial rate not measurable
P waves: Fibrillatory waves are present
PR interval: Not measurable
QRS: 0.06 to 0.08 seconds
Rhythm interpretation: Atrial fibrillation; some flutter waves are noted

## Strip 7-15

Rhythm: First rhythm regular; second rhythm regular
Rate: 167 first rhythm; 100 second rhythm
P waves: Obscured in T waves in first rhythm; sinus P waves in second rhythm
PR interval: Not measurable in first rhythm; 0.16–0.18 seconds in second rhythm
QRS: 0.08 seconds (both rhythms)
Rhythm interpretation: Paroxysmal atrial tachycardia converting to normal sinus rhythm

## Strip 7-16

Rhythm: Regular
Rate: Atrial, 300; ventricular, 100
P waves: Three flutter waves before each QRS
PR interval: Not measurable
QRS: 0.08 seconds
Rhythm interpretation: Atrial flutter with 3:1 AV conduction

## Strip 7-17

Rhythm: Irregular
Rate: 40
P waves: Fibrillatory waves
PR interval: Not measurable
QRS: 0.08 seconds
Rhythm interpretation: Atrial fibrillation

**Strip 7-18**

Rhythm: Irregular
Rate: Atrial, 320; ventricular, 90
P waves: Flutter waves (varying ratios)
PR interval: Not discernible
QRS: 0.04 to 0.06 seconds
Rhythm interpretation: Atrial flutter with variable AV conduction

**Strip 7-19**

Rhythm: Basic rhythm regular; irregular following nonconducted PAC
Rate: Basic rate 107
P waves: Sinus P waves with basic rhythm; premature abnormal P wave with nonconducted PAC
PR interval: 0.16–0.18 seconds
QRS: 0.08–0.10 seconds
Rhythm interpretation: Sinus tachycardia with nonconducted PAC

**Strip 7-20**

Rhythm: Regular
Rate: 167
P waves: Pointed abnormal P wave
PR interval: 0.16–0.18 seconds
QRS: 0.06–0.08 seconds
Rhythm interpretation: Paroxysmal atrial tachycardia

**Strip 7-21**

Rhythm: Basic rhythm regular; irregular with nonconducted PAC
Rate: Basic rhythm 75—rate slows to 72 for 2 cycles following pause; temporary rate suppression is common following a pause in the underlying rhythm
P waves: Sinus in basic rhythm; premature, pointed P wave without QRS complex follows 3rd QRS
PR interval: 0.16 seconds
QRS: 0.08 seconds
Rhythm interpretation: Normal sinus rhythm with one non-conducted PAC (following 3rd QRS); a U wave is present

**Strip 7-22**

Rhythm: Regular
Rate: Atrial: 290 Ventricular: 58
P waves: 5 flutter waves to each QRS
PR interval: Not measurable
QRS: 0.06–0.08 seconds
Rhythm interpretation: Atrial flutter with 5:1 AV conduction

**Strip 7-23**

Rhythm: Basic rhythm regular; irregular with pause
Rate: Basic rhythm rate 79
P waves: Sinus with basic rhythm; premature abnormal P wave without QRS follows 4th QRS
PR interval: 0.16–0.18 seconds basic rhythm
QRS: 0.06–0.08 seconds basic rhythm
Rhythm interpretation: Normal sinus rhythm with 1 nonconducted PAC (follows 4th QRS) ST segment depression and T wave inversion is present

**Strip 7-24**

Rhythm: Irregular
Rate: Ventricular rate: 170; atrial rate not measurable
P waves: Fibrillatory waves present
PR interval: Not measurable
QRS: 0.06–0.08 seconds
Rhythm interpretation: Atrial fibrillation

**Strip 7-25**

Rhythm: Regular
Rate: 84
P waves: Vary in size, shape, and position
PR interval: 0.12 to 0.14 seconds
QRS: 0.06 to 0.08 seconds
Rhythm interpretation: Wandering atrial pacemaker; T wave inversion is present

**Strip 7-26**

Rhythm: Basic rhythm regular; irregular with PACs
Rate: Basic rhythm rate 68
P waves: Sinus with basic rhythm; premature, inverted P wave with PAC
PR interval: 0.12–0.14 seconds (basic rhythm); 0.12 seconds (PAC)
QRS: 0.06–0.08 seconds (basic rhythm); 0.08 seconds (PAC)
Rhythm interpretation: Normal sinus rhythm with 1 PAC (4th complex) a U wave is present

**Strip 7-27**

Rhythm: Regular
Rate: Atrial: 232 Ventricular: 58
P waves: 4 flutter waves to each QRS
PR interval: Not measurable
QRS: 0.06–0.08 seconds
Rhythm interpretation: Atrial flutter with 4:1 AV conduction

**Strip 7-28**
Rhythm: Basic rhythm regular; irregular with PACs
Rate: Basic rhythm 42
P waves: Sinus P waves with basic rhythm; premature, abnormal P waves with PACs
PR interval: 0.12 to 0.14 seconds (basic rhythm); 0.16 seconds (PACs)
QRS: 0.08 to 0.10 seconds
Rhythm interpretation: Sinus bradycardia with four PACs (2nd, 4th, 7th and 9th complexes)

**Strip 7-29**
Rhythm: Regular
Rate: 150
P waves: Obscured in preceding T wave
PR interval: Not measurable
QRS: 0.08 seconds
Rhythm interpretation: Paroxysmal atrial tachycardia

**Strip 7-30**
Rhythm: Regular
Rate: Atrial: 272 Ventricular: 136
P waves: 2 flutter waves to each QRS
PR interval: Not measurable
QRS: 0.06 seconds
Rhythm interpretation: Atrial flutter with 2:1 AV conduction

**Strip 7-31**
Rhythm: Basic rhythm regular; irregular with PACs and atrial fibrillation
Rate: Basic rhythm rate 68; Atrial fibrillation rate 140
P waves: Sinus P waves are present with basic rhythm; premature, abnormal P waves with PACs; fibrillation waves with atrial fibrillation
PR interval: 0.12 to 0.14 seconds (basic rhythm)
QRS: 0.08 to 0.10 seconds
Rhythm interpretation: Normal sinus rhythm with two PACs, (2nd and 5th complex); last PAC initiates atrial fibrillation; ST segment depression is present

**Strip 7-32**
Rhythm: Basic rhythm regular; irregular with nonconducted PAC
Rate: Basic rate 94—rate slows to 84 for one cycle following pause (temporary rate suppression can occur following a pause in the basic rhythm)
P waves: Sinus P waves in basic rhythm; premature, abnormal P wave without a QRS is hidden in T wave following 7th QRS complex
PR interval: 0.16–0.18 seconds
QRS: 0.06–0.08 seconds
Rhythm interpretation: Normal sinus rhythm with one nonconducted PAC (following 7th QRS)

**Strip 7-33**
Rhythm: Basic rhythm regular; irregular with PAC
Rate: Basic rhythm rate 47
P waves: Sinus with basic rhythm; premature, pointed P wave associated with PAC
PR interval: 0.18–0.20 seconds
QRS: 0.08 seconds
Rhythm interpretation: Sinus bradycardia with one PAC (5th complex); a U wave is present

**Strip 7-34**
Rhythm: Irregular
Rate: Ventricular rate: 50; Atrial rate not measurable
P waves: Fibrillatory waves are present
PR interval: Not measurable
QRS: 0.06 to 0.08 seconds
Rhythm interpretation: Atrial fibrillation; ST segment depression and T wave inversion are present

**Strip 7-35**
Rhythm: Regular
Rate: 188
P waves: Obscured in T waves
PR interval: Unmeasurable
QRS: 0.04–0.08 seconds
Rhythm interpretation: Paroxysmal atrial tachycardia; ST segment depression is present

**Strip 7-36**
Rhythm: Irregular
Rate: 60
P waves: Vary in size, shape, direction across strip
PR interval: 0.12–0.16 seconds
QRS: 0.06–0.08 seconds
Rhythm interpretation: Wandering atrial pacemaker

**Strip 7-37**
Rhythm: Irregular
Rate: Atrial, 260; ventricular, 70
P waves: Flutter waves (varying ratios)
PR interval: Not measurable
QRS: 0.08 seconds
Rhythm interpretation: Atrial flutter with variable AV conduction

**Strip 7-38**
Rhythm: Regular
Rate: 150
P waves: Obscured in T wave
PR interval: Not measurable
QRS: 0.04–0.06 seconds
Rhythm interpretation: Paroxysmal atrial tachycardia; ST segment depression is present

## Strip 7-39

Rhythm: Basic rhythm regular; irregular with PAC
Rate: Basic rhythm rate 136
P waves: Sinus with basic rhythm; premature, pointed P wave with PAC
PR interval: 0.16–0.18 (basic rhythm); 0.18 seconds (PAC)
QRS: 0.06–0.08 seconds (basic rhythm); 0.06 seconds (PAC)
Rhythm interpretation: Sinus tachycardia with 1 PAC (11th complex)

## Strip 7-40

Rhythm: Irregular
Rate: Ventricular rate: 130; Atrial rate not measurable
P waves: Fibrillatory waves present
PR interval: Not measurable
QRS: 0.04–0.06 seconds
Rhythm interpretation: Atrial fibrillation (uncontrolled rate)

## Strip 7-41

Rhythm: Basic rhythm regular; irregular with nonconducted PAC
Rate: Basic rhythm rate 79
P waves: Sinus P waves with basic rhythm; premature, abnormal P waves hidden in T wave following 7th QRS
PR interval: 0.20 seconds
QRS: 0.08–0.10 seconds
Rhythm interpretation: Normal sinus rhythm with one nonconducted PAC (hidden in T wave following 7th QRS) a U wave is present

## Strip 7-42

Rhythm: Basic rhythm regular; irregular with nonconducted PAC
Rate: 72
P waves: Sinus P waves are present; one premature, abnormal P wave without a QRS (follows 5th QRS)
PR interval: 0.16 seconds
QRS: 0.08 seconds
Rhythm interpretation: Normal sinus rhythm with one nonconducted PAC (follows 5th QRS); T wave inversion is present

## Strip 7-43

Rhythm: Regular
Rate: 68
P waves: Vary in size, shape, and position
PR interval: 0.12 seconds
QRS: 0.06–0.08 seconds
Rhythm interpretation: Wandering atrial pacemaker; ST segment depression is present

## Strip 7-44

Rhythm: Regular
Rate: Atrial: 428 Ventricular: 214
P waves: 2 flutter waves to each QRS
PR interval: Not measurable
QRS: 0.06–0.08 seconds
Rhythm interpretation: Atrial flutter with 2:1 AV conduction

## Strip 7-45

Rhythm: Regular
Rate: 188
P waves: Hidden in T waves
PR interval: Not measurable
QRS: 0.04 to 0.06 seconds
Rhythm interpretation: Paroxysmal atrial tachycardia; ST segment depression is present

## Strip 7-46

Rhythm: Basic rhythm regular; irregular with premature beat
Rate: Basic rhythm rate 79
P waves: Sinus with basic rhythm; premature pointed P wave with PAC
PR interval: 0.14–0.16 seconds (basic rhythm); 0.12 seconds (PAC)
QRS: 0.06–0.08 seconds
Rhythm interpretation: Normal sinus rhythm with 1 PAC (5th complex)

## Strip 7-47

Rhythm: Basic rhythm regular; irregular with PAC
Rate: Basic rhythm rate 84
P waves: Sinus P waves present; premature, pointed P wave with PAC
PR interval: 0.14 to 0.16 (basic rhythm); 0.16 seconds (PAC)
QRS: 0.06 to 0.08 seconds (basic rhythm) 0.08 seconds (PAC)
Rhythm interpretation: Normal sinus rhythm with one PAC (7th complex); ST segment depression is present

## Strip 7-48

Rhythm: Irregular
Rate: 40
P waves: Fibrillatory waves are present
PR interval: Not measurable
QRS: 0.08 seconds
Rhythm interpretation: Atrial fibrillation (controlled rate)

**Strip 7-49**
Rhythm: Irregular
Rate: Atrial, 280; ventricular, 50
P waves: Flutter waves present (varying ratios)
PR interval: Not measurable
QRS: 0.06 to 0.08 seconds
Rhythm interpretation: Atrial flutter with variable AV conduction

**Strip 7-50**
Rhythm: Irregular
Rate: Atrial, 300; ventricular, 100
P waves: Flutter waves (varying ratios)
PR interval: Not measurable
QRS: 0.04–0.06 seconds
Rhythm interpretation: Atrial flutter with variable AV conduction

**Strip 7-51**
Rhythm: Regular
Rate: 150
P waves: Hidden in T waves
PR interval: Not measurable
QRS: 0.08 to 0.10 seconds
Rhythm interpretation: Paroxysmal atrial tachycardia

**Strip 7-52**
Rhythm: Basic rhythm regular; irregular with nonconducted PAC
Rate: Basic rhythm rate 88—rate slows to 79 following each nonconducted PAC (temporary rate suppression is common following a pause in the basic rhythm)
P waves: Sinus with basic rhythm; two premature abnormal P waves without a QRS complex follows 5th QRS and 7th QRS
PR interval: 0.18–0.20 seconds
QRS: 0.06–0.08 seconds
Rhythm interpretation: Normal sinus rhythm with two nonconducted PACs (following 5th and 7th QRS)

**Strip 7-53**
Rhythm: Irregular
Rate: 70
P waves: Fibrillatory waves
PR interval: Not measurable
QRS: 0.06–0.08 seconds
Rhythm interpretation: Atrial fibrillation; ST segment depression is present

**Strip 7-54**
Rhythm: Basic rhythm regular; irregular with PAC
Rate: Basic rhythm rate 94
P waves: Sinus in basic rhythm; premature pointed P wave with PAC
PR interval: 0.12–0.16 seconds
QRS: 0.06–0.08 seconds
Rhythm interpretation: Normal sinus rhythm with one PAC (8th complex); ST segment depression is present

**Strip 7-55**
Rhythm: Irregular
Rate: Ventricular rate 140; atrial rate not measurable
P waves: Fibrillatory waves 1st part of strip; sinus P waves last part of strip
PR interval: Not measurable 1st part of strip; 0.14 seconds (with the two sinus beats last part of strip)
QRS: 0.04–0.06 seconds
Rhythm interpretation: Atrial fibrillation converting to a sinus rhythm (one PAC follows 1st sinus beat)

**Strip 7-56**
Rhythm: Basic rhythm regular; irregular with PAC
Rate: Basic rhythm rate 84
P waves: Sinus in basic rhythm; premature, pointed P wave with PAC
PR interval: 0.12–0.14 seconds (basic rhythm); 0.12 seconds (PAC)
QRS: 0.06–0.08 seconds (basic rhythm) 0.08 seconds (PAC)
Rhythm interpretation: Normal sinus rhythm with 1 PAC (5th complex); baseline artifact is present (baseline artifact should not be confused with atrial fibrillation)

**Strip 7-57**
Rhythm: Regular
Rate: Atrial, 300; ventricular, 75
P waves: Four flutter waves to each QRS
PR interval: Not measurable
QRS: 0.04 seconds
Rhythm interpretation: Atrial flutter with 4:1 AV conduction

**Strip 7-58**

Rhythm: Basic rhythm regular; irregular with nonconducted PAC

Rate: Basic rhythm rate 88—rate slows to 72 following pause (temporary rate suppression is common following a pause in the basic rhythm)

P waves: Sinus with basic rhythm; premature abnormal P wave (without associated QRS) hidden in T wave following 7th QRS

PR interval: 0.12–0.14 seconds (basic rhythm)

QRS: 0.08–0.10 seconds

Rhythm interpretation: Normal sinus rhythm with one nonconducted PAC (follows 7th QRS)

**Strip 7-59**

Rhythm: Irregular

Rate: 70

P waves: Vary in size, shape, direction

PR interval: 0.14–0.16 seconds

QRS: 0.06–0.08 seconds

Rhythm interpretation: Wandering atrial pacemaker; T wave inversion is present

**Strip 7-60**

Rhythm: Irregular

Rate: Atrial: 300 Ventricular: 80

P waves: Flutter waves are present before each QRS in varying ratios

PR interval: Not measurable

QRS: 0.04–0.06 seconds

Rhythm interpretation: Atrial flutter with variable AV conduction

**Strip 7-61**

Rhythm: Irregular

Rate: 50

P waves: Fibrillatory waves are present

PR interval: Not measurable

QRS: 0.06–0.08 seconds

Rhythm interpretation: Atrial fibrillation; some flutter waves are present

**Strip 7-62**

Rhythm: Regular with basic rhythm; irregular with PAC

Rate: Basic rhythm rate 58

P waves: Sinus with basic rhythm; premature, abnormal P wave with PAC

PR interval: 0.16–0.18 seconds (basic rhythm)

QRS: 0.06–0.08 seconds

Rhythm interpretation: Sinus bradycardia with one PAC (5th complex); a U wave is present

**Strip 7-63**

Rhythm: Irregular

Rate: Ventricular rate: 80 Atrial rate not measurable

P waves: Fibrillatory waves present

PR interval: Not measurable

QRS: 0.04 to 0.06 seconds

Rhythm interpretation: Atrial fibrillation; ST segment depression is present

**Strip 7-64**

Rhythm: Regular

Rate: 214

P waves: Hidden in T waves

PR interval: Not measurable

QRS: 0.08 seconds

Rhythm interpretation: Paroxysmal atrial tachycardia

**Strip 7-65**

Rhythm: Basic rhythm regular; irregular with PAC

Rate: Basic rhythm rate 52

P waves: Sinus with basic rhythm; premature pointed P wave associated with PAC (abnormal P wave hidden in T wave following 4th QRS)

PR interval: 0.16–0.18 seconds

QRS: 0.06–0.08 seconds

Rhythm interpretation: Sinus bradycardia with one PAC (5th complex); a U wave is present

**Strip 7-66**

Rhythm: Basic rhythm regular; irregular with nonconducted PAC

Rate: Basic rhythm rate 75

P waves: Sinus with basic rhythm; premature, abnormal P wave hidden in T wave following 4th QRS

PR interval: 0.20 seconds

QRS: 0.06–0.08 seconds

Rhythm interpretation: Normal sinus rhythm with one nonconducted PAC (follows 4th QRS); a U wave is present

**Strip 7-67**

Rhythm: Regular (off by 2 squares)

Rate: 79

P waves: Vary in size, shape, direction

PR interval: 0.12–0.18 seconds

QRS: 0.08–0.10 seconds

Rhythm interpretation: Wandering atrial pacemaker

**Strip 7-68**
Rhythm: Regular
Rate: 150
P waves: Hidden (possibly in preceding T waves)
PR interval: Not measurable
QRS: 0.04–0.06 seconds
Rhythm interpretation: Paroxysmal atrial tachycardia; ST segment depression is present

**Strip 7-69**
Rhythm: Irregular
Rate: Atrial: 250 Ventricular: 70
P waves: Flutter waves before each QRS in varying ratios
PR interval: Not measurable
QRS: 0.06–0.08 seconds
Rhythm interpretation: Atrial flutter with variable AV conduction

**Strip 7-70**
Rhythm: Irregular
Rate: Ventricular rate: 130; Atrial rate not measurable
P waves: Fibrillatory waves; some flutter waves are seen
PR interval: Not measurable
QRS: 0.04 seconds
Rhythm interpretation: Atrial fibrillation; some flutter waves are noted; ST segment depression is present

**Strip 7-71**
Rhythm: Basic rhythm regular; irregular with PACs
Rate: Basic rhythm rate 88
P waves: Sinus P waves with basic rhythm; premature, abnormal P waves with PACs
PR interval: 0.14 to 0.16 seconds (basic rhythm)
QRS: 0.06 to 0.08 seconds
Rhythm interpretation: Normal sinus rhythm with paired PACs (3rd and 4th complexes)

**Strip 7-72**
Rhythm: Regular
Rate: 54
P waves: Varying in size and shape
PR interval: 0.12
QRS: 0.08 to 0.10 seconds
Rhythm interpretation: Wandering atrial pacemaker; ST segment depression is present

**Strip 7-73**
Rhythm: Regular
Rate: Atrial: 272; Ventricular: 136
P waves: 2 flutter waves to each QRS
PR interval: Not measurable
QRS: 0.08 seconds
Rhythm interpretation: Atrial flutter with 2:1 AV conduction

**Strip 7-74**
Rhythm: Basic rhythm regular; irregular with PAC
Rate: Basic rhythm rate 63
P waves: Sinus in basic rhythm; premature, abnormal P wave with PAC
PR interval: 0.12–0.14 seconds (basic rhythm); 0.14 seconds (PAC)
QRS: 0.06–0.08 seconds (basic rhythm) 0.08 seconds (PAC)
Rhythm interpretation: Normal sinus rhythm with 1 PAC (4th complex); a small U wave is present

**Strip 7-75**
Rhythm: Regular
Rate: 150
P waves: Hidden in T waves
PR interval: Not measurable
QRS: 0.06 to 0.08 seconds
Rhythm interpretation: Paroxysmal atrial tachycardia; ST segment depression is present

**Strip 7-76**
Rhythm: Irregular
Rate: Ventricular rate: 80; Atrial rate not measurable
P waves: Fibrillatory waves present
PR interval: Not measurable
QRS: 0.04 seconds
Rhythm interpretation: Atrial fibrillation; ST segment depression and T wave inversion are present

**Strip 7-77**
Rhythm: Regular
Rate: 88
P waves: Vary in size, shape, position
PR interval: 0.12 to 0.14 seconds
QRS: 0.06 to 0.08 seconds
Rhythm interpretation: Wandering atrial pacemaker; T wave inversion is present

## Strip 7-78

Rhythm: Irregular
Rate: 50
P waves: Vary in size, shape, and position
PR interval: 0.12 to 0.16 seconds
QRS: 0.08 seconds
Rhythm interpretation: Wandering atrial
pacemaker; ST segment depression is present

## Strip 7-79

Rhythm: Regular
Rate: Atrial: 232; Ventricular: 58
P waves: 4 flutter waves to each QRS
PR interval: Not measurable
QRS: 0.08 seconds
Rhythm interpretation: Atrial flutter with 4:1 AV
conduction

## Strip 7-80

Rhythm: Basic rhythm regular; irregular with
nonconducted PACs
Rate: Basic rhythm rate 107
P waves: Sinus with basic rhythm; premature
abnormal P waves with nonconducted PACs
PR interval: 0.16–0.18 seconds
QRS: 0.06–0.08 seconds
Rhythm interpretation: Sinus tachycardia with two
nonconducted PACs (following 3rd and 8th QRS
complex)

## Strip 7-81

Rhythm: Regular
Rate: 68
P waves: Vary in size, shape, direction
PR interval: 0.12–0.16 seconds
QRS: 0.08 seconds
Rhythm interpretation: Wandering atrial
pacemaker; a U wave is present

## Strip 7-82

Rhythm: Regular
Rate: Atrial: 240; Ventricular: 60
P waves: 4 flutter waves to each QRS
PR interval: Not measurable
QRS: 0.06 seconds
Rhythm interpretation: Atrial flutter with 4:1 AV
conduction

## Strip 7-83

Rhythm: Regular
Rate: 167
P waves: Hidden in preceding T wave
PR interval: Not measurable
QRS: 0.08–0.10 seconds
Rhythm interpretation: Paroxysmal atrial tachycardia

## Strip 7-84

Rhythm: Irregular
Rate: 50
P waves: Fibrillatory waves
PR interval: Not measurable
QRS: 0.08–0.10 seconds
Rhythm interpretation: Atrial fibrillation

## Strip 7-85

Rhythm: Irregular
Rate: 40
P waves: Vary in size, shape, direction
PR interval: 0.14–0.16 seconds
QRS: 0.08 seconds
Rhythm interpretation: Wandering atrial pacemaker

## Strip 7-86

Rhythm: Basic rhythm regular; irregular with PACs
Rate: Basic rhythm rate 107
P waves: Sinus with basic rhythm; premature,
pointed P waves with PACs
PR interval: 0.16 seconds (basic rhythm)
QRS: 0.06 seconds
Rhythm interpretation: Sinus tachycardia with 3
PACs (4th, 9th, 11th complex)

## Strip 7-87

Rhythm: Irregular
Rate: Atrial: 250; Ventricular: 40
P waves: Flutter waves before each QRS in varying
ratios
PR interval: Not measurable
QRS: 0.06–0.08 seconds
Rhythm interpretation: Atrial flutter with variable
AV conduction

## Strip 7-88

Rhythm: Irregular
Rate: Ventricular rate: 40; atrial rate not measurable
P waves: Fibrillatory waves present
PR interval: Not measurable
QRS: 0.04–0.06 seconds
Rhythm interpretation: Atrial fibrillation;
ST segment depression is present

## Strip 7-89

Rhythm: Basic rhythm regular; irregular with
nonconducted PAC
Rate: Basic rhythm rate 84
P waves: Sinus in basic rhythm; premature, pointed
P wave with nonconducted PAC
PR interval: 0.16–0.20 seconds
QRS: 0.06–0.08 seconds
Rhythm interpretation: Normal sinus rhythm with
one nonconducted PAC (follows 5th QRS); ST
segment depression is present

**Strip 7-90**

Rhythm: Basic rhythm regular; irregular with PAC

Rate: Basic rhythm rate: 54

P waves: Sinus with basic rhythm; premature abnormal P wave with PAC

PR interval: 0.16–0.18 seconds

QRS: 0.06 seconds

Rhythm interpretation: Sinus bradycardia with one PAC (4th complex)

**Strip 7-91**

Rhythm: Basic rhythm regular; irregular with PAC

Rate: Basic rhythm 63

P waves: Sinus P waves with basic rhythm; premature, abnormal P waves with PAC

PR interval: 0.14 to 0.16 seconds

QRS: 0.06 seconds

Rhythm interpretation: Normal sinus rhythm with one PAC (5th complex); a U wave is present

**Strip 7-92**

Rhythm: Regular

Rate: Atrial, 235; ventricular, 47

P waves: Five flutter waves to each QRS

PR interval: Not discernible

QRS: 0.08 seconds

Rhythm interpretation: Atrial flutter with 5:1 block; T wave inversion is present

**Strip 7-93**

Rhythm: Regular

Rate: 150

P waves: Pointed

PR interval: Not measurable

QRS: 0.06–0.08 seconds

Rhythm interpretation: Paroxysmal atrial tachycardia

**Strip 7-94**

Rhythm: Irregular

Rate: 50

P waves: Wavy

PR interval: Not measurable

QRS: 0.04–0.06 seconds

Rhythm interpretation: Atrial fibrillation

**Strip 7-95**

Rhythm: Basic rhythm regular; irregular following burst of PAT

Rate: Basic rhythm rate 84

P waves: Sinus P waves with basic rhythm; abnormal premature P waves with run of PAT

PR interval: 0.16–0.18 seconds in basic rhythm not measurable in PAT

QRS: 0.04–0.06 seconds basic rhythm and PAT

Rhythm interpretation: Normal sinus rhythm with burst of PAT (3 PACs following 4th QRS complex)

**Strip 8-1**

Rhythm: Basic rhythm regular; irregular with PJC

Rate: Basic rhythm rate 58

P waves: Sinus with basic rhythm; premature inverted P wave with PJC

PR interval: 0.14–0.16 (basic rhythm); 0.08 (PJC)

QRS: 0.06 seconds (basic rhythm and PJC)

Rhythm interpretation: Sinus bradycardia with 1 PJC (5th complex); a U wave is present

**Strip 8-2**

Rhythm: Regular

Rate: 60

P waves: Sinus P waves present

PR interval: 0.24

QRS: 0.06 to 0.08 seconds

Rhythm interpretation: Normal sinus rhythm with first-degree AV block; ST segment elevation and T wave inversion are present

**Strip 8-3**

Rhythm: Regular atrial and ventricular rhythm

Rate: Atrial: 46 Ventricular: 23

P waves: 2 Sinus P waves before each QRS

PR interval: 0.22–0.24 seconds (remains constant)

QRS: 0.08–0.10 seconds

Rhythm interpretation: Second-Degree AV Block, Mobitz II; clinical correlation is suggested to diagnose Mobitz II when 2:1 conduction is present; ST segment elevation is present

**Strip 8-4**

Rhythm: Basic rhythm regular; irregular with junctional beat

Rate: Basic rhythm rate 58

P waves: Sinus P waves with basic rhythm; hidden P wave with junctional beat

PR interval: 0.16 to 0.18 seconds (basic rhythm)

QRS: 0.08 to 0.10 seconds (basic rhythm and junctional beat)

Rhythm interpretation: Sinus bradycardia with junctional escape beat (4th complex) following pause in basic rhythm; ST segment depression is present

**Strip 8-5**
Rhythm: Regular
Rate: 115
P waves: Inverted
PR interval: 0.08 seconds
QRS: 0.04–0.06 seconds
Rhythm interpretation: Junctional tachycardia

**Strip 8-6**
Rhythm: Regular
Rate: 84
P waves: Sinus
PR interval: 0.22–0.24 seconds
QRS: 0.08–0.10 seconds
Rhythm interpretation: Normal sinus rhythm with first-degree AV block

**Strip 8-7**
Rhythm: Regular
Rate: 65
P waves: Inverted before each QRS
PR interval: 0.08 seconds
QRS: 0.06 to 0.08 seconds
Rhythm interpretation: Accelerated junctional rhythm; ST segment elevation and T wave inversion are present

**Strip 8-8**
Rhythm: Regular atrial rhythm; irregular ventricular rhythm
Rate: Atrial, 75; ventricular, 70
P waves: Sinus P waves present; one P wave without QRS
PR interval: Progresses from 0.28 to 0.32 seconds
QRS: 0.04 to 0.08 seconds
Rhythm interpretation: Second-degree AV block, Mobitz I; ST segment depression and T wave inversion are present

**Strip 8-9**
Rhythm: Regular
Rate: 47
P waves: Hidden in QRS
PR interval: Not measurable
QRS: 0.08 seconds
Rhythm interpretation: Junctional rhythm; ST segment depression is present

**Strip 8-10**
Rhythm: Atrial rhythm regular; Ventricular rhythm irregular
Rate: Atrial: 75; Ventricular: 30
P waves: 2 Sinus P waves before each QRS
PR interval: 0.20–0.22 seconds
QRS: 0.08–0.10 seconds
Rhythm interpretation: Second-degree AV block, Mobitz II (clinical correlation is suggested to diagnose Mobitz II when 2:1 conduction is present) ST segment depression is present

**Strip 8-11**
Rhythm: Atrial rhythm regular; ventricular rhythm regular
Rate: Atrial 63; Ventricular: 33
P waves: Sinus P waves are present; P waves have no relationship to QRS (found hidden in QRS and T waves)
PR interval: Varies greatly
QRS: 0.12 seconds
Rhythm interpretation: Third-degree AV block; ST segment depression and T wave inversion are present

**Strip 8-12**
Rhythm: Regular
Rate: 84
P waves: Hidden in QRS
PR interval: Not measurable
QRS: 0.06–0.08 seconds
Rhythm interpretation: Accelerated junctional rhythm; ST segment depression is present

**Strip 8-13**
Rhythm: Regular
Rate: 65
P waves: Sinus
PR interval: 0.44–0.48 seconds
QRS: 0.08–0.10 seconds
Rhythm interpretation: Normal sinus rhythm with first-degree AV block; an elevated ST segment is present

**Strip 8-14**
Rhythm: Basic rhythm regular; irregular with PJC
Rate: Basic rhythm rate 136
P waves: Sinus P waves with basic rhythm; hidden P wave with PJC
PR interval: 0.12 to 0.14 seconds
QRS: 0.04–0.06 seconds
Rhythm interpretation: Sinus tachycardia with PJC (13th complex)

## Strip 8-15
Rhythm: Regular
Rate: 94
P waves: Sinus
PR interval: 0.26–0.28 seconds
QRS: 0.06 seconds
Rhythm interpretation: Normal sinus rhythm with first-degree AV block

## Strip 8-16
Rhythm: Basic rhythm regular; irregular with premature beat
Rate: Basic rate 58
P waves: Sinus with basic rhythm; inverted P wave with premature beat
PR interval: Basic rhythm 0.16–0.18 seconds; PJC 0.08 seconds
QRS: 0.06–0.08 seconds
Rhythm interpretation: Sinus bradycardia with 1 PJC (4th complex); ST segment depression is present

## Strip 8-17
Rhythm: Regular atrial and ventricular rhythm
Rate: Atrial: 108; ventricular: 54
P waves: Two P waves to each QRS complex
PR interval: 0.20 and constant
QRS: 0.08 to 0.10 seconds
Rhythm interpretation: Second-degree AV block Mobitz II. Clinical correlation is suggested to diagnose Mobitz II when 2:1 conduction is present; ST segment elevation and T wave inversion are present

## Strip 8-18
Rhythm: Irregular ventricular rhythm; regular atrial rhythm
Rate: Atrial: 65; ventricular: 50
P waves: Sinus P waves present; one P wave without QRS
PR interval: Progresses from 0.20 to 0.48 seconds
QRS: 0.04 seconds
Rhythm interpretation: Second-degree AV block, Mobitz I

## Strip 8-19
Rhythm: Regular
Rate: 125
P waves: Inverted before each QRS
PR interval: 0.08 to 0.10 seconds
QRS: 0.06 seconds
Rhythm interpretation: Junctional tachycardia

## Strip 8-20
Rhythm: Regular atrial and ventricular rhythm
Rate: Atrial: 100 Ventricular: 38
P waves: Sinus P waves present; bear no relationship to QRS (found hidden in QRS and T waves)
PR interval: Varies greatly
QRS: 0.06–0.08 seconds
Rhythm interpretation: Third-degree AV block; ST segment depression is present

## Strip 8-21
Rhythm: Basic rhythm regular; irregular with PJC
Rate: Basic rhythm rate 60
P waves: Sinus P waves with basic rhythm; premature, inverted P wave with PJC
PR interval: 0.12 to 0.14 seconds (basic rhythm); 0.08 seconds (PJC)
QRS: 0.08 seconds (basic rhythm and PJC)
Rhythm interpretation: Normal sinus rhythm with one PJC (4th complex)

## Strip 8-22
Rhythm: Regular atrial and ventricular rhythm
Rate: Atrial, 100; ventricular, 50
P waves: Two sinus P waves before each QRS complex
PR interval: 0.16 and constant
QRS: 0.08 seconds
Rhythm interpretation: Second-degree AV block, Mobitz II. Clinical correlation is suggested to diagnose Mobitz II when 2:1 conduction is present

## Strip 8-23
Rhythm: Regular
Rate: 35
P waves: Sinus
PR interval: 0.60–0.62 seconds (remains constant)
QRS: 0.06 seconds
Rhythm interpretation: Sinus bradycardia with first-degree AV block

## Strip 8-24
Rhythm: Irregular ventricular rhythm; regular atrial rhythm
Rate: Atrial, 68; ventricular, 60
P waves: Sinus P waves present; one without a QRS
PR interval: Progresses from 0.28 to 0.36 seconds
QRS: 0.08 seconds
Rhythm interpretation: Second-degree AV block, Mobitz I; a U wave is present

**Strip 8-25**
Rhythm: Regular
Rate: 75
P waves: Sinus P waves
PR interval: 0.28
QRS: 0.08 seconds
Rhythm interpretation: Sinus rhythm with first-degree AV block

**Strip 8-26**
Rhythm: Basic rhythm regular; irregular with PJCs
Rate: Basic rhythm rate 100
P waves: Sinus P waves with basic rhythm; premature, inverted P waves with PJCs
PR interval: 0.20 seconds (basic rhythm); 0.06 seconds (PJC)
QRS: 0.06 to 0.08 seconds (basic rhythm and PJC)
Rhythm interpretation: Normal sinus rhythm with paired PJCs; (8th and 9th complexes); ST segment depression is present

**Strip 8-27**
Rhythm: Regular
Rate: 65
P waves: Inverted before each QRS
PR interval: 0.08 seconds
QRS: 0.08 seconds
Rhythm interpretation: Accelerated junctional rhythm; ST segment is present

**Strip 8-28**
Rhythm: Basic rhythm regular; irregular with nonconducted PAC
Rate: Basic rhythm rate 56
P waves: Sinus P waves with basic rhythm; premature, abnormal P wave without QRS
PR interval: 0.24–0.26 seconds (remains constant)
QRS: 0.08 seconds
Rhythm interpretation: Sinus bradycardia with first-degree AV block and nonconducted PAC (follows 4th QRS); ST segment depression is present

**Strip 8-29**
Rhythm: Regular atrial rhythm; irregular ventricular rhythm
Rate: Atrial: 63; Ventricular: 50
P waves: Sinus P waves are present
PR interval: Progressively lengthens from 0.28–0.32 seconds
QRS: 0.06–0.08 seconds
Rhythm interpretation: Second-degree AV block, Mobitz I; ST segment depression is present

**Strip 8-30**
Rhythm: Regular atrial and ventricular rhythm
Rate: Atrial: 79; Ventricular: 32
P waves: Sinus P waves which have no constant relationship to QRS (found hidden in QRS complexes and T waves)
PR interval: Varies greatly
QRS: 0.12 seconds
Rhythm interpretation: Third-degree AV block

**Strip 8-31**
Rhythm: Regular atrial and ventricular rhythm
Rate: Atrial, 84; ventricular, 28
P waves: Three sinus P waves to each QRS
PR interval: 0.28 to 0.32 (remains constant)
QRS: 0.08 seconds
Rhythm interpretation: Second-degree AV block, Mobitz II

**Strip 8-32**
Rhythm: Regular atrial and ventricular rhythm
Rate: Atrial: 75; Ventricular: 34
P waves: Sinus P waves present with no relationship to QRS complexes (found hidden in QRS and T waves)
PR interval: Varies greatly
QRS: 0.12–0.14 seconds
Rhythm interpretation: Third-degree AV block; ST segment elevation is present

**Strip 8-33**
Rhythm: Basic rhythm regular; irregular with PAC
Rate: Basic rhythm rate 100
P waves: Inverted before QRS in basic rhythm; upright and premature with PAC
PR interval: 0.08 seconds (basic rhythm); 0.12 seconds (PAC)
QRS: 0.08 seconds (basic rhythm and PAC)
Rhythm interpretation: Accelerated junctional rhythm with one PAC (6th complex); ST segment depression is present

**Strip 8-34**
Rhythm: Irregular ventricular rhythm; regular atrial rhythm
Rate: Atrial: 75; ventricular: 50
P waves: Sinus P waves present; two P waves without QRS
PR interval: Progresses from 0.28 to 0.40 seconds
QRS: 0.08 to 0.10 seconds
Rhythm interpretation: Second-degree AV block, Mobitz I

**Strip 8-35**
Rhythm: Regular
Rate: 60
P waves: Sinus
PR interval: 0.24–0.26 seconds
QRS: 0.06–0.08 seconds
Rhythm interpretation: Normal sinus rhythm with first-degree AV block

**Strip 8-36**
Rhythm: Regular
Rate: 41
P waves: Inverted after QRS
PR interval: 0.04 to 0.06 seconds
QRS: 0.06 to 0.08 seconds
Rhythm interpretation: Junctional rhythm

**Strip 8-37**
Rhythm: Basic rhythm regular; irregular with PJC
Rate: Basic rhythm rate 58
P waves: Sinus P waves with basic rhythm; premature, inverted P waves with PJCs
PR interval: 0.16 seconds (basic rhythm); 0.08 to 0.10 seconds (PJC)
QRS: 0.08 seconds (basic rhythm and PJC)
Rhythm interpretation: Sinus bradycardia with two PJCs (4th complex and 6th complex); a U wave is present

**Strip 8-38**
Rhythm: Regular atrial and ventricular rhythm
Rate: Atrial: 66; Ventricular: 33
P waves: 2 Sinus P waves to each QRS
PR interval: 0.44 seconds (remains constant)
QRS: 0.14–0.16 seconds
Rhythm interpretation: Second-degree AV block, Mobitz II; clinical correlation is suggested to diagnose Mobitz II when 2:1 conduction is present

**Strip 8-39**
Rhythm: Regular atrial and ventricular rhythm
Rate: Atrial: 52; ventricular: 26
P waves: Two sinus P waves present before each QRS complex
PR interval: 0.22 (remains constant)
QRS: 0.12 seconds
Rhythm interpretation: Second-degree AV block, Mobitz II. Clinical correlation is suggested to diagnose Mobitz II when 2:1 conduction is present

**Strip 8-40**
Rhythm: Regular atrial rhythm; irregular ventricular rhythm
Rate: Atrial: 107; Ventricular: 50
P waves: Sinus P waves present—bear no relationship to QRS complexes (found hidden in QRS and T waves)
PR interval: Varies greatly
QRS: 0.08 seconds
Rhythm interpretation: Third-degree AV block

**Strip 8-41**
Rhythm: Regular
Rate: 68
P waves: Inverted before each QRS
PR interval: 0.08 seconds
QRS: 0.06–0.08 seconds
Rhythm interpretation: Accelerated junctional rhythm

**Strip 8-42**
Rhythm: Regular atrial and ventricular rhythm
Rate: Atrial: 104; Ventricular: 52
P waves: Two sinus P waves to each QRS complex
PR interval: 0.24 and constant
QRS: 0.06 to 0.08 seconds
Rhythm interpretation: Second-degree AV block, Mobitz II. Clinical correlation is suggested to diagnose Mobitz II when 2:1 conduction is present; ST segment elevation and T wave inversion are present

**Strip 8-43**
Rhythm: First rhythm irregular; second rhythm regular
Rate: First rhythm about 80; second rhythm 42
P waves: Fibrillatory waves in first rhythm; hidden P waves in second rhythm
PR interval: Not measurable in either rhythm
QRS: 0.06–0.08 seconds
Rhythm interpretation: Atrial fibrillation to junctional rhythm; ST segment depression is present

**Strip 8-44**
Rhythm: Basic rhythm regular; irregular with premature beats
Rate: Basic rhythm rate 60
P waves: Sinus P waves with basic rhythm; premature, abnormal P waves with premature beats
PR interval: 0.12 to 0.16 seconds (basic rhythm); 0.12 seconds (PAC); 0.08 seconds (PJC)
QRS: 0.06 to 0.08 seconds
Rhythm interpretation: Normal sinus rhythm with one PAC (4th complex) and one PJC (5th complex); ST segment depression and T wave inversion are present

**Strip 8-45**

Rhythm: Regular atrial and ventricular rhythm
Rate: Atrial: 72; Ventricular: 32
P waves: Sinus P waves present; bear no relationship to QRS complexes (hidden in QRS and T waves)
PR interval: Varies greatly
QRS: 0.12 seconds
Rhythm interpretation: Third-degree AV block; ST segment elevation is present

**Strip 8-46**

Rhythm: Irregular
Rate: 40
P waves: Sinus P waves are present
PR interval: 0.28 seconds (remains constant)
QRS: 0.08 to 0.10 seconds
Rhythm interpretation: Sinus arrhythmia with first-degree AV block; a U wave is present

**Strip 8-47**

Rhythm: Regular atrial rhythm; irregular ventricular rhythm
Rate: Atrial: 79; Ventricular: 50
P waves: Sinus P waves present
PR interval: Lengthens 0.24–0.40 seconds
QRS: 0.08–0.10 seconds
Rhythm interpretation: Second-degree AV block, Mobitz I

**Strip 8-48**

Rhythm: Regular atrial and ventricular rhythm
Rate: Atrial: 108; ventricular: 54
P waves: Two sinus P waves before each QRS complex
PR interval: 0.18 to 0.20 seconds (remains constant)
QRS: 0.08 seconds
Rhythm interpretation: Second-degree AV block, Mobitz II. Clinical correlation is suggested to diagnose Mobitz II when 2:1 conduction is present. ST segment elevation and T wave inversion are present

**Strip 8-49**

Rhythm: Irregular
Rate: 40
P waves: Inverted before each QRS
PR interval: 0.04 to 0.06 seconds
QRS: 0.08 to 0.10 seconds
Rhythm interpretation: Junctional rhythm; ST segment depression is present

**Strip 8-50**

Rhythm: Basic rhythm regular; irregular with escape beat
Rate: Basic rhythm rate 84; rate slows to 75 after escape beat; rate suppression can occur following premature or escape beats; after several cycles rate will return to basic rate
P waves: Sinus P waves present; P wave hidden with escape beat
PR interval: 0.14 to 0.16 seconds
QRS: 0.06 to 0.08 seconds
Rhythm interpretation: Normal sinus rhythm with junctional escape beat (5th complex) following a pause in the basic rhythm; a U wave is present

**Strip 8-51**

Rhythm: Regular ventricular rhythm; irregular atrial rhythm
Rate: Atrial: 70; ventricular: 25
P waves: Sinus P waves present; bear no relationship to QRS
PR interval: Varies greatly
QRS: 0.12 seconds
Rhythm interpretation: Third-degree AV block

**Strip 8-52**

Rhythm: Regular
Rate: 63
P waves: Hidden in QRS
PR interval: Not measurable
QRS: 0.08 seconds
Rhythm interpretation: Accelerated junctional rhythm

**Strip 8-53**

Rhythm: Regular atrial and ventricular rhythm
Rate: Atrial: 76; ventricular: 38
P waves: Two sinus P waves before each QRS complex
PR interval: 0.24–0.26 seconds
QRS: 0.12–0.14 seconds
Rhythm interpretation: Second-degree AV block, Mobitz II. Clinical correlation is suggested to diagnose Mobitz II when 2:1 conduction is present

**Strip 8-54**

Rhythm: Regular
Rate: 94
P waves: Inverted before QRS
PR interval: 0.08 seconds
QRS: 0.06 to 0.08 seconds
Rhythm interpretation: Accelerated junctional rhythm

**Strip 8-55**
Rhythm: Basic rhythm regular
Rate: 55 (basic rhythm)
P waves: Sinus P waves with basic rhythm (notched P waves usually indicate left atrial hypertrophy); no P wave seen with 4th complex; 5th complex has P wave on top of preceding T wave
PR interval: 0.20 seconds (basic rhythm); 0.40 seconds (PAC)
QRS: 0.06–0.08 seconds
Rhythm interpretation: Sinus bradycardia with 1 junctional escape beat (4th complex) and 1 PAC (5th complex) (Both follow a pause in the basic rhythm)

**Strip 8-56**
Rhythm: Both rhythms regular
Rate: 72 (first rhythm) about 140 (second rhythm)
P waves: Sinus P waves (first rhythm); inverted P waves (second rhythm)
PR interval: 0.12 seconds (first rhythm); 0.08 to 0.10 seconds (second rhythm)
QRS: 0.08 seconds
Rhythm interpretation: Normal sinus rhythm changing to junctional tachycardia; ST segment depression is present

**Strip 8-57**
Rhythm: Regular
Rate: 84
P waves: Sinus P waves present
PR interval: 0.30 to 0.32 seconds (remains constant)
QRS: 0.04–0.06 seconds
Rhythm interpretation: Normal sinus rhythm with first-degree AV block; ST segment elevation is present

**Strip 8-58**
Rhythm: Regular atrial and ventricular rhythm
Rate: Atrial: 75; ventricular: 30
P waves: Sinus P waves present; bear no relationship to QRS
PR interval: Varies greatly
QRS: 0.12 to 0.14 seconds
Rhythm interpretation: Third-degree AV block

**Strip 8-59**
Rhythm: Regular atrial and ventricular rhythm
Rate: Atrial: 93; ventricular: 31
P waves: 3 Sinus P waves to each QRS (one hidden in T-wave)
PR interval: 0.32 to 0.36 seconds
QRS: 0.08 seconds
Rhythm interpretation: Second-degree AV block, Mobitz II; ST segment depression is present

**Strip 8-60**
Rhythm: Basic rhythm regular; irregular with premature beats
Rate: Basic rhythm rate 60
P waves: Sinus P waves present with basic rhythm; premature, abnormal P waves with premature beats
PR interval: 0.12 seconds (basic rhythm); 0.12 seconds (PAC); 0.08 to 0.10 seconds (PJCs)
QRS: 0.08 seconds
Rhythm interpretation: Normal sinus rhythm with one PAC (3rd complex) and paired PJCs (6th and 7th complexes)

**Strip 8-61**
Rhythm: Regular
Rate: 47
P waves: Hidden in QRS
PR interval: Not measurable
QRS: 0.08 seconds
Rhythm interpretation: Junctional rhythm

**Strip 8-62**
Rhythm: Basic rhythm regular; irregular with nonconducted PAC
Rate: Basic rhythm rate 79—rate slows to 63 following pause (temporary rate suppression is common following a pause in the basic rhythm
P waves: Sinus with basic rhythm; premature, pointed P wave distorting T wave following 6th QRS
PR interval: 0.24 seconds (remains constant)
QRS: 0.08 seconds
Rhythm interpretation: Normal sinus rhythm with first-degree AV block; a nonconducted PAC is present following 6th QRS

**Strip 8-63**
Rhythm: Irregular ventricular rhythm; regular atrial rhythm
Rate: Atrial: 75; ventricular: 50
P waves: Sinus P waves are present
PR interval: Progresses from 0.24 to 0.32 seconds
QRS: 0.08 seconds
Rhythm interpretation: Second-degree AV block, Mobitz I

**Strip 8-64**
Rhythm: Regular atrial and ventricular rhythm
Rate: Atrial: 72; ventricular: 31
P waves: Sinus P waves present; bear no relationship to QRS (hidden in QRS complexes and T waves)
PR interval: Varies greatly
QRS: 0.12 seconds
Rhythm interpretation: Third-degree AV block

**Strip 8-65**
Rhythm: Regular atrial and ventricular rhythm
Rate: Atrial: 90; ventricular: 45
P waves: Two sinus P waves to each QRS
PR interval: 0.26–0.28 seconds (remains constant)
QRS: 0.12 seconds
Rhythm interpretation: Second-degree AV block, Mobitz II; clinical correlation is suggested to diagnose Mobitz II when 2:1 conduction is present; ST segment elevation is present

**Strip 8-66**
Rhythm: Regular
Rate: 79
P waves: Inverted P waves before each QRS
PR interval: 0.08–0.10 seconds
QRS: 0.06–0.08 seconds
Rhythm interpretation: Accelerated junctional rhythm

**Strip 8-67**
Rhythm: Regular
Rate: 94
P waves: Sinus
PR interval: 0.24 seconds
QRS: 0.08 seconds
Rhythm interpretation: Normal sinus rhythm with first-degree AV block

**Strip 8-68**
Rhythm: Basic rhythm regular; irregular with premature beats
Rate: Basic rhythm rate 72
P waves: Sinus P waves with basic rhythm; premature, abnormal P waves with premature beats
PR interval: 0.14 to 0.16 seconds (basic rhythm); 0.12 seconds (PACs); 0.10 seconds (PJCs)
QRS: 0.06 to 0.08 seconds
Rhythm interpretation: Normal sinus rhythm with two PACs (3rd and 8th complex) and one PJC (5th complex); a U wave is present

**Strip 8-69**
Rhythm: Basic rhythm regular; irregular with premature beats
Rate: Basic rhythm rate 52
P waves: Hidden with basic rhythm; premature, abnormal with premature beats
PR interval: Not measurable in basic rhythm; 0.12–0.14 seconds (PACs)
QRS: 0.06 to 0.08 seconds
Rhythm interpretation: Junctional rhythm with two PACs (2nd and 5th complex); ST segment depression is present

**Strip 8-70**
Rhythm: Irregular ventricular rhythm; regular atrial rhythm
Rate: Atrial: 79; ventricular: 70
P waves: Sinus P waves present
PR interval: Progresses from 0.24 to 0.28 seconds
QRS: 0.08 seconds
Rhythm interpretation: Second-degree AV block, Mobitz I

**Strip 8-71**
Rhythm: Regular atrial and ventricular rhythm
Rate: Atrial: 80; ventricular: 40
P waves: Two sinus P waves to each QRS
PR interval: 0.24 seconds (remain constant)
QRS: 0.04 to 0.06 seconds
Rhythm interpretation: Second-degree AV block, Mobitz II; clinical correlation is suggested to diagnose Mobitz II when 2:1 conduction is present; ST segment depression is present

**Strip 8-72**
Rhythm: Regular atrial and ventricular rhythm
Rate: Atrial: 94; ventricular: 40
P waves: Sinus P waves are present; bear no relationship to QRS (hidden in QRS complexes and T waves)
PR interval: Varies greatly
QRS: 0.10 seconds
Rhythm interpretation: Third-degree AV block

**Strip 8-73**
Rhythm: Regular
Rate: 84
P waves: Hidden in QRS complexes
PR interval: Not measurable
QRS: 0.06 seconds
Rhythm interpretation: Accelerated junctional rhythm; ST segment depression and T wave inversion are present

**Strip 8-74**
Rhythm: Regular atrial rhythm; irregular ventricular rhythm
Rate: Atrial: 54 Ventricular: 50
P waves: Sinus P waves are present
PR interval: Lengthens from 0.34–0.44 seconds
QRS: 0.08 seconds
Rhythm interpretation: Second-degree AV block, Mobitz I

**Strip 8-75**
Rhythm: Basic rhythm regular; irregular with escape beat
Rate: Basic rhythm rate 58
P waves: Sinus P waves with basic rhythm; hidden P wave with escape beat
PR interval: 0.16 to 0.18 seconds
QRS: 0.08 to 0.10 seconds
Rhythm interpretation: Sinus bradycardia with junctional escape beat (4th complex) following a pause in the basic rhythm

**Strip 8-76**
Rhythm: Regular
Rate: 47
P waves: Hidden in QRS
PR interval: Not measurable
QRS: 0.06–0.08 seconds
Rhythm interpretation: Junctional rhythm; ST segment depression is present

**Strip 8-77**
Rhythm: Regular atrial and ventricular rhythm
Rate: Atrial: 94; ventricular: 44
P waves: Sinus P waves are present; P waves bear no relationship to QRS (found hidden in QRS complexes and T waves)
PR interval: Varies greatly
QRS: 0.14–0.16 seconds
Rhythm interpretation: Third-degree AV block; ST segment elevation is present

**Strip 8-78**
Rhythm: Basic rhythm regular; irregular with premature beats
Rate: Basic rhythm rate 68
P waves: Sinus with basic rhythm; premature abnormal P waves with premature beats
PR interval: 0.12–0.14 seconds (basic rhythm); 0.14 seconds (PAC); 0.10 seconds (PJC)
QRS: 0.06–0.08 seconds
Rhythm interpretation: Normal sinus rhythm with 1 PAC (3rd complex) and 1 PJC (7th complex); a U wave is present

**Strip 8-79**
Rhythm: Regular atrial and ventricular rhythm
Rate: Atrial: 80; ventricular: 40
P waves: Two P waves to each QRS
PR interval: 0.12 to 0.14 seconds (remain constant)
QRS: 0.06–0.08 seconds
Rhythm interpretation: Second-degree AV block, Mobitz II; clinical correlation is suggested to diagnose Mobitz II when 2:1 conduction is present

**Strip 8-80**
Rhythm: Basic rhythm regular; irregular with nonconducted PAC
Rate: Basic rhythm rate 72
P waves: Sinus with basic rhythm; premature, pointed P wave without QRS follows 6th QRS
PR interval: 0.22–0.24 seconds (remains constant)
QRS: 0.04–0.06 seconds
Rhythm interpretation: Normal sinus rhythm with first-degree AV block and 1 nonconducted PAC (follows 6th QRS); ST segment depression and T wave inversion are present

**Strip 8-81**
Rhythm: Regular
Rate: 88
P waves: Inverted before each QRS
PR interval: 0.08 seconds
QRS: 0.06–0.08 seconds
Rhythm interpretation: Accelerated junctional rhythm

**Strip 8-82**
Rhythm: Irregular ventricular rhythm; regular atrial rhythm
Rate: Atrial: 75; ventricular: 50
P waves: Sinus P waves are present
PR interval: Progresses from 0.26 to 0.40 seconds
QRS: 0.06 to 0.08 seconds
Rhythm interpretation: Second-degree AV block, Mobitz I; ST depression is present

**Strip 8-83**
Rhythm: Regular
Rate: 107
P waves: Inverted before each QRS
PR interval: 0.08 seconds
QRS: 0.08–0.10 seconds
Rhythm interpretation: Junctional tachycardia

**Strip 8-84**
Rhythm: There are two separate rhythms, both regular
Rate: 79 (1st rhythm); 84 (2nd rhythm)
P waves: Sinus (1st rhythm); inverted (2nd rhythm)
PR interval: 0.14–0.16 seconds (1st rhythm); 0.08 seconds (2nd rhythm)
QRS: 0.06–0.08 seconds (both rhythms)
Rhythm interpretation: Normal sinus rhythm changing to accelerated junctional rhythm

**Strip 8-85**
Rhythm: Regular atrial and ventricular rhythm
Rate: Atrial: 79; ventricular: 31
P waves: Sinus P waves present; bear no relationship to QRS; hidden in QRS complexes and T waves
PR interval: Varies greatly
QRS: 0.12 seconds
Rhythm interpretation: Third-degree AV block

**Strip 8-86**
Rhythm: Regular
Rate: 60
P waves: Sinus P waves present
PR interval: 0.24 seconds
QRS: 0.08 seconds
Rhythm interpretation: Normal sinus rhythm with first-degree AV block; ST segment depression and T wave inversion are present

**Strip 8-87**
Rhythm: Regular atrial and ventricular rhythm
Rate: Atrial: 88; ventricular: 33
P waves: Sinus P waves present—bear no relationship to QRS (found hidden in QRS and T waves)
PR interval: Varies greatly
QRS: 0.12–0.14 seconds
Rhythm interpretation: Third-degree AV block

**Strip 8-88**
Rhythm: Basic rhythm regular; irregular with premature and escape beats
Rate: Basic rate is 60
P waves: Sinus P waves with basic rhythm; pointed P wave with atrial beat and inverted P wave with junctional beats
PR interval: 0.12–0.14 seconds (basic rhythm); 0.14 seconds (atrial beat); 0.08–0.10 seconds (junctional beats)
QRS: 0.06 to 0.08 seconds
Rhythm interpretation: Normal sinus rhythm with one PJC (3rd complex), one atrial escape beat (4th complex), and one junctional escape beat (5th complex)

**Strip 8-89**
Rhythm: Irregular ventricular rhythm; regular atrial rhythm
Rate: Atrial, 65; ventricular, 50
P waves: Sinus P waves present
PR interval: Progresses from 0.32 to 0.40 seconds
QRS: 0.08–0.10 seconds
Rhythm interpretation: Second-degree AV block, Mobitz I

**Strip 8-90**
Rhythm: Regular
Rate: 107
P waves: Inverted before each QRS
PR interval: 0.08 to 0.10 seconds
QRS: 0.06 seconds
Rhythm interpretation: Junctional tachycardia

**Strip 8-91**
Rhythm: Basic rhythm regular; irregular with nonconducted PAC
Rate: Basic rhythm rate 88
P waves: Sinus with basic rhythm; premature pointed P wave deforming T wave following 6th QRS; pointed abnormal P wave with 7th QRS
PR interval: 0.22–0.24 seconds (remains constant)
QRS: 0.06–0.08 seconds
Rhythm interpretation: Normal sinus rhythm with First-Degree AV Block; Nonconducted PAC (following 6th QRS); an atrial escape beat (7th complex) occurs during the pause following the nonconducted PAC (note different P wave when compared with that of underlying rhythm)

**Strip 8-92**
Rhythm: Irregular ventricular rhythm; regular atrial rhythm
Rate: Atrial: 75; ventricular: 30
P waves: Sinus P waves present (two to three P waves before each QRS)
PR interval: 0.16 seconds (remains constant)
QRS: 0.12 seconds
Rhythm interpretation: Second-degree AV block, Mobitz II; ST segment depression is present

**Strip 8-93**
Rhythm: Regular
Rate: 65
P waves: Inverted before each QRS
PR interval: 0.08–0.10 seconds
QRS: 0.06 seconds
Rhythm interpretation: Accelerated junctional rhythm; ST segment elevation is present

**Strip 8-94**
Rhythm: Regular with basic rhythm; irregular with PJCs
Rate: Basic rhythm rate 72
P waves: Sinus P waves with basic rhythm; inverted P waves with PJCs
PR interval: 0.14 seconds (basic rhythm); 0.08 seconds (PJCs)
QRS: 0.08 seconds
Rhythm interpretation: Normal sinus rhythm with 2 PJCs (4th and 6th complex)

**Strip 8-95**
Rhythm: Regular atrial and ventricular rhythm
Rate: Atrial: 90; ventricular: 45
P waves: Two sinus P waves before each QRS complex
PR interval: 0.16 seconds (remains constant)
QRS: 0.12 seconds
Rhythm interpretation: Second-degree AV block, Mobitz II. Clinical correlation is suggested to diagnose Mobitz II when 2:1 conduction is present. T wave inversion is present

**Strip 8-96**
Rhythm: Regular atrial rhythm; irregular ventricular rhythm
Rate: Atrial: 75 Ventricular: 70
P waves: Sinus P waves present
PR interval: Lengthens from 0.32–0.40 seconds
QRS: 0.04–0.06 seconds
Rhythm interpretation: Second-degree AV block, Mobitz I

**Strip 8-97**
Rhythm: Regular
Rate: 40
P waves: Hidden in QRS
PR interval: Not measurable
QRS: 0.10 seconds
Rhythm interpretation: Junctional rhythm; ST segment elevation is present

**Strip 8-98**
Rhythm: Regular atrial and ventricular rhythm
Rate: Atrial; 80; Ventricular: 40
P waves: 2 sinus P waves to each QRS
PR interval: 0.22–0.24 seconds (remain constant)
QRS: 0.10 seconds
Rhythm interpretation: Second-degree AV block, Mobitz II; clinical correlation is suggested to diagnose Mobitz II when 2:1 conduction is present; ST segment elevation is present

**Strip 8-99**
Rhythm: Basic rhythm regular; irregular with PJC
Rate: Basic rhythm rate 84
P waves: Sinus P waves with basic rhythm; inverted P waves with PJC
PR interval: 0.12 seconds (basic rhythm); 0.08 seconds (PJC)
QRS: 0.06 to 0.08 seconds
Rhythm interpretation: Normal sinus rhythm with one PJC

**Strip 8-100**
Rhythm: Basic rhythm regular; irregular following PJC and run of PJT
Rate: Basic rhythm rate: 100; PJT rate: 136
P waves: Sinus with basic rhythm; inverted P waves with PJC and PJT
PR interval: 0.12–0.14 seconds (basic rhythm); 0.08 seconds (PJC and PJT)
QRS: 0.06–0.08 seconds (basic rhythm); 0.08–0.10 seconds (PJC and PJT)
Rhythm interpretation: Normal sinus rhythm with one PJC (fifth complex) and run of PJT (8th, 9th, 10th complexes)

**Strip 8-101**
Rhythm: Regular
Rate: 44
P waves: Hidden in QRS complex
PR interval: Not measurable
QRS: 0.08–0.10 seconds
Rhythm interpretation: Junctional rhythm

**Strip 9-1**
Rhythm: Regular
Rate: 167
P waves: Absent
PR interval: Not measurable
QRS: 0.12–0.14 seconds
Rhythm interpretation: Ventricular tachycardia

**Strip 9-2**
Rhythm: Regular
Rate: 65
P waves: Sinus; notched P waves usually indicate left atrial hypertrophy
PR interval: 0.14–0.16 seconds
QRS: 0.12–0.14 seconds
Rhythm interpretation: Normal sinus rhythm with bundle branch block; an elevated ST segment is present

**Strip 9-3**
Rhythm: Basic rhythm regular; irregular with PVCs
Rate: Basic rhythm rate 75
P waves: Sinus P waves with basic rhythm; no P waves associated with PVCs; sinus P waves can be seen after the PVCs
PR interval: 0.18 to 0.20 seconds
QRS: 0.08 seconds (basic rhythm); 0.12 seconds (PVCs)
Rhythm interpretation: Normal sinus rhythm with two unifocal PVCs (5th complex and 8th complex)

### Strip 9-4
Rhythm: Irregular
Rate: 30
P waves: Absent
PR interval: Not measurable
QRS: 0.16 seconds
Rhythm interpretation: Idioventricular rhythm

### Strip 9-5
Rhythm: 0
Rate: Not measurable
P waves: Chaotic wave deflection of varying height, size, and shape
PR interval: Not measurable
QRS: Absent
Rhythm interpretation: Ventricular fibrillation

### Strip 9-6
Rhythm: Basic rhythm regular; irregular with PVCs
Rate: Basic rhythm 100
P waves: Sinus P waves present with basic rhythm
PR interval: 0.14 to 0.16 seconds (basic rhythm)
QRS: 0.08 seconds (basic rhythm); 0.12 seconds (PVCs)
Rhythm interpretation: Normal sinus rhythm with unifocal PVCs in a bigeminal pattern (2nd, 4th, 6th, 8th complex)

### Strip 9-7
Rhythm: First rhythm (cannot be determined for sure; only one cardiac cycle); second rhythm: irregular
Rate: First rhythm 54; second rhythm 80
P waves: Sinus P waves present with basic rhythm
PR interval: 0.16 seconds (basic rhythm)
QRS: 0.08 seconds (basic rhythm); 0.12 seconds (ventricular beats)
Rhythm interpretation: Sinus bradycardia changing to accelerated idioventricular rhythm; ST segment depression is present (basic rhythm)

### Strip 9-8
Rhythm: 1st rhythm: irregular; 2nd rhythm: irregular
Rate: 1st rhythm: 60; 2nd rhythm: about 200
P waves: 1st rhythm: fibrillation waves; 2nd rhythm: none identified
PR interval: Not measurable
QRS: 1st rhythm: 0.06–0.08 seconds; 2nd rhythm: 0.12–0.14 seconds
Rhythm interpretation: Atrial fibrillation with burst of ventricular tachycardia; ST segment depression is noted with basic rhythm

### Strip 9-9
Rhythm: Ventricular rhythm regular; atrial rhythm slightly irregular
Rate: Atrial, about 36; ventricular, 38
P waves: Sinus P waves present; bear no relationship to QRS
PR interval: Varies
QRS: 0.12 seconds
Rhythm interpretation: Third-degree AV block changing to ventricular standstill, ST segment elevation is present

### Strip 9-10
Rhythm: Basic rhythm regular; irregular with PVCs
Rate: Basic rhythm rate 79
P waves: Sinus P waves present with basic rhythm
PR interval: 0.16 seconds
QRS: 0.06 seconds (basic rhythm); 0.14 to 0.16 seconds (PVCs)
Rhythm interpretation: Normal sinus rhythm with paired unifocal PVCs (6th and 7th complex)

### Strip 9-11
Rhythm: Regular
Rate: 42
P waves: Absent
PR interval: Not measurable
QRS: 0.12 to 0.14 seconds
Rhythm interpretation: Idioventricular rhythm

### Strip 9-12
Rhythm: Regular
Rate: 125
P waves: Sinus
PR interval: 0.12 seconds
QRS: 0.12 seconds
Rhythm interpretation: Sinus tachycardia with bundle branch block; an elevated ST segment is present

### Strip 9-13
Rhythm: Cannot be determined
Rate: 0
P waves: None identified
PR interval: Not measurable
QRS: 0.12 seconds
Rhythm interpretation: One QRS complex followed by ventricular standstill

### Strip 9-14
Rhythm: Regular
Rate: 214
P waves: None identified
PR interval: Not measurable
QRS: 0.16 seconds
Rhythm interpretation: Ventricular tachycardia

**Strip 9-15**
Rhythm: Basic rhythm regular
Rate: Basic rhythm 50
P waves: Sinus in basic rhythm
PR interval: 0.16–0.18 seconds
QRS: 0.08 seconds (basic rhythm) 0.14 seconds (PVC)
Rhythm interpretation: Sinus bradycardia with one PVC (3rd complex); ST segment depression is present

**Strip 9-16**
Rhythm: Chaotic
Rate: 0
P waves: Absent; wave deflections are irregular and vary in height, size, and shape
PR interval: Not measurable
QRS: Absent
Rhythm interpretation: Ventricular fibrillation

**Strip 9-17**
Rhythm: Chaotic
Rate: 0
P waves: Wave deflections are chaotic and vary in height, size, and shape
PR interval: Not measurable
QRS: Absent
Rhythm interpretation: Ventricular fibrillation followed by electrical shock and return to ventricular fibrillation

**Strip 9-18**
Rhythm: Regular
Rate: 107
P waves: Sinus
PR interval: 0.16–0.18 seconds
QRS: 0.12 seconds
Rhythm interpretation: Sinus tachycardia with bundle branch block

**Strip 9-19**
Rhythm: Irregular
Rate: Atrial: 300; Ventricular: 50
P waves: Flutter waves before each QRS
PR interval: Not measurable
QRS: 0.06–0.08 seconds (basic rhythm) 0.12 seconds (PVC)
Rhythm interpretation: Atrial flutter with variable AV conduction and 1 PVC (5th complex)

**Strip 9-20**
Rhythm: Regular atrial rhythm
Rate: Atrial, 136; ventricular, 0 (no QRS complexes)
P waves: Sinus P waves are present
PR interval: Not measurable
QRS: Absent
Rhythm interpretation: Ventricular standstill

**Strip 9-21**
Rhythm: Irregular
Rate: 40
P waves: Absent
PR interval: Not measurable
QRS: 0.16 seconds
Rhythm interpretation: Idioventricular rhythm

**Strip 9-22**
Rhythm: Chaotic
Rate: 0 (no QRS complexes)
P waves: None identified
PR interval: Not measurable
QRS: Absent
Rhythm interpretation: Ventricular fibrillation

**Strip 9-23**
Rhythm: Regular
Rate: 100
P waves: Absent
PR interval: Not measurable
QRS: 0.12 seconds
Rhythm interpretation: Accelerated idioventricular rhythm

**Strip 9-24**
Rhythm: Irregular
Rate: 60
P waves: Fibrillation waves present
PR interval: Not measurable
QRS: 0.12 seconds
Rhythm interpretation: Atrial fibrillation with bundle branch block; ST segment depression and T wave inversion are present

**Strip 9-25**
Rhythm: Basic rhythm regular
Rate: 1st rhythm (100); 2nd rhythm (188)
P waves: Sinus with basic rhythm
PR interval: 0.14–0.16 seconds
QRS: 0.08 seconds (basic rhythm); 0.12–0.16 seconds (ventricular beats)
Rhythm interpretation: Normal sinus rhythm with burst of ventricular tachycardia and paired PVCs

**Strip 9-26**
Rhythm: Basic rhythm regular; irregular with PVC
Rate: Basic rhythm rate 107
P waves: Sinus with basic rhythm
PR interval: 0.18–0.20 seconds
QRS: 0.08–0.10 seconds (basic rhythm); 0.16 seconds (PVC)
Rhythm interpretation: Sinus tachycardia with 1 PVC (R-on-T pattern); an elevated ST segment is present

### Strip 9-27
Rhythm: Regular
Rate: 43
P waves: Absent
PR interval: Not measurable
QRS: 0.16 to 0.18 seconds
Rhythm interpretation: Idioventricular rhythm

### Strip 9-28
Rhythm: Regular
Rate: 250
P waves: None identified
PR interval: Not measurable
QRS: 0.12–0.16 seconds (QRS complexes change in polarity from negative to positive across strip)
Rhythm interpretation: Ventricular tachycardia (torsades de pointes)

### Strip 9-29
Rhythm: Regular
Rate: 84
P waves: None identified
PR interval: Not measurable
QRS: 0.14–0.16 seconds
Rhythm interpretation: Accelerated idioventricular rhythm

### Strip 9-30
Rhythm: Chaotic
Rate: 0
P waves: Absent; wave deflections are irregular and vary in height, size, and shape
PR interval: Not measurable
QRS: Absent
Rhythm interpretation: Ventricular fibrillation

### Strip 9-31
Rhythm: Basic rhythm regular; irregular with PVCs
Rate: Basic rhythm rate 115
P waves: Sinus P waves with basic rhythm
PR interval: 0.14 to 0.16 seconds
QRS: 0.04 to 0.06 seconds (basic rhythm); 0.12 seconds (PVCs)
Rhythm interpretation: Sinus tachycardia with two unifocal PVCs (4th complex and 12th complex)

### Strip 9-32
Rhythm: Basic rhythm regular; irregular with PVCs
Rate: Basic rhythm rate 125
P waves: Sinus with basic rhythm
PR interval: 0.14–0.16 seconds
QRS: 0.08–0.10 seconds (basic rhythm); 0.12 seconds (PVCs)
Rhythm interpretation: Sinus tachycardia with multifocal paired PVCs (8th and 9th complex)

### Strip 9-33
Rhythm: Basic rhythm regular
Rate: Basic rate 37
P waves: Sinus with basic rhythm
PR interval: 0.14–0.16 seconds
QRS: 0.06–0.08 seconds (basic rhythm); 0.12 seconds (PVC)
Rhythm interpretation: Sinus bradycardia with 1 ventricular escape beat (3rd complex)

### Strip 9-34
Rhythm: 1st rhythm regular; 2nd rhythm regular
Rate: 1st rhythm (72); 2nd rhythm (150)
P waves: Sinus with basic rhythm
PR interval: 0.18–0.20 seconds
QRS: 0.08 seconds (basic rhythm); 0.12 seconds (ventricular beats)
Rhythm interpretation: Normal sinus rhythm with burst of ventricular tachycardia; an inverted T wave is present in basic rhythm

### Strip 9-35
Rhythm: Chaotic
Rate: 0
P waves: Absent; wave deflections vary in height, size, and shape
PR interval: Not measurable
QRS: Absent
Rhythm interpretation: Ventricular fibrillation

### Strip 9-36
Rhythm: Irregular
Rate: About 30
P waves: Absent
PR interval: Not measurable
QRS: 0.12 seconds
Rhythm interpretation: Idioventricular rhythm; ST segment elevation is present

### Strip 9-37
Rhythm: Not measurable
Rate: Not measurable (1 complex present)
P waves: None identified
PR interval: Not measurable
QRS: 0.28 seconds or wider
Rhythm interpretation: One ventricular complex followed by ventricular standstill

**Strip 9-38**
Rhythm: Regular
Rate: 84
P waves: None identified
PR interval: Not measurable
QRS: 0.14–0.16 seconds
Rhythm interpretation: Accelerated idioventricular rhythm

**Strip 9-39**
Rhythm: Basic rhythm regular
Rate: Basic rhythm rate 115
P waves: Inverted before each QRS in basic rhythm
PR interval: 0.08 seconds (basic rhythm)
QRS: 0.06 to 0.08 seconds (basic rhythm); 0.12 seconds (PVC)
Rhythm interpretation: Junctional tachycardia with one PVC (10th complex)

**Strip 9-40**
Rhythm: Regular atrial rhythm
Rate: Atrial, 30; ventricular, 0 (no QRS complexes)
P waves: Sinus P waves present
PR interval: Not measurable
QRS: Absent
Rhythm interpretation: Ventricular standstill

**Strip 9-41**
Rhythm: Basic rhythm regular; irregular with PVCs
Rate: Basic rhythm rate 65
P waves: Sinus P waves present with basic rhythm
PR interval: 0.16 seconds
QRS: 0.06 to 0.08 seconds (basic rhythm); 0.12 seconds (PVC)
Rhythm interpretation: Normal sinus rhythm with two unifocal PVCs (3rd and 6th complex); ST segment depression is present

**Strip 9-42**
Rhythm: Basic rhythm irregular
Rate: Basic rhythm rate 100
P waves: Basic rhythm (fibrillation waves)
PR interval: Not measurable
QRS: 0.08 seconds (basic rhythm); 0.12 seconds (PVCs)
Rhythm interpretation: Atrial fibrillation with a burst of ventricular tachycardia

**Strip 9-43**
Rhythm: 1st rhythm (regular); 2nd rhythm (irregular)
Rate: 1st rhythm (100); 2nd rhythm (100)
P waves: Sinus with basic rhythm
PR interval: 0.12 seconds
QRS: 1st rhythm (0.12–0.14 seconds); 2nd rhythm (0.12 seconds)
Rhythm interpretation: Normal sinus rhythm with bundle branch block with transient episode of accelerated idioventricular rhythm

**Strip 9-44**
Rhythm: First rhythm (cannot be determined for sure; only one cardiac cycle present); second rhythm (regular)
Rate: First rhythm 50; second rhythm 41
P waves: Sinus P waves with first rhythm
PR interval: 0.12 seconds (first rhythm)
QRS: 0.06 to 0.08 seconds (first rhythm); 0.12 to 0.14 seconds (second rhythm)
Rhythm interpretation: Sinus bradycardia changing to idioventricular rhythm; a U wave is present

**Strip 9-45**
Rhythm: Regular
Rate: 214
P waves: Not identified
PR interval: Not measurable
QRS: 0.16–0.18 seconds or wider
Rhythm interpretation: Ventricular tachycardia

**Strip 9-46**
Rhythm: Basic rhythm slightly irregular; irregular with ventricular beats
Rate: Basic rhythm is about 58
P waves: Sinus P waves with basic rhythm
PR interval: 0.20 seconds
QRS: 0.06 seconds (basic rhythm); 0.16 seconds (1st ventricular beat); 0.12 seconds (2nd ventricular beat)
Rhythm interpretation: Sinus bradycardia, with one PVC (4th complex) and 1 ventricular escape beat (5th complex); ST segment depression is present

**Strip 9-47**
Rhythm: Basic rhythm regular; irregular with PVC
Rate: Basic rhythm rate 94
P waves: Sinus with basic rhythm
PR interval: 0.20 seconds
QRS: 0.08 seconds (basic rhythm); 0.12 seconds (PVC)
Rhythm interpretation: Normal sinus rhythm with 1 PVC (5th complex)

### Strip 9-48
Rhythm: Not measurable
Rate: Not measurable (1 complex present)
P waves: None identified
PR interval: Not measurable
QRS: 0.12 seconds
Rhythm interpretation: 1 ventricular complex
followed by ventricular standstill

### Strip 9-49
Rhythm: Regular
Rate: 56
P waves: Sinus P waves present
PR interval: 0.12 to 0.16 seconds
QRS: 0.12 seconds
Rhythm interpretation: Sinus bradycardia with
bundle branch block; ST segment depression is
present

### Strip 9-50
Rhythm: Regular
Rate: 188
P waves: Not identified
PR interval: Not measurable
QRS: 0.12 seconds
Rhythm interpretation: Ventricular tachycardia

### Strip 9-51
Rhythm: Regular atrial rhythm; irregular ventricular
rhythm
Rate: Atrial, 58; ventricular, about 40
P waves: Sinus P waves present
PR interval: Progresses from 0.30 to 0.36 seconds
QRS: 0.08 seconds (basic rhythm); 0.12 seconds
(escape beat)
Rhythm interpretation: Second-degree AV block,
Mobitz I with one ventricular escape beat

### Strip 9-52
Rhythm: 1st rhythm regular; 2nd rhythm regular
Rate: 1st rhythm: 72; 2nd rhythm: 72
P waves: Sinus in 1st rhythm
PR interval: 0.12–0.14 seconds (1st rhythm)
QRS: 0.08 seconds (1st rhythm); 0.12–0.14 seconds
(2nd rhythm)
Rhythm interpretation: Normal sinus rhythm with a
transient episode of accelerated idioventricular
rhythm

### Strip 9-53
Rhythm: Slightly irregular atrial rhythm
Rate: Atrial: about 40 ventricular: 0 (no QRS
complexes)
P waves: Sinus P waves present
PR interval: Not measurable
QRS: Absent
Rhythm interpretation: Ventricular standstill

### Strip 9-54
Rhythm: Regular
Rate: 84
P waves: Sinus
PR interval: 0.16 seconds
QRS: 0.12–0.14 seconds
Rhythm interpretation: Normal sinus rhythm with
bundle branch block; a depressed ST segment is
present

### Strip 9-55
Rhythm: Regular
Rate: 41
P waves: Absent
PR interval: Not measurable
QRS: 0.16 seconds
Rhythm interpretation: Idioventricular rhythm

### Strip 9-56
Rhythm: Regular
Rate: 75
P waves: Sinus P waves present
PR interval: 0.12 seconds
QRS: 0.16–0.18 seconds
Rhythm interpretation: Normal sinus rhythm
with bundle branch block. T wave inversion is
present

### Strip 9-57
Rhythm: Basic rhythm regular; irregular with
PVCs
Rate: Basic rhythm rate 72
P waves: Sinus with basic rhythm
PR interval: 0.12 seconds
QRS: 0.08 seconds (basic rhythm); 0.12–0.14
seconds (PVCs)
Rhythm interpretation: Normal sinus rhythm with
unifocal PVCs (4th, 8th complex) in a
quadrigeminal pattern

### Strip 9-58
Rhythm: Atrial: regular P waves; Ventricular: not
measurable—only 1 QRS complex present
Rate: Atrial: 29; Ventricular: not measurable—only
1 QRS complex
P waves: Sinus P waves present
PR interval: Not measurable
QRS: 0.08 seconds
Rhythm interpretation: One QRS complex followed
by ventricular standstill

**Strip 9-59**
Rhythm: Chaotic
Rate: 0
P waves: Absent; wave deflections are irregular and chaotic and vary in size, shape, height
PR interval: Not measurable
QRS: Absent
Rhythm interpretation: Ventricular fibrillation

**Strip 9-60**
Rhythm: Not measurable (only 1 QRS)
Rate: Not measurable (only 1 QRS)
P waves: None identified
PR interval: Not measurable
QRS: 0.12 seconds or greater
Rhythm interpretation: One QRS complex followed by ventricular standstill

**Strip 9-61**
Rhythm: Regular (first rhythm); regular (second rhythm)
Rate: 100 (first rhythm); 100 (second rhythm)
P waves: Sinus P waves with first rhythm; no P waves with second rhythm
PR interval: 0.14 to 0.16 seconds (first rhythm)
QRS: 0.06 to 0.08 seconds (first rhythm); 0.12 seconds (second rhythm)
Rhythm interpretation: Normal sinus rhythm changing to accelerated idioventricular rhythm

**Strip 9-62**
Rhythm: Regular
Rate: 40
P waves: Absent
PR interval: Not measurable
QRS: 0.16 seconds
Rhythm interpretation: Idioventricular rhythm

**Strip 9-63**
Rhythm: Regular
Rate: 167
P waves: Not identified
PR interval: Not measurable
QRS: 0.16–0.18 seconds
Rhythm interpretation: Ventricular tachycardia

**Strip 9-64**
Rhythm: Regular
Rate: 88
P waves: Sinus
PR interval: 0.22–0.24 seconds
QRS: 0.12 seconds
Rhythm interpretation: Normal sinus rhythm with bundle branch block and first-degree AV block

**Strip 9-65**
Rhythm: Irregular
Rate: Basic rhythm rate 80
P waves: Fibrillation waves present
PR interval: Not measurable
QRS: 0.06–0.08 seconds (basic rhythm); 0.12 seconds (PVCs)
Rhythm interpretation: Atrial fibrillation with paired PVCs

**Strip 9-66**
Rhythm: Basic rhythm regular
Rate: Basic rhythm rate 84
P waves: Sinus P waves present
PR interval: 0.24 seconds
QRS: 0.08 seconds
Rhythm interpretation: Normal sinus rhythm with first-degree AV block changing to ventricular standstill

**Strip 9-67**
Rhythm: Chaotic
Rate: 0
P waves: None identified
PR interval: Not measurable
QRS: Absent
Rhythm interpretation: Ventricular fibrillation

**Strip 9-68**
Rhythm: Regular
Rate: 167
P waves: None identified
PR interval: Not measurable
QRS: 0.14–0.16 seconds
Rhythm interpretation: Ventricular tachycardia

**Strip 9-69**
Rhythm: 1st rhythm regular; 2nd rhythm slightly irregular
Rate: 1st rhythm (115); 2nd rhythm (about 214)
P waves: Sinus in first rhythm; none identified in 2nd rhythm
PR interval: 0.12–0.14 seconds (1st rhythm)
QRS: 0.10 seconds (1st rhythm); 0.12–0.16 seconds (2nd rhythm)
Rhythm interpretation: Sinus tachycardia with burst of ventricular tachycardia returning to sinus tachycardia; an inverted T wave is present

**Strip 9-70**
Rhythm: Regular
Rate: 40
P waves: Absent
PR interval: Not measurable
QRS: 0.16 seconds
Rhythm interpretation: Idioventricular rhythm

**Strip 9-71**
Rhythm: Regular
Rate: 100
P waves: Absent
PR interval: Not measurable
QRS: 0.12 seconds
Rhythm interpretation: Accelerated idioventricular rhythm

**Strip 9-72**
Rhythm: 0 (only 1 QRS complex)
Rate: 0 (only 1 QRS complex)
P waves: None identified
PR interval: Not measurable
QRS: 0.24–0.26 seconds
Rhythm interpretation: One QRS complex followed by ventricular standstill

**Strip 9-73**
Rhythm: Regular
Rate: 188
P waves: Not identified
PR interval: Not measurable
QRS: 0.16–0.20 seconds or wider
Rhythm interpretation: Ventricular tachycardia followed by electrical shock and return to ventricular tachycardia

**Strip 9-74**
Rhythm: Basic rhythm regular; irregular with PVC
Rate: Basic rhythm rate 100
P waves: Sinus P waves with basic rhythm
PR interval: 0.14 to 0.16 seconds
QRS: 0.08 seconds (basic rhythm); 0.12 seconds (PVC)
Rhythm interpretation: Normal sinus rhythm with one PVC (5th complex)

**Strip 9-75**
Rhythm: Regular
Rate: 50
P waves: Sinus
PR interval: 0.16–0.18 seconds
QRS: 0.12–0.14 seconds
Rhythm interpretation: Sinus bradycardia with bundle branch block

**Strip 9-76**
Rhythm: 0
Rate: 0 (no QRS complexes)
P waves: Sinus P waves present
PR interval: Not measurable
QRS: Absent
Rhythm interpretation: Ventricular standstill

**Strip 9-77**
Rhythm: Regular
Rate: 41
P waves: Absent
PR interval: Not measurable
QRS: 0.12 seconds
Rhythm interpretation: Idioventricular rhythm

**Strip 9-78**
Rhythm: 0 (only 1 QRS complex)
Rate: 0 (only 1 QRS complex)
P waves: None identified
PR interval: Not measurable
QRS: 0.14 seconds
Rhythm interpretation: One ventricular complex followed by ventricular standstill

**Strip 9-79**
Rhythm: 0
Rate: 0
P waves: Absent; wave deflections are chaotic and vary in height, size, and shape
PR interval: Not measurable
QRS: Absent
Rhythm interpretation: Ventricular fibrillation changing to ventricular standstill

**Strip 9-80**
Rhythm: First rhythm regular; second rhythm regular
Rate: 94 (first rhythm); 75 (second rhythm)
P waves: Sinus P waves present with first rhythm
PR interval: 0.16 seconds
QRS: 0.12 seconds (first rhythm); 0.12 seconds (second rhythm)
Rhythm interpretation: Normal sinus rhythm with bundle branch block changing to accelerated idioventricular rhythm and back to NSR; T wave inversion is present

**Strip 9-81**
Rhythm: Regular atrial rhythm; ventricular rhythm cannot be determined for sure (only one cardiac cycle)
Rate: Atrial: 94; Ventricular: 40
P waves: Sinus P waves present; bear no relationship to QRS
PR interval: Varies greatly
QRS: 0.14 seconds
Rhythm interpretation: Third-degree AV block changing to ventricular standstill

## Strip 9-82
Rhythm: Regular
Rate: 72
P waves: Sinus P waves are present
PR interval: 0.16 seconds
QRS: 0.12 seconds
Rhythm interpretation: Normal sinus rhythm with bundle branch block

## Strip 9-83
Rhythm: First rhythm regular; second rhythm irregular, chaotic
Rate: 214 (first rhythm)
P waves: None identified
PR interval: Not measurable
QRS: 0.16 to 0.18 seconds (first rhythm)
Rhythm interpretation: Ventricular tachycardia changing to ventricular fibrillation

## Strip 9-84
Rhythm: Regular
Rate: 32
P waves: Absent
PR interval: Not measurable
QRS: 0.20 seconds
Rhythm interpretation: Idioventricular rhythm

## Strip 9-85
Rhythm: Regular with basic rhythm; irregular with PVCs
Rate: Basic rhythm rate 125
P waves: Sinus with basic rhythm
PR interval: 0.12 seconds
QRS: 0.06–0.08 seconds (basic rhythm); 0.12 seconds (PVCs)
Rhythm interpretation: Sinus tachycardia with multifocal paired PVCs (8th, 9th complexes)

## Strip 9-86
Rhythm: P waves are regular; (no QRS complexes)
Rate: Atrial: 52; Ventricular: 0
P waves: Sinus P waves present
PR interval: Not measurable
QRS: Absent
Rhythm interpretation: Ventricular standstill

## Strip 9-87
Rhythm: First rhythm regular; second rhythm irregular
Rate: 68 (first rhythm); about 80 (second rhythm)
P waves: Sinus P waves with first rhythm
PR interval: 0.12 to 0.14 seconds
QRS: 0.08 seconds (first rhythm); 0.12 seconds (second rhythm)
Rhythm interpretation: Normal sinus rhythm changing to accelerated idioventricular rhythm

## Strip 9-88
Rhythm: Regular
Rate: 167
P waves: Not identified
PR interval: Not measurable
QRS: 0.16 to 0.20 seconds
Rhythm interpretation: Ventricular tachycardia (torsades de pointes)

## Strip 9-89
Rhythm: Basic rhythm regular; irregular with PVCs
Rate: Basic rhythm rate 125
P waves: Sinus with basic rhythm
PR interval: 0.12 seconds
QRS: 0.06–0.08 seconds (basic rhythm); 0.12 seconds (PVCs)
Rhythm interpretation: Sinus tachycardia with paired PVCs (7th and 8th complexes)

## Strip 9-90
Rhythm: Regular atrial rhythm
Rate: Atrial: 72; ventricular: 0 (no QRS complexes)
P waves: Sinus P waves present
PR interval: Not measurable
QRS: Absent
Rhythm interpretation: Ventricular standstill

## Strip 9-91
Rhythm: Regular
Rate: 188
P waves: Sinus P waves seen between QRS complexes but not associated with QRS
PR interval: Not measurable
QRS: 0.18–0.20 seconds or wider
Rhythm interpretation: Ventricular tachycardia

## Strip 9-92
Rhythm: Chaotic
Rate: 0
P waves: Wave deflections chaotic—vary in size, shape, direction
PR interval: Not measurable
QRS: Absent
Rhythm interpretation: Ventricular fibrillation; 60-cycle (electrical) interference is noted on baseline

## Strip 9-93
Rhythm: Regular
Rate: 28
P waves: None
PR interval: Not measurable
QRS: 0.20 seconds or wider
Rhythm interpretation: Idioventricular rhythm

**Strip 9-94**
Rhythm: Regular
Rate: 79
P waves: Sinus P waves present
PR interval: 0.18 to 0.20 seconds
QRS: 0.12 seconds
Rhythm interpretation: Normal sinus rhythm with bundle branch block

**Strip 9-95**
Rhythm: Basic rhythm regular
Rate: Basic rhythm rate 68
P waves: Sinus P waves with basic rhythm
PR interval: 0.16 to 0.18 seconds
QRS: 0.06 to 0.08 seconds
Rhythm interpretation: Normal sinus rhythm with one interpolated PVC (7th complex). Interpolated PVCs are sandwiched between two sinus beats and have no compensatory pause. ST segment depression and T wave inversion are present

**Strip 9-96**
Rhythm: Basic rhythm regular; irregular with PVCs
Rate: Basic rhythm rate 72
P waves: Sinus P waves are present with basic rhythm
PR interval: 0.12 to 0.14 seconds
QRS: 0.08 seconds (basic rhythm); 0.12–0.14 seconds (PVCs)
Rhythm interpretation: Normal sinus rhythm with PVCs in a trigeminal pattern

**Strip 9-97**
Rhythm: Irregular
Rate: 80
P waves: Wavy fib waves present
PR interval: Not measurable
QRS: 0.14–0.16 seconds
Rhythm interpretation: Atrial fibrillation with bundle branch block

**Strip 9-98**
Rhythm: Not enough complete cycles to measure with basic rhythm; AIVR rhythm is regular
Rate: 72 estimated rates for basic rhythm; AIVR rate is 75
P waves: Sinus P waves with basic rhythm; no P waves with AIVR
PR interval: 0.16 seconds (basic rhythm)
QRS: 0.08 seconds (basic rhythm); 0.12 seconds AIVR
Rhythm interpretation: Sinus rhythm with episode of accelerated idioventricular rhythm

**Strip 9-99**
Rhythm: Basic rhythm is regular; irregular during pause
Rate: 79 (basic rhythm)
P waves: P waves are present with basic rhythm; absent during pause
PR interval: 0.20 seconds
QRS: 0.14–0.16 seconds
Rhythm interpretation: Normal sinus rhythm with bundle branch block and sinus exit block

**Strip 9-100**
Rhythm: None
Rate: 0
P waves: None identified; wavy baseline
PR interval: Not measurable
QRS: Absent
Rhythm interpretation: Ventricular fibrillation changing to ventricular standstill

**Strip 10-1**
Automatic interval rate: 72
Analysis: The first four beats are paced beats followed by one patient beat and three paced beats
Interpretation: Normal pacemaker function

**Strip 10-2**
Automatic interval rate: 84
Analysis: The first three beats are paced beats, followed by two patient beats, a pacer spike occuring too early, a patient beat, a fusion beat, and two paced beats
Interpretation: Undersensing malfunction

**Strip 10-3**
Automatic interval rate: 72
Analysis: All beats are pacemaker-induced
Interpretation: Pacemaker rhythm

**Strip 10-4**
Automatic interval rate: 68
Analysis: First two beats are paced followed by a failure to capture spike, paced beat, failure to capture spike, pt beat, paced beat, failure to capture spike, and patient beat
Interpretation: Frequent failure to capture

**Strip 10-5**
Automatic interval rate: 72
Analysis: No patient or paced beats are seen
Interpretation: Failure to capture in the presence of ventricular standstill (asystole)

**Strip 10-6**
Automatic interval rate: 72
Analysis: First five beats are patient beats followed by two paced beats, two patient beats and one paced beat
Interpretation: Normal pacemaker function: Underlying rhythm is NSR with frequent PVCs (multifocal)

**Strip 10-7**
Automatic interval rate: 50
Analysis: The first two beats are pacemaker induced, followed by a pseudofusion beat, two patient beats, and one paced beat
Interpretation: Normal pacemaker function

**Strip 10-8**
Automatic interval rate: 72
Analysis: All beats are pacemaker induced
Interpretation: Pacemaker rhythm

**Strip 10-9**
Automatic interval rate: 63
Analysis: The first two beats are paced beats followed by a pacing spike that occurs on time but doesn't capture, a native beat, three paced beats, and a native beat
Interpretation: Failure to capture

**Strip 10-10**
Automatic interval rate: 72
Analysis: All beats are pacemaker induced
Interpretation: Pacemaker rhythm

**Strip 10-11**
Automatic interval rate: 72
Analysis: First three beats are paced beats followed by one patient beat, a pacing spike that occurs too early, one patient beat, a paced beat that occurs too early and 3 paced beats
Interpretation: Undersensing malfunction

**Strip 10-12**
Automatic interval rate: 72
Analysis: First six beats are patient beats followed by two paced beats and two patient beats
Interpretation: Normal pacemaker function; underlying rhythm is atrial fibrillation

**Strip 10-13**
Automatic interval rate: 60
Analysis: All beats are pacemaker induced
Interpretation: Pacemaker rhythm

**Strip 10-14**
Automatic interval rate: 72
Analysis: The first three beats are paced beats followed by two patient beats, and two paced beats, one patient beat, and one paced beat
Interpretation: Normal pacemaker function

**Strip 10-15**
Automatic interval rate: 84
Analysis: The first three beats are paced beats; when the pacemaker is turned off the underlying rhythm is ventricular standstill. Two paced beats are seen when the pacemaker is turned back on
Interpretation: This strip shows an indication for permanent pacemaker implantation, if the underlying rhythm does not resolve

**Strip 10-16**
Automatic interval rate: 72
Analysis: First two beats are paced beats followed by one patient beat, a pacing spike that occurs on time but doesn't capture, two paced beats, two patient beats and one paced beat
Interpretation: Failure to capture

**Strip 10-17**
Automatic interval rate: 72
Analysis: The first two beats are paced followed by a fusion beat (note spike in native QRS with decrease in height); two native beats; a spike that occurs too early; a native beat; a spike that occurs too early; a native beat; a paced beat that occurs too early; and a paced beat
Interpretation: Undersensing malfunction (spikes too early following 5th and 6th complex and a paced beat too early following 7th complex)

**Strip 10-18**
Automatic interval rate: 72
Analysis: The first two beats are patient beats followed by a spike that occurs on time but doesn't capture, a patient beat, and five paced beats
Interpretation: Failure to capture

**Strip 10-19**
Automatic interval rate: 60
Analysis: First four beats are paced beats followed by one patient beat (PVC) and three paced beats
Interpretation: Normal pacemaker function

**Strip 10-20**
Automatic interval rate: 72
Analysis: All beats are pacemaker induced
Interpretation: Pacemaker rhythm

## Strip 10-21
Automatic interval rate: 72
Analysis: All beats are pacemaker induced
Interpretation: Pacemaker rhythm

## Strip 10-22
Automatic interval rate: Cannot be determined (only one paced beat)
Analysis: One paced beat with rhythm changing to ventricular tachycardia
Interpretation: One paced beat changing to ventricular tachycardia (torsades de pointes)

## Strip 10-23
Automatic interval rate: 63
Analysis: The first four beats are paced beats followed by a patient beat (PVC), a pacing spike that occurs too early, a fusion beat, and a paced beat
Interpretation: Undersensing malfunction (pacing spike occurs too early following 5th complex)

## Strip 10-24
Automatic interval rate: 72
Analysis: The first beat is paced followed by one failure to capture spike, one patient beat, one failure to capture spike, one patient beat, one paced beat, one failure to capture spike, one patient beat, one failure to capture spike, and one patient beat
Interpretation: Frequent failure to capture

## Strip 10-25
Automatic interval rate: 63
Analysis: All beats are pacemaker induced
Interpretation: Pacemaker rhythm

## Strip 10-26
Automatic interval rate: 72
Analysis: The first two beats are paced beats followed by one PVC, two paced beats, one pseudofusion beat, one patient beat, and two paced beats
Interpretation: Normal pacemaker function

## Strip 10-27
Automatic interval rate: 72
Analysis: The first two beats are paced beats followed by a spike, which occurs on time but does not capture, a patient beat, a spike that occurs on time but doesn't capture, a patient beat, a spike that occurs on time but doesn't capture, a patient beat, a spike that occurs on time but doesn't capture, and a patient beat.
Interpretation: Loss of capture malfunction (loss of capture spikes occur after 2nd, 3rd, 4th, and 5th complexes)

## Strip 10-28
Automatic interval rate: 72
Analysis: The first three beats are paced beats followed by one patient beat, two paced beats, one pseudofusion beat (spike superimposed on R wave), and two paced beats
Interpretation: Normal pacemaker function

## Strip 10-29
Automatic interval rate: 72
Analysis: The first two beats are paced beats followed by three patient beats (second a PVC), and three paced beats
Interpretation: Normal pacemaker function; underlying rhythm is atrial fibrillation

## Strip 10-30
Automatic interval rate: 65
Analysis: The first two beats are patient beats followed by three pseudofusion beats, and four patient beats
Interpretation: Normal pacemaker function

## Strip 10-31
Automatic interval rate: Cannot be determined for sure since there aren't two consecutively paced beats present
Analysis: Strip shows six patient beats and 5 failure to capture spikes. No paced beats are seen
Interpretation: Complete failure to capture

## Strip 10-32
Automatic interval rate: 68
Analysis: The first beat is a patient beat followed by a pacing spike that occurs too early, a patient beat, a paced beat that occurs too early, 3 paced beats that sense and capture appropriately, a pseudofusion beat, a patient beat, a pacing spike that occurs too early, and two patient beats
Interpretation: Undersensing malfunction (pacing spikes occur too early following 1st and 8th complex; paced beat occurs too early following 2nd complex)

## Strip 10-33
Automatic interval rate: 65
Analysis: First two beats are paced beats followed by two patient beats, one fusion beat and two paced beats
Interpretation: Normal pacemaker function

## Strip 10-34
Automatic interval rate: 72
Analysis: All beats are pacemaker induced
Interpretation: Pacemaker rhythm

## Strip 10-35
Automatic interval rate: 56
Analysis: The first two beats are paced beats followed by one patient beat, one paced beat, one patient beat, one paced beat that occurs too early, two paced beats, and one patient beat
Interpretation: Undersensing malfunction

## Strip 10-36
Automatic interval rate: 68
Analysis: The first beat is a patient beat followed by a pacing spike that occurs too early, a patient beat, a pacing spike that occurs too early, a patient beat, a paced beat that occurs too early, a paced beat that paces and senses appropriately, a pseudofusion beat, two patient beats, a pacing spike that occurs too early, a patient beat, and another paced beat that occurs too early.
Interpretation: Frequent undersensing malfunction (pacing spikes that occur too early following 1st, 2nd, and 8th complexes; paced beats which occur too early following 3rd and 9th complex)

## Strip 10-37
Automatic interval rate: 72
Analysis: All beats are pacemaker induced
Interpretation: Pacemaker rhythm

## Strip 10-38
Automatic interval rate: 72
Analysis: No patient beats or paced beats are seen
Interpretation: Failure to capture in the presence of ventricular standstill (asystole)

## Strip 10-39
Automatic interval rate: 60
Analysis: All beats are pacemaker produced
Interpretation: Pacemaker rhythm

## Strip 10-40
Automatic interval rate: 72
Analysis: The first four beats are patient beats followed by a ventricular capture beat that occurs too early, three ventricular capture beats that occur on time and sense appropriately, and two patient beats
Interpretation: Undersensing malfunction (ventricular capture beat occurs too early following 4th complex)

## Strip 11-1
Rhythm: Regular
Rate: 107
P waves: Sinus P waves are present
PR interval: 0.12 seconds
QRS: 0.06 to 0.08 seconds
Rhythm interpretation: Sinus tachycardia

## Strip 11-2
Rhythm: Regular
Rate: 58
P waves: Sinus P waves are present
PR interval: 0.12 to 0.14 seconds
QRS: 0.12 seconds
Rhythm interpretation: Sinus bradycardia with bundle branch block; ST segment depression is present

## Strip 11-3
Rhythm: Regular atrial and ventricular rhythm
Rate: Atrial: 42; Ventricular: 21
P waves: Two sinus P waves to each QRS
PR interval: 0.32 to 0.36 seconds (remain constant)
QRS: 0.12 seconds
Rhythm interpretation: Second-degree AV block, Mobitz II; clinical correlation is suggested to diagnose Mobitz II when 2 : 1 conduction is present; ST segment elevation is present

## Strip 11-4
Rhythm: Irregular
Rate: 100
P waves: Fibrillatory waves are present—some flutter waves are seen mixed with the fibrillatory waves
PR interval: Not measurable
QRS: 0.04 seconds
Rhythm interpretation: Atrial fibrillation; ST segment depression is present

## Strip 11-5
Rhythm: Regular
Rate: 48
P waves: Hidden in QRS
PR interval: Not measurable
QRS: 0.08 seconds
Rhythm interpretation: Junctional rhythm; ST segment depression is present

**Strip 11-6**
Rhythm: Regular
Rate: 188
P waves: Hidden in preceding T waves
PR interval: Not measurable
QRS: 0.10 seconds
Rhythm interpretation: Paroxysmal atrial tachycardia

**Strip 11-7**
Automtic interval rate: 72
Analysis: First four beats are paced followed by two patient beats, one paced beat, and two patient beats
Rhythm interpretation: Normal pacemaker function

**Strip 11-8**
Rhythm: Regular atrial and ventricular rhythm
Rate: Atrial: 75; Ventricular: 26
P waves: Sinus P waves present—bear no constant relationship to QRS complexes
PR interval: Varies
QRS: 0.14–0.16 seconds
Rhythm interpretation: Third-degree AV block; ST segment elevation is present

**Strip 11-9**
Rhythm: Regular
Rate: 188
P waves: Not discernible
PR interval: Not discernible
QRS: 0.16 to 0.20 seconds
Rhythm interpretation: Ventricular tachycardia

**Strip 11-10**
Rhythm: Regular
Rate: 42
P waves: Absent
PR interval: Not measurable
QRS: 0.16 seconds
Rhythm interpretation: Idioventricular rhythm

**Strip 11-11**
Rhythm: Basic rhythm regular
Rate: Basic rhythm rate 56
P waves: Sinus P waves present (appear notched which may indicate left atrial hypertrophy)
PR interval: 0.16 seconds
QRS: 0.06 seconds (basic rhythm); 0.16 seconds (PVC)
Rhythm interpretation: Sinus bradycardia with one interpolated PVC; ST segment depression is present

**Strip 11-12**
Rhythm: Regular
Rate: 84
P waves: Inverted before each QRS
PR interval: 0.10 seconds
QRS: 0.06–0.08 seconds
Rhythm interpretation: Accelerated junctional rhythm

**Strip 11-13**
Rhythm: Regular
Rate: Atrial: 232; Ventricular: 58
P waves: Four flutter waves before each QRS
PR interval: Not measurable
QRS: 0.06–0.08 seconds
Rhythm interpretation: Atrial flutter with 4 : 1 AV conduction

**Strip 11-14**
Rhythm: Regular
Rate: 88
P waves: Sinus
PR interval: 0.20 seconds
QRS: 0.08–0.10 seconds
Rhythm interpretation: Normal sinus rhythm

**Strip 11-15**
Rhythm: Regular
Rate: 88
P waves: Absent
PR interval: Not measurable
QRS: 0.14–0.16 seconds
Rhythm interpretation: Accelerated idioventricular rhythm

**Strip 11-16**
Rhythm: Basic rhythm regular; irregular with pause
Rate: Basic rhythm 75
P waves: Sinus P waves present with basic rhythm; one premature, abnormal P wave with QRS (after 5th QRS)
PR interval: 0.24 to 0.28 seconds
QRS: 0.06 to 0.08 seconds
Rhythm interpretation: Normal sinus rhythm with first-degree AV block and one nonconducted PAC (follows 5th QRS)

**Strip 11-17**
Rhythm: Regular
Rate: 115
P waves: Sinus P waves are present
PR interval: 0.14 to 0.16 seconds
QRS: 0.06 seconds
Rhythm interpretation: Sinus tachycardia

**Strip 11-18**
Rhythm: Regular
Rate: 48
P waves: Sinus
PR interval: 0.12 seconds
QRS: 0.08–0.10 seconds
Rhythm interpretation: Sinus bradycardia; ST segment elevation is present

**Strip 11-19**
Rhythm: Basic rhythm regular; irregular with premature beats
Rate: Basic rhythm rate 72
P waves: Sinus with basic rhythm; inverted with premature beats
PR interval: 0.12–0.14 seconds (basic rhythm); 0.08 seconds (premature beats)
QRS: 0.08 seconds
Rhythm interpretation: Normal sinus rhythm with two premature junctional contractions (4th and 6th complexes)

**Strip 11-20**
Rhythm: Regular
Rate: 63
P waves: Vary in size, shape, and position
PR interval: 0.12 to 0.14 seconds
QRS: 0.06 to 0.08 seconds
Rhythm interpretation: Wandering atrial pacemaker; ST segment depression is present

**Strip 11-21**
Rhythm: Chaotic
Rate: 0 (no QRS complexes)
P waves: No P waves; wave deflections are chaotic, irregular and vary in height, size, and shape
PR interval: Not measurable
QRS: Absent
Rhythm interpretation: Ventricular fibrillation

**Strip 11-22**
Rhythm: Regular
Rate: 107
P waves: Inverted before each QRS
PR interval: 0.08 seconds
QRS: 0.04 to 0.06 seconds
Rhythm interpretation: Junctional tachycardia

**Strip 11-23**
Rhythm: Irregular atrial rhythm
Rate: Atrial, 40; ventricular, 0
P waves: Sinus P waves are present
PR interval: Not measurable
QRS: Absent
Rhythm interpretation: Ventricular standstill

**Strip 11-24**
Rhythm: Irregular
Rate: 70
P waves: Sinus
PR interval: 0.44–0.48 seconds
QRS: 0.08–0.10 seconds
Rhythm interpretation: Sinus arrhythmia with first-degree AV block; ST segment elevation is present

**Strip 11-25**
Rhythm: Regular
Rate: 188
P waves: Not discernible
PR interval: Unmeasurable
QRS: 0.16 to 0.20 seconds
Rhythm interpretation: Ventricular tachycardia; ST segment elevation is present

**Strip 11-26**
Rhythm: Atrial: regular; Ventricular: irregular
Rate: Atrial (72); Ventricular (40)
P waves: Sinus
PR interval: Lengthens from 0.20–0.28 seconds
QRS: 0.04–0.06 seconds
Rhythm interpretation: Second-degree AV block, Mobitz I; ST segment depression is present

**Strip 11-27**
Rhythm: Regular
Rate: 72
P waves: Sinus
PR interval: 0.20 seconds
QRS: 0.08–0.10 seconds
Rhythm interpretation: Normal sinus rhythm; ST segment depression and T wave inversion is present

**Strip 11-28**
Rhythm: Basic rhythm regular; irregular with pause
Rate: Basic rhythm 72 (rate slows to 63 during first cycle following pause; rate suppression can occur for several cycles following an interruption in the basic rhythm)
P waves: Sinus P waves are present
PR interval: 0.16 to 0.18 seconds
QRS: 0.04 to 0.06 seconds
Rhythm interpretation: Normal sinus rhythm with sinus arrest

**Strip 11-29**
Rhythm: Basic rhythm regular; irregular with premature beats
Rate: Basic rhythm rate 63
P waves: Sinus with basic rhythm; premature, pointed P wave with premature beat
PR interval: 0.14–0.16 seconds (basic rhythm); 0.12 seconds (Premature beat)
QRS: 0.08 seconds
Rhythm interpretation: Normal sinus rhythm with one PAC (5th complex)

**Strip 11-30**
Rhythm: Basic rhythm regular; irregular with PVCs
Rate: Basic rhythm rate 72
P waves: Sinus P waves are present
PR interval: 0.12 to 0.14 seconds
QRS: 0.12 seconds (basic rhythm and PVCs)
Rhythm interpretation: Normal sinus rhythm with bundle branch block and paired PVCs; a U wave is present

**Strip 11-31**
Rhythm: Atrial: regular; Ventricular: regular
Rate: Atrial: 240; Ventricular: 60
P waves: 4 Flutter waves to each QRS
PR interval: Not measurable
QRS: 0.04–0.06 seconds
Rhythm interpretation: Atrial flutter with 4 : 1 AV conduction

**Strip 11-32**
Rhythm: Basic rhythm regular; irregular with pause
Rate: Basic rhythm rate 54
P waves: Sinus with basic rhythm; no P waves with 4th and 5th complexes
PR interval: 0.18–0.20 seconds (basic rhythm)
QRS: 0.06–0.08 seconds
Rhythm interpretation: Sinus bradycardia with sinus arrest and 2 junctional escape beats during pause

**Strip 11-33**
Rhythm: Regular
Rate: 25
P waves: None identified
PR interval: Not measurable
QRS: 0.24 seconds or greater
Rhythm interpretation: Idioventricular rhythm

**Strip 11-34**
Automatic interval rate: 63
Analysis: The first three beats are paced beats followed by a pacing spike that doesn't capture, one patient beat, and 2 paced beats
Rhythm interpretation: Failure to capture

**Strip 11-35**
Rhythm: Regular
Rate: 84
P waves: Not identified
PR interval: Not measurable
QRS: 0.12–0.14 seconds
Rhythm interpretation: Accelerated idioventricular rhythm

**Strip 11-36**
Rhythm: Chaotic
Rate: 0
P waves: Absent; wave deflections are chaotic, irregular and vary in size, shape, and height
PR interval: Not measurable
QRS: Absent
Rhythm interpretation: Ventricular fibrillation followed by electrical shock and return to ventricular fibrillation

**Strip 11-37**
Rhythm: Regular
Rate: 52
P waves: Sinus P waves are present
PR interval: 0.18 to 0.20 seconds
QRS: 0.06 to 0.08 seconds
Rhythm interpretation: Sinus bradycardia; a U wave is present

**Strip 11-38**
Rhythm: Regular
Rate: 94
P waves: Inverted before each QRS
PR interval: 0.08–0.10 seconds
QRS: 0.08 seconds
Rhythm interpretation: Accelerated junctional rhythm; baseline artifact is present

**Strip 11-39**
Rhythm: Irregular
Rate: 60
P waves: Fibrillatory waves are present
PR interval: Not measurable
QRS: 0.12 seconds
Rhythm interpretation: Atrial fibrillation with bundle branch block; ST segment depression and T wave inversion are present

**Strip 11-40**
Automatic interval rate: 72
Analysis: All beats are pacemaker induced
Rhythm interpretation: Pacemaker rhythm

**Strip 11-41**
Rhythm: P waves occur regularly
Rate: Atrial: 88; Ventricular: 0
P waves: P waves present
PR interval: Not measurable
QRS: Absent
Rhythm interpretation: Ventricular standstill

**Strip 11-42**
Rhythm: Basic rhythm regular; irregular with premature beats
Rate: Basic rhythm rate 63
P waves: Sinus with basic rhythm
PR interval: 0.12–0.14 seconds
QRS: 0.08 seconds (basic rhythm); 0.12–0.16 seconds (PVCs)
Rhythm interpretation: Normal sinus rhythm with paired multifocal PVCs (4th, 5th complexes)

**Strip 11-43**
Rhythm: Basic rhythm regular; irregular with PAC
Rate: Basic rhythm rate 136
P waves: Sinus with basic rhythm; premature pointed P waves with premature beats
PR interval: 0.16–0.20 seconds
QRS: 0.06–0.08 seconds
Rhythm interpretation: Sinus tachycardia with 2 PACs (4th and 8th complexes)

**Strip 11-44**
Rhythm: Basic rhythm regular; irregular with pause
Rate: Basic rhythm rate 84—rate slows after pause but returns to basic rate after 4 cycles
P waves: Sinus
PR interval: 0.20 seconds
QRS: 0.08 seconds
Rhythm interpretation: Normal sinus rhythm with sinus arrest; ST segment depression and T wave inversion are present

**Strip 11-45**
Rhythm: 0
Rate: 0
P waves: No P waves present; pacing spikes seen
PR interval: Not measurable
QRS: No QRS complexes are present
Rhythm interpretation: Failure to capture in presence of ventricular standstill (asystole)

**Strip 11-46**
Automatic interval rate: 72
Analysis: First four beats are paced beats, followed by one patient beat, a pacing spike that occurs too early, a patient beat, a fusion beat, and two paced beats
Rhythm interpretation: Sensing malfunction

**Strip 11-47**
Rhythm: Regular
Rate: 42
P waves: Hidden in QRS
PR interval: Not measurable
QRS: 0.08 to 0.10 seconds
Rhythm interpretation: Junctional rhythm

**Strip 11-48**
Rhythm: Atrial: regular; Ventricular: irregular
Rate: Atrial: 79; Ventricular: 50
P waves: Sinus P waves present
PR interval: Lengthens from 0.20–0.32 seconds
QRS: 0.08–0.10 seconds
Rhythm interpretation: Second-degree AV block, Mobitz I

**Strip 11-49**
Rhythm: Basic rhythm regular; irregular with premature beat
Rate: 107
P waves: Inverted before each QRS (except 9th QRS which has a premature, pointed P wave)
PR interval: 0.08–0.10 seconds (basic rhythm); 0.10 seconds (premature beat)
QRS: 0.08–0.10 seconds
Rhythm interpretation: Junctional tachycardia with one PAC (9th complex)

**Strip 11-50**
Rhythm: Regular atrial and ventricular rhythm
Rate: Atrial: 84; Ventricular: 28
P waves: Sinus P waves are present; bear no relationship to QRS complexes
PR interval: Varies greatly
QRS: 0.12 seconds
Rhythm interpretation: Third-degree AV block; ST segment depression is present

**Strip 11-51**
Rhythm: Irregular
Rate: 50
P waves: Sinus P waves are present
PR interval: 0.12 to 0.14 seconds
QRS: 0.08 seconds
Rhythm interpretation: Sinus arrhythmia; sinus bradycardia; a U wave is present

**Strip 11-52**
Rhythm: Basic rhythm regular; irregular with premature beats
Rate: Basic rhythm rate 72
P waves: Sinus with basic rhythm
PR interval: 0.16 seconds
QRS: 0.10 seconds
Rhythm interpretation: Normal sinus rhythm with unifocal PVCs in a trigeminal pattern. ST segment depression and T wave inversion are present

**Strip 11-53**
Rhythm: Regular
Rate: Atrial 93; ventricular 31
P waves: 3 sinus P waves to each QRS (one hidden in T wave)
PR interval: 0.36 seconds (remains constant)
QRS: 0.08 seconds
Rhythm interpretation: Second-degree AV block, Mobitz II

**Strip 11-54**
Rhythm: Basic rhythm regular; irregular with PVCs
Rate: Basic rhythm rate 72
P waves: Sinus P waves present with basic rhythm
PR interval: 0.12 to 0.14 seconds
QRS: 0.08 seconds (basic rhythm); 0.14–0.16 seconds (PVCs)
Rhythm interpretation: Normal sinus rhythm with multifocal PVCs

**Strip 11-55**
Rhythm: Regular atrial and ventricular rhythm
Rate: Atrial: 62; Ventricular: 31
P waves: Two sinus P waves before each QRS
PR interval: 0.44 seconds (remains constant)
QRS: 0.14–0.16 seconds
Rhythm interpretation: Second-degree AV block, Mobitz II

**Strip 11-56**
Rhythm: Regular
Rate: 65
P waves: Inverted before each QRS
PR interval: 0.10 seconds
QRS: 0.04 seconds
Rhythm interpretation: Accelerated junctional rhythm; ST segment elevation is present

**Strip 11-57**
Rhythm: Basic rhythm regular; irregular with pause
Rate: Basic rhythm rate 68
P waves: Sinus P waves
PR interval: 0.22–0.24 seconds
QRS: 0.08–0.10 seconds
Rhythm interpretation: Normal sinus rhythm with first-degree AV block and sinus arrest; ST segment elevation is present

**Strip 11-58**
Automatic Interval Rate: Cannot be determined for sure since there are no two consecutive paced beats or two consecutive pacing spikes (estimated to be 75 when measured from beat immediately preceding each spike)
Analysis: All beats are patient beats—four pacing spikes appear at appropriate intervals for capture to occur but capture doesn't occur
Rhythm interpretation: Complete failure to capture

**Strip 11-59**
Rhythm: Regular
Rate: 188
P waves: Not identified
PR interval: Not measurable
QRS: 0.06 to 0.08 seconds
Rhythm interpretation: Paroxysmal atrial tachycardia

**Strip 11-60**
Rhythm: Irregular
Rate: 30
P waves: None present
PR interval: Not measurable
QRS: 0.16 seconds
Rhythm interpretation: Idioventricular rhythm; ST segment depression is present

**Strip 11-61**
Rhythm: Atrial: regular; Ventricular: irregular
Rate: Atrial: 125; Ventricular: 80
P waves: Sinus
PR interval: Lengthens from 0.12–0.24 seconds
QRS: 0.06–0.08 seconds
Rhythm interpretation: Second-degree AV block, Mobitz I; T wave inversion is present

## Strip 11-62

Rhythm: Basic rhythm regular; irregular with nonconducted PAC
Rate: Basic rhythm rate 100
P waves: Sinus P waves present; two premature abnormal P waves without QRS (following 4th and 8th complexes)
PR interval: 0.12 seconds
QRS: 0.06 to 0.08 seconds
Rhythm interpretation: Normal sinus rhythm with two nonconducted PACs; T wave inversion is present

## Strip 11-63

Rhythm: Regular
Rate: 75
P waves: Sinus
PR interval: 0.16–0.18 seconds
QRS: 0.12–0.14 seconds
Rhythm interpretation: Normal sinus rhythm with bundle branch block; ST segment elevation is present

## Strip 11-64

Rhythm: Regular
Rate: 50
P waves: Sinus
PR interval: 0.16 seconds
QRS: 0.06–0.08 seconds
Rhythm interpretation: Sinus bradycardia; a U wave is present

## Strip 11-65

Automatic Interval rate: 72
Analysis: All beats are pacemaker induced
Rhythm interpretation: Pacemaker rhythm

## Strip 11-66

Rhythm: Regular
Rate: Atrial, 78; ventricular, 39
P waves: Two sinus P waves to each QRS complex
PR interval: 0.24 with a constant relationship to the QRS complexes
QRS: 0.12 to 0.14 seconds
Rhythm interpretation: Second-degree AV block, Mobitz II. Clinical correlation is suggested to diagnose Mobitz II when 2 : 1 conduction is present

## Strip 11-67

Rhythm: Basic rhythm regular
Rate: Basic rhythm rate: 54
P waves: Sinus P waves with basic rhythm; no P waves seen with 3rd, 4th complexes
PR interval: 0.20 seconds
QRS: 0.06–0.08 seconds
Rhythm interpretation: Sinus bradycardia with two junctional escape beats (3rd, 4th beat)

## Strip 11-68

Rhythm: Irregular and chaotic
Rate: 0
P waves: Absent
PR interval: Unmeasurable
QRS: Absent
Rhythm interpretation: Loss of pacemaker capture in the presence of ventricular fibrillation

## Strip 11-69

Rhythm: Regular
Rate: 115
P waves: Inverted before each QRS
PR interval: 0.08 to 0.10 seconds
QRS: 0.06 to 0.08 seconds
Rhythm interpretation: Junctional tachycardia

## Strip 11-70

Rhythm: Basic rhythm regular; irregular with PJC
Rate: Basic rhythm rate 58
P waves: Sinus P waves present (basic rhythm); inverted P waves with PJC
PR interval: 0.14 to 0.16 seconds (basic rhythm); 0.10 seconds (PJC)
QRS: 0.08 seconds
Rhythm interpretation: Sinus bradycardia with one PJC

## Strip 11-71

Rhythm: Basic rhythm regular; irregular with nonconducted PAC
Rate: Basic rhythm rate 63
P waves: Sinus P waves (basic rhythm); one premature, abnormal P wave without QRS complex (follows 4th complex)
PR interval: 0.28 to 0.32 seconds
QRS: 0.12 seconds
Rhythm interpretation: Normal sinus rhythm with first-degree AV block and bundle branch block with one nonconducted PAC following 4th QRS; ST segment elevation and T wave inversion are present

## Strip 11-72

Rhythm: Basic rhythm regular; irregular with PVC
Rate: Basic rate: 50
P waves: Sinus with basic rhythm
PR interval: 0.12–0.14 seconds
QRS: 0.08 seconds (basic rhythm); 0.18 seconds (PVC)
Rhythm interpretation: Sinus bradycardia with one PVC (follows 3rd QRS); ST segment elevation is present

**Strip 11-73**
Automatic interval rate: 79
Analysis: First two beats are paced beats followed by one fusion beat, one pseudofusion beat (note spike at beginning of R wave), three patient beats, pacing spike that occurs too early, a patient beat followed by a pacing spike that occurs too early, and another patient beat followed by an early pacing spike
Rhythm interpretation: Sensing malfunction

**Strip 11-74**
Rhythm: Regular
Rate: 50
P waves: None identified
PR interval: Not measurable
QRS: 0.04–0.06 seconds
Rhythm interpretation: Junctional rhythm; ST segment depression and T wave inversion is present

**Strip 11-75**
Rhythm: Irregular atrial rhythm
Rate: Atrial: 40 ventricular 0
P waves: Sinus P waves are present
PR interval: Not measurable
QRS: Absent
Rhythm interpretation: Ventricular standstill

**Strip 11-76**
Rhythm: Irregular
Rate: 60
P waves: Sinus
PR interval: 0.12–0.14 seconds
QRS: 0.08–0.10 seconds
Rhythm interpretation: Sinus arrhythmia; ST segment elevation is present

**Strip 11-77**
Rhythm: Regular
Rate: 68
P waves: P waves vary in size, shape and position
PR interval: 0.14 to 0.16 seconds
QRS: 0.06 to 0.08 seconds
Rhythm interpretation: Wandering atrial pacemaker; T wave inversion is present

**Strip 11-78**
Rhythm: Regular
Rate: 214
P waves: Hidden
PR interval: Not measurable
QRS: 0.06–0.08 seconds
Rhythm interpretation: Paroxysmal atrial tachycardia

**Strip 11-79**
Rhythm: First rhythm regular; second rhythm regular
Rate: 94 (first rhythm); 136 (second rhythm)
P waves: Sinus P waves (first rhythm)
PR interval: 0.18 to 0.20 seconds (first rhythm)
QRS: 0.06 to 0.08 seconds (first rhythm); 0.12 seconds (second rhythm)
Rhythm interpretation: Normal sinus rhythm changing to ventricular tachycardia

**Strip 11-80**
Rhythm: Basic rhythm regular
Rate: Basic rhythm rate 107
P waves: Sinus with basic rhythm
PR interval: 0.14–0.16 seconds
QRS: 0.06–0.08 seconds (basic rhythm); 0.12 seconds (ventricular beats)
Rhythm interpretation: Sinus tachycardia with a four-beat burst of ventricular tachycardia and paired, unifocal PVCs

**Strip 11-81**
Rhythm: Irregular
Rate: Atrial, 260; ventricular, 70
P waves: Flutter waves present
PR interval: Not measurable
QRS: 0.06 to 0.08 seconds
Rhythm interpretation: Atrial flutter with variable block

**Strip 11-82**
Rhythm: Regular
Rate: 88
P waves: Sinus
PR interval: 0.12 seconds
QRS: 0.04–0.06 seconds
Rhythm interpretation: Normal sinus rhythm

**Strip 11-83**
Automatic interval rate: 63
Analysis: First two beats are paced beats followed by one patient beat, two paced beats, one patient beat, and two paced beats
Rhythm interpretation: Normal pacemaker function

**Strip 11-84**
Rhythm: Regular
Rate: 136
P waves: Sinus
PR interval: 0.12–0.14 seconds
QRS: 0.06–0.08 seconds
Rhythm interpretation: Sinus tachycardia

**Strip 11-85**
Rhythm: Regular
Rate: 54
P waves: Sinus
PR interval: 0.24–0.26 seconds
QRS: 0.04–0.06 seconds
Rhythm interpretation: Sinus bradycardia with first-degree AV block

**Strip 11-86**
Rhythm: Regular atrial and ventricular rhythm
Rate: Atrial: 94; Ventricular: 37
P waves: Sinus P waves present—bear no relationship to QRS complexes
PR interval: Varies
QRS: 0.12–0.14 seconds
Rhythm interpretation: Third-degree AV block

**Strip 11-87**
Rhythm: Regular
Rate: 150
P waves: None identified
PR interval: Not measurable
QRS: 0.12–0.14 seconds
Rhythm interpretation: Ventricular tachycardia

**Strip 11-88**
Rhythm: Basic rhythm regular; irregular with pause
Rate: Basic rhythm rate: 56
P waves: Sinus with basic rhythm; absent during pause
PR interval: 0.16–0.18 seconds
QRS: 0.08–0.10 seconds
Rhythm interpretation: Sinus bradycardia with sinus arrest; ST segment depression and T wave inversion are present

**Strip 11-89**
Rhythm: 0
Rate: 0
P waves: Absent
PR interval: Not measurable
QRS: Absent
Rhythm interpretation: Ventricular standstill

**Strip 11-90**
Rhythm: Regular
Rate: 88
P waves: Sinus
PR interval: 0.16 seconds
QRS: 0.06–0.08 seconds
Rhythm interpretation: Normal sinus rhythm; ST segment depression and T wave inversion are present

**Strip 11-91**
Rhythm: Basic rhythm regular; irregular with PVC
Rate: 115 (basic rhythm)
P waves: Inverted before each QRS
PR interval: 0.08 to 0.10 seconds
QRS: 0.04 to 0.06 seconds; 0.12 (premature beat)
Rhythm interpretation: Junctional tachycardia with one premature ventricular contraction

**Strip 11-92**
Rhythm: Regular
Rate: 188
P waves: Hidden in T waves
PR interval: Not measurable
QRS: 0.06 to 0.08 seconds
Rhythm interpretation: Paroxysmal atrial tachycardia; ST segment depression is present

**Strip 11-93**
Rhythm: Chaotic
Rate: 0
P waves: Absent—fibrillatory waves present
PR interval: Not measurable
QRS: Absent
Rhythm interpretation: Ventricular fibrillation

**Strip 11-94**
Rhythm: Irregular
Rate: 80
P waves: Vary in size, shape, and position
PR interval: 0.14 to 0.16 seconds
QRS: 0.06 to 0.08 seconds
Rhythm interpretation: Wandering atrial pacemaker; T wave inversion is present

**Strip 11-95**
Rhythm: Regular
Rate: 100
P waves: Inverted before each QRS
PR interval: 0.08 seconds
QRS: 0.06 to 0.08 seconds
Rhythm interpretation: Accelerated junctional rhythm

**Strip 11-96**
Rhythm: Regular atrial rhythm; irregular ventricular rhythm
Rate: Atrial: 84; Ventricular: 70
P waves: Sinus
PR interval: Lengthens from 0.20–0.36 seconds
QRS: 0.08–0.10 seconds
Rhythm interpretation: Second-degree AV block, Mobitz I; ST segment depression is present

**Strip 11-97**
Rhythm: Irregular
Rate: 100
P waves: Fibrillatory waves present
PR interval: Not measurable
QRS: 0.06–0.08 seconds (basic rhythm); 0.12 seconds (PVC)
Rhythm interpretation: Atrial fibrillation with one PVC

**Strip 11-98**
Automatic interval rate: 63
Analysis: First two beats are paced beats followed by one patient beat, two paced beats, loss of capture spike, one patient beat, and 1 paced beat
Rhythm interpretation: Loss of capture

**Strip 11-99**
Rhythm: Basic rhythm regular; irregular with premature beat
Rate: Basic rhythm rate 125
P waves: Sinus
PR interval: 0.12 seconds
QRS: 0.04–0.06 seconds
Rhythm interpretation: Sinus tachycardia with one PAC (12th complex)

**Strip 11-100**
Rhythm: Regular
Rate: Atrial: 272; Ventricular: 136
P waves: Two flutter waves to each QRS
PR interval: Not measurable
QRS: 0.04 seconds
Rhythm interpretation: Atrial flutter with 2 : 1 AV conduction

**Strip 11-101**
Rhythm: Irregular
Rate: 60
P waves: Sinus
PR interval: 0.14–0.16 seconds
QRS: 0.08 seconds
Rhythm interpretation: Sinus arrhythmia

**Strip 11-102**
Rhythm: Regular
Rate: 48
P waves: Sinus
PR interval: 0.14–0.16 seconds
QRS: 0.08 seconds
Rhythm interpretation: Sinus bradycardia; a U wave is present

**Strip 11-103**
Rhythm: Regular
Rate: 214
P waves: None identified
PR interval: Not measurable
QRS: 0.16 seconds or greater
Rhythm interpretation: Ventricular tachycardia

**Strip 11-104**
Rhythm: Irregular
Rate: 60
P waves: Fibrillatory waves present
PR interval: Not measurable
QRS: 0.06–0.08 seconds
Rhythm interpretation: Atrial fibrillation

**Strip 11-105**
Rhythm: Basic rhythm regular
Rate: Basic rhythm rate 72
P waves: Sinus P waves present
PR interval: 0.16 to 0.18 seconds
QRS: 0.06 to 0.08 seconds (basic rhythm); 0.12 seconds (PVC)
Rhythm interpretation: Normal sinus rhythm with one interpolated PVC; ST segment depression is present

**Strip 11-106**
Rhythm: Basic rhythm regular; irregular with PJC
Rate: Basic rhythm rate 65
P waves: Sinus P waves with basic rhythm; inverted P wave with PJC
PR interval: 0.12 to 0.16 seconds (basic rhythm); 0.10 seconds (PJC)
QRS: 0.06 to 0.08 seconds
Rhythm interpretation: Normal sinus rhythm with one PJC; a U wave is present

**Strip 11-107**
Rhythm: Basic rhythm regular; irregular with PVC
Rate: Basic rhythm rate 88
P waves: Sinus
PR interval: 0.12–0.14 seconds
QRS: 0.04–0.06 seconds
Rhythm interpretation: Normal sinus rhythm with three PVCs